The Therapeutic
Perspective

The Therapeutic Perspective

Medical Practice, Knowledge, and Identity in America, 1820–1885

John Harley Warner

PRINCETON UNIVERSITY PRESS
PRINCETON, NEW JERSEY

Originally published in 1986 by Harvand University Press and
reprinted by arrangement with the author

Library of Congress Cataloging-in-Publication Data

Warner, John Harley, 1953–
The therapeutic perspective : medical practice, knowledge, and
identity in America, 1820–1885 / John Harley Warner.
p. cm.
Originally published: Cambridge, Mass. : Harvard University Press, 1986.
Includes bibliographical references and index.
ISBN 0-691-01209-1 (PB : alk. paper)
1. Therapeutics—United States—History—19th century.
2. Medicine—United States—History—19th century.
I. Title.
[DNLM: 1. Therapeutics—history—United States.
2. History of Medicine, 19th Cent.—United States. Not acquired]
RM47.U6W37 1997
610'.973'09034—dc21
DNLM/DLC
for Library of Congress 97-31326

First Princeton paperback printing, 1997

http://pup.princeton.edu

Printed in the United States of America

1 3 5 7 9 10 8 6 4 2

For
John G. Warner
and
Dorothy Nies Warner

Preface

At the core of this book is the contention that neither ideology nor behavior can be understood adequately except in relation to the other. To understand how nineteenth-century American physicians fashioned individual and collective identities, why they represented their knowledge and practices as they did, and how they transformed their professional world, we need to connect their rhetoric in medical journals, textbooks, and ceremonial orations with what they actually *did* at the bedside.

When I began writing this book at the start of the 1980s, a growing historical consensus encouraged this approach. Yet, in the history of medicine and science it was more often encountered in programmatic statements voiced around the seminar table than in the literature of the field. It has been satisfying, therefore, to have watched during the past decade as practice has moved to center stage in historical work. Just as historians of science have looked increasingly at the practice of experimentation, in part to move away from theory-dominated accounts of the construction of knowledge in the laboratory, so historians of medicine have turned their attention to the workaday acts of healing by physicians and other practitioners. The rise of the new cultural history has furthered this transformation in the attention of historians, in which the technical activities of medicine and science have joined other cultural practices such as appropriation, representation, the construction of identity, and the deployment of language as historiographic preoccupations.

As a graduate student in the late 1970s and early 1980s, at a moment when intellectual history was struggling to find a reconfigured, viable identity and when the new social history was in full ascendence, it was perhaps overdetermined that I was inclined to turn to cliometric analyses of previously unexplored records of everyday behavior. The pivotal sources I used in my reconstruction of nineteenth-century therapeutic practice—patient records from private and especially hospital practice—have also come into vogue in the decade since this book was first published in 1986. Like historians of science who have turned increasingly to laboratory and field notebooks, historians of medicine have recognized patient records as particularly rich sources for reconstructing not only therapeutic interventions but also diagnostic practices, the uses of technologies, and so on. These records do not give the historian privileged access to reality—a somehow true account of what happened—but they offer an invaluable source of insight into what doctors actually did in managing both diseases and patients and enacting their identity as professionals. What can emerge from comparing clinical behavior with its portrayal in other texts are reconstructions that draw together ideology and behavior, technical content with institutional context, the professional agendas of physicians and the realities of patient experiences.[1]

In retrospect, I wish I had been bolder in spelling out not so much the novelty of my methods and arguments as some of my premises. Reviewing *The Therapeutic Perspective*, Steven Shapin commented that it was "an important and radical book." Yet he went on to note critically that I had been "regrettably timid on the question of relativism" and that the book was "written in a way that masks its radicalism."[2] Although I briefly acknowledged my methodological relativism in the Introduction, I have grown convinced that, especially in a study focused on medical therapeutics, I should have made more of it. I am not suggesting that in trying to understand the past we should, or can, set aside what we know now. But historians have proven themselves to be vastly more comfortable holding in abeyance judgments based on a positivism informed by hindsight in analyzing past medical beliefs and theories than in dealing with medical practices, particularly therapeutics. By the 1970s, instead of judging past theories in the light of modern scientific knowledge, historians increasingly had set out to understand their construction in the context of their own times and to assess what gave them meaning; during the 1980s, this approach was assimilated into the mainstream. Yet, remarkably, many of the same historians continue to be cavalierly dismissive in treating the therapies of the past.

This asymmetrical historical management of medical theory and medical practice has enabled historians to avoid fully confronting an argument of Charles Rosenberg that I made one of my fundamental premises in this book: namely, that during the first half of the nineteenth century therapies like bloodletting *worked*.[3] His wonderfully insightful depiction of nineteenth-century therapeutics has been widely influential and widely cited, but his most daring contention—

that, properly understood, antebellum therapies were efficacious—has been vastly less integrated into historical understanding and treatments of American medicine than it should be. Using relativism as an historical tool in no way implies that therapeutics today are no better than a century and a half ago: when my toddler has an ear infection I expect that our doctor probably will prescribe antibiotics, which I believe are likely to help, and I would be appalled if she proposed bloodletting instead. But I am invested in belief systems prevalent in America at the end of the twentieth century, not those of the nineteenth. Methodological relativism is an indispensable starting point for understanding what, at a particular historical moment, empowered letting blood or administering calomel as cultural practices—for comprehending what made such treatments "work" in the eyes of the many healers who employed such therapies and in those of the patients who demanded them. That Shapin's call for a more assertive relativism was warranted is borne out, I believe, by the fact that not only for the nineteenth century but equally for the centuries that preceded and followed it, the problem of *efficacy*—a central focus of this book—remains one of the least satisfactorily engaged and historicized issues in the history of medicine.

There are other ways I wish I had been blunter. For example, in this book I tried to move away from the tendency to see the emergence of laboratory medicine as the emergence of scientific medicine, for in the appraisal of physicians throughout the first two-thirds of the nineteenth century their medicine was already scientific; it was the notion of what constituted scientific medicine that changed over time. This point needs to be boldly and persistently underscored, for the tacit equation of scientific medicine with medicine rooted in the experimental laboratory stands as one of the sturdiest bastions of presentism in the field. So, too, in my discussion of "The Principle of Specificity" (chapter 3), I point out but do not make enough of how the reciprocal relationship between prevailing cultural values and the internal logic of medical theory was fundamental to the ways that class, gender, ethnicity, race, and region structured physicians' perceptions of patients and of appropriate therapeutic behavior. These connections are made plainly, especially in the case of regionalism, but I presented their implications too timidly. Further, as a study of medical, scientific, and technological change, I wish I had been more explicit about the critical role that creating and recreating stories about medical history played for nineteenth-century doctors as a medical practice that enabled them to laud tradition while applauding innovation.

While the main currents of my research have taken me away

from therapeutics—to explore the wider French impulse in nine-teenth-century American medicine, the shifting place of science in medicine, and the clinical practice of narrative—in the years since this book was first published I have followed some of its themes. For example, while I depicted the role of alternative healers as crucial to understanding the world of nineteenth-century regular medicine, I now would go a step further to argue that during the second quarter of the century the growing power of organized groups such as homeo-pathy was the primary force propelling the creation of medical ortho-doxy. That ideology of orthodoxy, which became deeply infused into the cognitive and institutional structures of the regular medical pro-fession, took therapeutics as its most distinctive emblem, a marker of the boundaries by which regular physicians sought to demarcate and maintain their separateness. Equally, while my final two chapters ad-dressed the sea change that began in the 1870s and 1880s, I touched only lightly on the extent to which the ideal of science for which some physicians began to proselytize in those decades posited a new relationship not only between science and medical practice but also between science and professional identity and between science and professional integrity. Other physicians contested the wide-ranging social and moral implications of this emerging ideal of science, which in the 1880s—as the ideology of orthodoxy that had been forged dur-ing the antebellum period began to disintegrate—cleaved apart the leadership of the regular medical profession, creating intellectual and organizational rifts that lasted into the twentieth century. These are issues I have explored further in subsequent essays.[4]

There is also one convention I followed throughout this book that I regret—namely, my under-problematized use of the terms med-ical "sect" and medical "sectarianism." In nineteenth-century Ameri-can medicine, "sect" was a label of derision, ordinarily used not by members of a group to refer collectively to themselves but rather by their opponents. Thomsonianism, homeopathy, and hydropathy often were dismissively called sects by regular physicians, while homeo-pathic physicians went far toward cementing the language and imag-ery of sectarianism in medical discourse by labeling regular medicine "allopathy," a term the newly designated allopaths scorned. My use of "sect," "sectarian," and "sectarianism" conforms to what remains a virtually universal practice among historians of medicine, but I have grown convinced that we need to rethink their use in distin-guishing among various systems of healing. As actors' categories these are key words that deserve serious historical explication, not least of all because their resonance with religious sectarianism sug-gests a promising framework for sorting out the pluralism and polarizations of the nineteenth-century medical marketplace. But as historians' terms they are highly freighted, and make it all too easy to essentialize the otherness of non-orthodox medical systems and to oversimplify their social, political, and cultural meanings.

Except for making very minor corrections, I have not tampered with the text. If I were writing this book now, though, I would be tempted to relate the shift that I trace from "natural" to "normal" in medical cognition to recent work on changing conceptions of the human body; to relate my argument that therapeutics is the key to understanding professional identity in antebellum American medicine to the sophisticated work emerging on performance and the construction of identities; and to relate recent theoretical work in gender studies to the ways that physicians used the language of gender in valorizing epistemological and therapeutic stances. Also, while this book recounts and explains the decline of heroic therapeutics, I would want to investigate the emergence of heroic therapy as a practice and as a category, and particularly to explore Laurel Thatcher Ulrich's hints that its origins in America might be traced partly in shifting gender relations and patterns of authority over medical practice in the late-eighteenth and early-nineteenth centuries.[5] In any event, much as I hope that this reissued book as it stands tells an important story worth reading, I hope that read in the light of the historiographic changes of the past decade it will be suggestive to other cultural and social historians taking the analysis of medical practice, knowledge, and identity in directions I did not imagine a decade ago.

New Haven, Connecticut
January 1997

Notes

1. See Guenter B. Risse and John Harley Warner, "Reconstructing Clinical Activities: Patient Records in Medical History," *Social History of Medicine* 5 (1992): 183–205.

2. Steven Shapin, "Practical Healers," review of Warner, *The Therapeutic Perspective*, in the (London) *Times Higher Education Supplement*, 31 July 1987, p. 19.

3. Charles E. Rosenberg, "The Therapeutic Revolution: Medicine, Meaning, and Social Change in Nineteenth-Century America," *Perspectives in Biology and Medicine* 20 (1977): 485–506.

4. See John Harley Warner, "The Fall and Rise of Professional Mystery: Epistemology, Authority, and the Emergence of Laboratory Medicine in Nineteenth-Century America," in *The Laboratory Revolution in Medicine*, ed.

Andrew Cunningham and Perry Williams (Cambridge: Cambridge University Press, 1992), pp. 310–41; "Ideals of Science and Their Discontents in Late Nineteenth-Century American Medicine," *Isis* 82 (1991): 454–78; "Medical Sectarianism, Therapeutic Conflict, and the Shaping of Orthodox Professional Identity in Antebellum American Medicine," in *Medical Fringe and Medical Orthodoxy, 1750–1850*, ed. W. F. Bynum and Roy Porter (London: Croom Helm, 1987), pp. 234–60; "Orthodoxy and Otherness: Homeopathy and Regular Medicine in Nineteenth-Century America," in *Culture, Knowledge, and Healing: Historical Perspectives of Homeopathic Medicine in Europe and North America*, ed. Robert Jütte, Guenter B. Risse, and John Woodward, (European Association for the History of Health and Medicine, in press); "Power, Conflict, and Identity in Mid-Nineteenth-Century American Medicine: Therapeutic Change at the Commercial Hospital in Cincinnati," *Journal of American History* 73 (1987): 934–56; and "Science, Healing, and the Physician's Identity: A Problem of Professional Character in Nineteenth-Century America," in *Essays in the History of Therapeutics*, ed. W. F. Bynum and V. Nutton, special issue of *Clio Medica* 22 (1991): 65–88.

5. Laurel Thatcher Ulrich, *A Midwife's Tale: The Life of Martha Ballard, Based on Her Diary, 1785–1812* (New York: Alfred A. Knopf, 1990), pp. 254–61. On the need for study of the rise of what became known as heroic medicine, see Robert B. Sullivan, "Sanguine Practices: A Historical and Historiographic Reconsideration of Heroic Therapy in the Age of Rush," *Bulletin of the History of Medicine* 68 (1994): 211–34.

Acknowledgments

Several organizations have been kind enough to provide the time and research support that have enabled me to think about, research, and write this book. A National Science Foundation Graduate Fellowship aided my early studies in the history of science and medicine between 1976 and 1979. The present project was funded in part by Dissertation Improvement Grant SES–8107609 from the National Science Foundation (1981–82), a Charlotte W. Newcombe Dissertation Fellowship (1982–83), a research award from an Arthur Vining Davis Foundation grant to the Department of Social Medicine and Health Policy at Harvard Medical School (1983–84), and National Institutes of Health Grant LM 03910–01, –02 from the National Library of Medicine (1982–84). I completed revisions to the manuscript while supported by a NATO Postdoctoral Fellowship in Science at the Wellcome Institute for the History of Medicine in London.

In the course of my manuscript research in some sixty-odd archives, many individual archivists assisted me beyond their duties; I should especially like to thank Cynthia Goldstein, Charles Isetts, Carol Pine, Mary Van Winkle, and Richard J. Wolfe. The study of hospital case records presented in Chapter 4 was aided by the computer programming of Elizabeth Allred at the Computing Center of the Harvard School of Public Health and by the graphics of Alice Vickery at the Educational Media Support Center of Boston University Medical Center.

A number of people have contributed in diverse ways to the shaping of this project. I am particularly grateful to Thomas Babor, Saul Benison, Harriet Boardman, William F. Bynum, I. Bernard Cohen, Harold J. Cook, Leon Eisenberg, J. Worth Estes, Drew Gilpin Faust, Daniel M. Fox, Faye Getz, Carl and Audrey Gutmann, Oscar Handlin, Judith Walzer Leavitt, Kenneth Ludmerer, Jane Maienschein, Everett Mendelsohn, Raymond Neff, Charles E. Rosenberg, Elizabeth Smith, Ginnie

Smith, and Maurice M. Vance. I owe a special debt to Guenter B. Risse, who recruited me to the history of therapeutics and guided my early efforts in the field. I also gained much from the students who participated in a seminar on the history of therapeutics that I taught at Harvard in the fall of 1980.

Donald Fleming has given me a model of exacting and creative scholarship. Ronald L. Numbers has been an unfailing source of guidance and friendship. This project would have been more of a burden and less of a joy without the support of these two men.

Barbara Gutmann Rosenkrantz has fundamentally molded both this work and its author by her knowledge, energy, forthrightness, and care. I am more in her debt than I can begin to say.

Margaret Warner brought to this project her knowledge of the history of medicine; her ability to spot hand waving and willingness to call it out; and the reminder that while our work is serious, it should not be taken too gravely.

Contents

The Therapeutic
Perspective

Introduction: Therapeutics and the Transformation of American Medicine

Between the 1820s and the 1880s medical therapeutics in America was fundamentally altered. Traditional medical practices, founded on assumptions about disease shared by doctor and patient and oriented toward visibly altering the symptoms of sick individuals, began to be supplanted by strategies grounded in experimental science that objectified disease while minimizing differences among patients. Concurrently the bases of physicians' professional identity were also transformed. Through the mid-nineteenth century professional identity was based on proper behavior and on a medical theory that stressed the principle of specificity, the notion that treatment had to be matched to the idiosyncratic characteristics of individual patients and their environments. During the last third of the century a new conception of professional identity, defined by allegiance to knowledge generated and validated by experimental science and characterized by universalized diagnostic and therapeutic categories, was clearly in ascendance.

I have elected to use the study of medical therapeutics as a context in which to evaluate these changes in professional identity, scientific knowledge, and medical practice. This is, then, a therapeutic perspective on the culture of orthodox medicine in America and its transformation between the 1820s and 1880s. As the core of medical activity, therapeutics was central to the professional image and legitimacy of physicians. Moreover, therapeutics, regarded as both a cognitive system and a set of social practices, is a useful indicator of the changing real and perceived roles of scientific knowledge in medicine. A study of therapeutic change, its determinants, and its meaning is thus a singularly productive means of assessing physicians' professional values and their perceptions of what constituted proper sources of knowledge.

Yet as Charles Rosenberg has cogently commented, "Historians have always found therapeutics an awkward piece of business. On the whole, they have responded by ignoring it."[1]

In part, the dearth of research in the history of therapeutics is a reflection of the methodological difficulties inherent in determining what nineteenth-century physicians actually did at the bedside. Therapeutic theory is readily accessible to the historian through an abundance of published and manuscript narrative sources that present not only normative statements by physicians but also exemplary case histories. Yet therapeutic behavior at times bore little resemblance to therapeutic theory or principle, and reliable knowledge about actual therapeutic practice must come from sources that are less conventional in historical research, such as medical case history records.[2]

Still, the self-conscious quest of historians during the past two decades for new types of sources in reconstructing the social experience of the past makes methodological impediments less than compelling as an explanation for lack of interest in the history of therapeutics. With some exceptions, the same investigators who have perceived much promise in studying the history of disease and health care have seen little in medical therapeutics that seems to meet their theoretical or personal agendas. Therapeutics has appeared to be ground too arid to warrant tilling either by the physician exploring his or her profession's past or by the professional historian interested in using medicine as one mirror of society, thought, and values. Nineteenth-century therapeutic practice is certainly an unappealing vehicle for hagiographic celebration, and its usefulness as a spade in the archaeology of values is far from obvious at first sight.

Identifying the boundaries of my study will spare the reader a search for something that is not here. My concern is with *medical* therapeutics, not with surgical and dental therapeutics.[3] I have further restricted my analysis to orthodox (also called regular) physicians, and I examine the beliefs and practices of irregular or sectarian practitioners only where they impinged upon the regular profession. Moreover, the endpoints of my study are not rigid. I have selected the opening date to include a time when speculative systems of practice were still influential and the turn toward empiricism was just beginning. My study closes when experimental laboratory science was ascendant but not yet hegemonic, and when bacteriology intrigued many American physicians but had yet to engender the frenetic activity of the 1890s.

I have made several assumptions about how medical therapeutics ought to be regarded in order to be productively exploited as a guide to the culture of nineteenth-century American medicine. What physicians actually *did* matters as much as their normative statements, and neither behavior nor ideology can be adequately interpreted without knowledge of the other. Erwin Ackerknecht called a decade and a half ago for what he termed a "behaviorist" approach to the history of medicine, in which the historian would focus on the behavior of physicians, not just on their ideas and institutions.[4] Such historical operationalism has been but little applied to the study of medical practice, and often therapeutic theory and principle have been represented as actual practice. Yet historical attention to the realities of daily events as distinguished from ordinarily elite perceptions of them is hardly novel in recent social history. The leading implication of Ackerknecht's advice for this study is that therapeutic activities must be reconstructed as a backdrop against which the knowledge, image, and values of the profession can be evaluated. To this end, I have used information about actual prescribing habits drawn from private practice case books and hospital case histories both to describe change in therapeutic practice and as a practical referent for assessing the meaning of what physicians said they did and told each other they ought to be doing.

One of the most striking impressions that emerges from a study of nineteenth-century practice records is the diversity of practice among various physicians at any particular time. Place was one important determinant, and accordingly I have been very sensitive to regional differences in formulating statements about medical therapeutics in America. In part this stems from my conviction that the history of American medicine has suffered from overgeneralizing the experience of a single region, the Northeast. More than this, the meaning of therapeutic regionalism was transformed during the period under study. Early in the century the notion that the physical and social environments were significant factors in determining appropriate therapeutic behavior made region a necessary consideration in planning a patient's treatment and in evaluating the applicability of knowledge from another place, but by the 1880s therapeutic regionalism and nationalism had by and large become stigmata of inferior practice and antiquated thinking.

Regional variation therefore figures prominently in my account of therapeutic change. In assessing therapeutic thought and practice I have given more attention to published and manuscript records produced in and for a particular region of the country than to, for example, the standardized pharmacopeias and dispensatories. The latter sources present a deceptively unified image of therapeutic thought that masks geographic (as well as generational and educational) differences in opinion. To appreciate such regional differences, I have looked especially hard at medical practice in the vicinities of three cities that were professional centers in different parts of the United States: Boston, Cincinnati, and New Orleans.

I have assumed that it is necessary to take the thought and actions of nineteenth-century physicians seriously in order to do more than confirm my initial expectations about their culture. Unmistakably, nineteenth-century medical therapeutics did work, though perhaps not when judged by criteria of efficacy satisfying to a twentieth-century pharmacologist. Physicians were not ordinarily simpleminded, passive, or duplicitous, nor were they unobservant of the results of their therapies. Instead of dismissing antebellum therapy as either risible or tragic, the historian should endeavor to understand what made it meaningful. Further, nineteenth-century physicians did not necessarily care about what I care about, and I have paid attention when it is clear that something seriously troubled them that seems trivial to me. If this suggests a relativism more fitting for an anthropologist than a historian, I can say only that I have been at least as interested in understanding nineteenth-century American culture as I have been in clarifying my own.

Any list of the causes of therapeutic change would obscure as much as it would illuminate. For example, at least in passing, historians have frequently listed the factors that contributed to the demise of therapeutic bloodletting. These include French skeptical empiricism, growing faith in the healing power of nature, pressure from patients, and the introduction of alternative treatments. Competition from such sectarian practitioners as homeopathists (who prescribed greatly diluted doses of drugs) and Thomsonians and eclectics (who used energetic botanical drugs), and their derision of heroically, aggressively used orthodox therapies such as bloodletting and mineral drugs, have also commonly been cited. All of these factors did indeed contribute to the decline in bloodletting. Yet at the same time each one also encouraged regular physicians to defend the practice even more stridently than before and to cling to it as a symbol of the orthodox profession. To understand why therapeutic change occurred and what it meant, therefore, the historian must scrutinize and explain the process of change, not merely describe its animi and end points.

The transformation of medical practice, knowledge, and professional identity followed no simple or consistent formula. Physicians' dual commitment to progress and to tradition persistently shaped the way that change occurred and was rationalized, but it affected various components of the medical ethos in different ways. In analyzing therapeutic change, I have concentrated on several particular dimensions of the framework that ordered the physician's practice. These are therapeutic epistemology, theory, and principle; actual medical treatment;

and professional identity. The general characteristics of change in each of these elements underscore the complexity of therapeutic change and at the same time identify several of its persistent features.

Therapeutic principle was broader and more stable than therapeutic theory. Physicians who vehemently opposed each other's theories often agreed in principle: two practitioners who explained the therapeutic action of bloodletting on the body in sharply divergent fashions might well agree that bloodletting was a good therapy. Neither principle nor theory necessarily bore much relation to actual therapeutic practice. By the 1860s regular physicians in America rarely employed bloodletting, for example, but the majority still maintained that it was—in principle—one of the most valuable therapies in the orthodox armamentarium.

Physicians bickered constantly about their favorite therapeutic theories, which changed frequently and sometimes abruptly, but they ordinarily assumed that therapeutic principle was established truth. The stability of therapeutic principle owed much to its symbolic function. In antebellum America the proposition that bloodletting was a good practice, for instance, was a cardinal tenet of the regular profession's therapeutic creed. An allegiance to that principle set members of the orthodox profession apart from sectarian practitioners, who proudly used their heretical condemnation of bloodletting as both a rallying point and a political tool. Shared faith in the value of bloodletting was a distinctive mark of the regular physician, and upholding this principle was a matter of professional ethics. When therapeutic principle changed, it did so gradually; unlike theory it was rarely overthrown.

Physicians were likewise conservative about altering what they actually did therapeutically at the bedside. But while continuity strongly characterized both principle and practice, the latter was by far the more malleable of the two. Change in practice over the long duration of time was dramatic. Between the early nineteenth century and the 1860s the use of aggressively lowering, depleting therapies like bloodletting and mineral cathartics declined and physicians came to prescribe stimulating treatments in their place, while at the same time many practitioners began to look less to cure and more to palliation and care. From the 1860s there was a marked move toward using fewer but more narrowly targeted drugs. Underlying these changes was a transformation in the way physicians conceived the objective of therapy: their aim shifted from restoring the balance that represented the individual patient's natural condition to correcting the body's abnormal state by bringing it back in line with fixed norms.

What is most striking, though, is that while the overall transformation in actual practice between the 1820s and 1880s was momentous, the process of change was almost invariably very gradual. Virtually the only circumstance that generated rapid change was the introduction of a new therapy. Change in therapeutic practice did not involve the violent overturning of the old that is characteristic of revolution. Established practices were not abruptly abandoned but rather passed gradually into disuse. Continuity was fostered both by habit and by the extent to which regular physicians identified themselves by their therapies, as well as by the fact that outright rejection of a once-esteemed therapy would have implied rejection of the supporting framework of professional tradition. The fundamental changes in practice that did occur were generally accommodated into existing frameworks of explanation and professional values.

Such transformation through the accretion of small, peaceful permutations did not characterize change in therapeutic epistemology, however. It is here that true revolutions, involving violent overturning of the old, are most readily found. Starting in the 1820s some physicians sought to reshape therapeutics radically using a skeptical medical empiricism derived in part from French teachings, a sharp contrast to their early-nineteenth-century fidelity to systems of practice cast in the mold of Enlightenment rationalism. A celebration of therapeutic empiricism and vilification of rationalism characterized the middle third of the century, but from the 1860s on the promise of experimental laboratory science incited other physicians to overturn the reign of empiricism. This group perceived in experimental science a solid foundation for erecting a New Rationalism that would lift the profession out of the therapeutic stagnancy empiricism had engendered.

Therapeutic epistemology mattered to thinking physicians, for they were convinced that it made a critical difference to the success of both the individual practitioner at the bedside and the profession as a whole in American society. They linked epistemology not only to the standing of therapeutics as a science and their own therapeutic power, but also to the cultural power of the orthodox profession. In both the early-nineteenth-century turn from rationalism toward empiricism and the later turn back toward rationalism, the epistemological iconoclasts in medicine justified the vehemence of their campaign by their belief that it would transform therapeutic thought and practice and uplift the profession. Epistemologies lacked the symbolic power invested in such emblems of the regular profession as bloodletting; thus the abrupt inversions of rationalism and empiricism were not intrinsically threatening to the profession in the way the prospect of revolution in principle or practice was. As physicians employed it, however, therapeutic epistemology was a powerful tool in professional reform, and often the crusading zeal of such reforms did open violence to the old order.

Coupled with these epistemological shifts were redefinitions of what constituted science in therapeutics. Certainly at the beginning of the century "the spirit of system" that informed rationalistic systems of practice affirmed medicine's claims to be scientific. From the 1820s on, intellectually active physicians turned more and more to empirical clinical observation, sometimes ordered by application of the numerical method, as the scientific foundation of therapeutics. Later, some began to see reductionist knowledge of physiological processes and drug action produced in the laboratory as the chief starting point for scientific reasoning in the clinic. While this remained a minority position in 1885, it plainly was gaining ascendancy. Medicine did not simply become more scientific during the nineteenth century; what was considered science, and what was not, changed. The notion of what constituted therapeutic science, like epistemology and theory, was more amenable to sharp redirections of allegiance than was either principle or practice.

Because medical therapeutics was so central to what defined a regular practitioner—and to what set the orthodox practitioner apart from the sectarian—it was closely linked to professional identity. Shifts in therapeutic thinking led to a reassessment of the various attributes that defined the proper physician, and thereby contributed to a remolding of professional identity. There was clear evidence by the 1870s for the beginning of a redefinition of the physician's principal therapeutic task. This is best characterized as a shift from the emphasis on the exercise of judgment to that on the application of knowledge. Experience became relatively less important (though never unimportant) as a source of authority, and expert knowledge more important. Advocates of this newer model believed the physician's identity should derive less from an interaction with patients and other practitioners, more from an allegiance to science (defined especially as that of the research laboratory). At the same time, the movement from proper behavior to expert knowledge as the principal support of professional identity began to transform professional morality.

The first section of this study analyzes the structure and functioning of antebellum medical therapeutics. Chapter 1 assesses what it meant to be a physician in pre–Civil War America and establishes the critical importance of therapeutic activity to professional identity. Chapter 2 describes the shift in physicians' allegiance from rationalism to empiricism, and evaluates the function that epistemological reorientation served for the profession. Chapter 3 establishes and analyzes the pervasive influence during the antebellum period of the therapeutic principle of specificity—that is, the insistent emphasis on the individuality of patient and environment in determining treatment.

The second section concentrates on the process of change. Chapter 4 describes the broad movements in therapeutic practice, then uses a computer-aided study of therapeutic practice at two hospitals to discern the fine structure of change. The reader unfamiliar with nineteenth-century therapeutics may wish to read the first portion of this chapter, which describes what physicians actually did therapeutically and what they expected from treatment, before turning to the first chapter. Chapter 5 uses the tension between the commitment to progress and the commitment to tradition as a framework for weighing the influences of such sources of change as the profession's institutions (medical schools, societies, literature) and the socioeconomic context of practice (especially pressure from competing sectarian practitioners). Chapter 6 evaluates the influence of European knowledge and method on therapeutic permutations in the United States, stressing how and why Americans eagerly took up the Paris clinical school's skeptical empiricism while eschewing the example of French practice. Chapter 7 scrutinizes the profession's debates on three therapies—bloodletting, calomel, and veratrum viride—to illustrate how physicians measured the authority of arguments calling for change and how they minimized the disruption that attended it.

The final section explicates the therapeutic reconstruction that some physicians believed was warranted by experimental laboratory science during the two decades following the Civil War. Chapter 8 describes the therapeutic gloom that had befallen the profession by the 1860s and the various pathways out that physicians advocated, and establishes why the proposal to ground therapeutics in experimental science appeared so promising to some and so radical to nearly all. Chapter 9 develops the implications of this plan for therapeutic knowledge, practice, and professional identity, and underscores the persistent ambivalence that most physicians retained toward the medical pretensions of science at least through the mid-1880s.

PART I

Antebellum Medical Therapeutics

— 1 —

Intervention and
Identity

IN A COMMENCEMENT ADDRESS to Cincinnati medical students in 1877
on "the dignity and sanctity of the medical profession," the speaker
asserted that "its chief excellence is, not that it is scientific, but that
it is redemptive." To understand and explain illness were important
parts of the physician's task, but did not constitute the whole of it.
The physician was more than a natural scientist; he was also a healer.
Dissenting from the emerging but still novel view that professional
identity in medicine should be defined chiefly by science, the speaker
admonished the graduates that "the physician is not only the inter-
preter of Nature."[1]

However necessary this admonition may have been by 1877, during the first two-thirds of the nineteenth century no American physician would have questioned it. The physician's "redemptive" role,
his active therapeutic intervention in an effort to redeem patients from
disease, was at the core of what it meant to be a physician in America.

Although Alexis de Tocqueville may have overstated Americans'
valuation of practice over theory, he nonetheless perceived correctly
their predilection for activity. His observation that the American was
above all a "man of action" closely matched the views American physicians held of their professional role and identity. In 1833, two years
before Tocqueville toured the United States, a young Bostonian studying medicine in Paris proposed to his father the idea that he pursue
the Parisian plan of clinical research for several years before starting
practice. Pierre Louis, the student's French mentor, endorsed this scheme,
and wrote to the boy's physician father, "I recommend this to you,
because no one is more capable than he is of cultivating the *science
and thereby* of making progress in the *practice*, for what is practice

11

but science put into operation?"[2] But the father, James Jackson, Sr., could not consent to this postponement of activity for the sake of observation. He rejected his son's proposal, arguing that for an American physician scientific investigation was not a legitimate substitute for practice. "In this country," the elder Jackson later explained, "his course would have been so singular, as in a measure to separate him from other men. We are a business doing people. We are new. We have, as it were, but just landed on these uncultivated shores; there is a vast deal to be done; and he who will not be doing, must be set down as a drone. If he is a drone in appearance only and not in fact, it will require a long time to prove it so, when his character has once been fixed in the public mind."[3]

The antebellum American physician derived his professional identity from practice, in which a primary imperative was to act therapeutically. Yet among the most persistent myths about medical therapeutics in America is the notion that from the 1820s through the 1860s therapeutic skeptics and nihilists appeared in the regular ranks to denounce and abandon traditional therapy. This myth matters, because it suggests incorrectly that a physician could preserve proper professional identity and at the same time reject active intervention. In the United States a truly noninterventionist posture either in normative statements or at the bedside was not an option. The physician had to do something; a "do-nothing" physician, as critics often caricatured skeptics, would be bereft of professional legitimacy, would in fact not be a physician at all.

Grasping the tight connection between therapeutic intervention and professional identity is the most important key to understanding the course and meaning of nineteenth-century therapeutics. Because therapeutics in part defined professional identity, therapeutic change involved the risk of destabilizing its supports. Therapeutic ideology and debate were dominated and constrained by their implications for the profession's image and standing. The integrity of regular therapeutics could not be radically challenged without an implicit threat to regular professional identity as well. Traditional remedies such as bloodletting, elements of the regular creed and identity, held a symbolic significance that transcended and added meaning to their use at the bedside. Orthodox practitioners were, after all, largely distinguishable from their sectarian competitors by their practices. The link between identity and intervention molded regular physicians' evaluation of knowledge and its sources, the ways the profession sought to portray itself and its practices, and the interactions among regular physicians, sectarian practitioners, and the public.

Medical treatment, the core of the physician's "redemptive" role, was the essence of what patients expected. Throughout the antebellum period "prescribing" for a patient was a widely used synonym for making a professional visit. The rural sick, who sometimes wrote to physicians in lieu of the more costly option of sending for them, ordinarily wanted drugs more than explanation or hygienic advice.[4] Yet the patient could obtain treatment from a variety of sources, among them home remedies and lay healers, so the provision of therapy was in itself insufficient to define a distinctive identity for the physician.

In the perception of physicians, what gave the proper practitioner of medicine a distinctive identity was his *profession*, his proclaimed worthiness of confidence in performing the task of healing. "Physic is not a trade," one New England physician declared in 1834. "It is a *profession* made by its members, that is, a declaration, an assertion, that the candidate possesses knowledge, skill, and integrity, sufficient to entitle him to confidence."[5] Among the elements of that profession, he continued, was the "moral obligation" to intervene. The physician professed, in effect, that he had faith in his ability to act, and that this merited in turn the confidence of the public.

Professional identity was principally based upon practice, not, as it became to a large extent after the late nineteenth century, upon a claim to special knowledge.[6] Knowledge was, to be sure, a necessary attribute of the competent physician. "By his profession," one physician observed, "he has already declared that he has done all, according to his best ability, to fit himself for the all-important and trust-worthy situation which he has assumed. In other words, he declares that he has a good medical education."[7] Extensive knowledge about the basic sciences was desirable, but not essential to proper professional identity. What was essential was that the physician be able to act, and to do so in accordance wih regular values. The common, defining body of learning that all regular practitioners shared was knowledge about practice. Further, it was practice that mattered most to physicians in assessing the orthodoxy of their fellows.

A professionally respectable practitioner could remain ignorant of much of basic medical science. While one physician traveling in the rural South in the mid-1840s could observe that the regular practitioners of the district "are not familiar with the minutiae of Anatomy, Physiology, and Pathology," he could nonetheless avow "that a more able and skilful set of practitioners is not to be found in any country . . . They are men of close observation, and sound judgment; above all they are well acquainted with the *peculiarities* of the malignant diseases with which they have to contend, and act with promptness and skilful decision."[8] Their deficiencies did not undermine their legitimacy as regular physicians. Similarly, in evaluating the qualifications of an applicant for a Confederate Army surgical post, one physician could advise the examining board that even though the candidate was "entirely ignorant of Anatomy, Surgery, Physiology, Pathology and Chemistry," he was nevertheless "a pretty fair practitioner in the ordinary acute diseases of the Country."[9] The knowledge required to sustain professional identity was of the sort that could be gained through experience, as in apprenticeship.

Conversely, the possession of extensive knowledge about medical science was insufficient to make a person a physician. There was little place in American society for a nonpracticing physician: the two terms were contradictory. Someone with medical training and perhaps an M.D. degree could and often did take up an occupation other than medical practice (such as business, farming, or teaching), but by doing so exclusively he lost his professional identity as a true physician and became something else. In antebellum America the physician was a practitioner.

Enthusiasm for scientific investigation could even diminish the practitioner's capability at the bedside by diverting his attention from the primary task of intervening, physicians maintained. "I almost think that a man may learn so much before he begins to practice as to prevent his doing well," an eminent Boston physician cautioned. "Too much knowledge of the dangers & difficulties tend to paralyze one's powers— or at least to check one's efforts."[10] Harvard medical professor John Ware was typical in continually reminding his classes that the final purpose of medical education was not the mere acquisition of knowledge but to prepare the student for practice. "He may be an excellent anatomist, pathologist, chemist—nay, he may be minutely acquainted with the history and treatment of disease, and yet be totally unfit to take charge of a single patient."[11] The useful physician, he urged, had to learn how to "apply this knowledge with a wisdom which is sometimes altogether beyond that which merely high attainments in science can confer."[12]

One of the attributes Ware had in mind was judgment, something informed by learning but developed through experience. Professional judgment came only from practice, and generated a confidence that knowledge alone could not command. A New Orleans practitioner wrote of his physician brother that although "his understanding of the theory and principles of his profession is superior to that of nine tenths of the physicians in the country," he "is too distrustful of his own abilities." He explained to their mother that "one thing is wanting in him & but one to ensure abundant success—confidence, self-confidence, the all indispensable prerequisite for an undertaking in our country."[13] More often than not, physicians elected to praise a colleague by characterizing him as a man of good judgment or sound experience rather than one of great learning. Still, cultivated experience and judgment were not so much essential ingredients in professional identity as signs of the practitioner's expected maturation.

More essential to proper professional identity was moral character. Being a moral man was deemed crucial not merely to the physician's standing in the community, but also to his effectiveness as a healer. A high standard of "moral excellence," the Committee on Ethics of an Ohio medical society declared, "is a duty every physician owes alike to his profession and to his patients. It is due to the latter as without it he cannot command respect and confidence and to both because no scientific attainments can compensate for the want of correct moral principles."[14] "Moral influence" was both a source and an expression of the physician's healing power and was regarded as an active force that daily made a difference in the sickroom. Partially for this reason physicians often perceived challenges to the regular profession's therapeutic acumen in moral terms. At the same time, anything that debased the practitioner's moral integrity threatened his professional identity and imperiled his therapeutic effectiveness.

Practical knowledge, morality, and interaction with patients (in accordance with the regular belief system) were, then, what physicians held to be the essence of their professional identity. The genre of medical literature that set exemplars for the profession, such as introductory lectures at medical schools, presidential addresses to medical society meetings, and medical theses, identified many other characteristics that were desirable in the physician. These included a sense of responsibility, duty, judgment, piety, intellectual achievement, patience, industry, Christian faith, and citizenship—in other words, an inventory of those qualities esteemed in contemporary American society.[15] And as women made incursions into regular practice from midcentury onward, most medical men added being male, hitherto assumed, to their list of important traits. Thinking physicians also urged that they, like lawyers and clerics, had a special responsibility and capacity for providing community leadership, particularly in the country's newer regions, and expressed this by participating in temperance movements, developing cultural institutions, and instigating public health measures.[16] But even though these admirable features made a more successful physician, they did not define professional identity, only enhanced it.

The physician looked to his profession for much of his identity but derived little of his status from that source. During a large part of the nineteenth century many practitioners enjoyed the public's high esteem at a time when the profession as a whole was in a degraded position. The simple fact of membership in the regular medical profession had little to do with the individual physician's status, which came more from his own interactions with patients and other practitioners and from such factors as family and community connections. But even though the practitioner's status was largely independent of his profession, the welding of his personal professional identity to that of the collective physician gave him reason to care about the position of the profession and motivation for defending and bettering its image. Thinking physicians sought to uplift the standing of the profession for reasons that transcended improving their individual socioeconomic positions.

Medical institutions had more to do with forming the image of the aggregate regular profession, and the status of some individuals, than they did with shaping the characteristics of the individual that determined whether or not he was a physician. Medical schools, licensing societies, and journals were all vehicles through which regular values could be affirmed and regular beliefs codified and transmitted. Institutions were also one means by which the individual physician could acquire esteem: a professorship, society membership, publication, and hospital appointment were all tools for improving a practitioner's status. Many a thinking physician recognized the potential of medical institutions as platforms to elevate the profession as a whole and thereby to enhance his personal professional identity; but for the unambitious rural practitioner's everyday activity, self-perception, and place within his community, such institutions might have little meaning. From the 1820s through the end of the antebellum period, a medical practitioner in America could lack an M.D. degree, be unlicensed, belong to no professional society, and not read (much less write for) a medical journal, yet still undeniably be a regular physician. Physician-intellectuals might deplore his ignorance and seek to distance themselves from him, but would still recognize him as a physician—legitimate, however regrettable.

All of the elements of professional identity pivoted upon action. Professional knowledge was of doubtful value if it did not direct activity. It was this emphasis on useful knowledge that informed the persistent ambivalence of nineteenth-century American physicians toward scientific knowledge, represented in turn by the products of speculative system building, pathoanatomical investigation, and laboratory research. Members of the medical profession vigorously debated the value of chemistry, physiology, and even anatomy for the practitioner, but no one questioned the value of knowledge about practice, knowledge that would guide action at the patient's bedside.

Professional morality was similarly welded to activity. It included an imperative to act, to do whatever was possible to cure or palliate the patient. "The moral duty of [the medical] man is to employ every means, which an enlightened mind, can perceive to have a bearing on the case," one practitioner urged in 1840.[17] The physician was not truly moral, and was therefore violating his profession, unless he was useful and active. This belief forcefully drew into question the moral status of the physician who became more interested in science for its own sake than in practice. A second, related sort of morality was also a part of the physician's moral duty: he was to act as a moral agent in a religious sense. Even in the case of the dying patient he had an important function to perform as "missionary to the bedside."[18]

Therapeutic action was, then, an essential element of professional identity. The physician who failed to act was reneging on his "profession" through his immoral behavior. One corollary to this bond between action and professional rectitude is particularly important for understanding the meaning of therapeutics and the dynamics of its shifting course: faith in action, not just action itself, was a necessary attribute of the proper physician. A practitioner who lacked or lost faith in the efficacy of his action, or in the precepts for therapeutic intervention that distinguished the regular physician, lost the justification for his profession. Without confidence in the capacity of regular medicine to heal the sick, he had no basis for asking the public to trust in him as a physician. His profession of faith was voided. As a result, programmatic statements that exemplified a loss of faith, such as advocacy of a true therapeutic nihilism, would nullify the physician's professional legitimacy.

The best way to understand and decisively establish the strength of the link between medical intervention and professional identity is to analyze closely the most forceful counterexample that can be brought forward to refute it. That is the notion widely held by some physicians and historians from the early nineteenth century on that American therapeutic skeptics and nihilists wrenched identity and intervention apart. According to this view, the skepticism that emerged in the 1820s and became especially strong in the 1850s and 1860s led some regular physicians to reject active drugs. Skepticism, those perpetuating this caricature have supposed, was especially fostered by the therapeutic philosophy of the Paris clinical school and by homeopathic and lay opposition to strong drugging. It coalesced around a belief in the *vis medicatrix naturae*, the healing power of nature. An account of the charges that critics brought against this movement, followed by an assessment of the so-called skeptics' actual thought and practice, illustrates why a noninterventionist posture was not possible in America. At the same time, the charges reveal the consequences for professional identity that some physicians envisioned if the bond between intervention and identity were to be ruptured.

Nineteenth-century arguments about skepticism were largely framed within the context of the debate waged since antiquity on the roles of nature and art in healing.[19] Whereas the putative skeptics placed considerable confidence in nature's healing force, the opposing view stressed the power of medical art. The teachings of Philadelphia medical professor Benjamin Rush epitomized this latter stance in early-nineteenth-century America. The hallmark of Rush's therapeutics was faith in the physician's power to aggressively cut short the natural course of a disease with bloodletting and large doses of drugs; it was this ability to master disease that gave the physician confidence and inspired it in patients. Nature, Rush believed, acted capriciously in disease, generally to the patient's detriment. "In all violent diseases nature is like a drunken man reeling to & fro & occasionally stumbl[ing] against a door with so much violence as to break it through," he told his students. "Always treat nature in a sick room as you would a noisy dog or cat[;] drive her out at the door & lock it upon her."[20] Even though many of the American physicians who criticized skepticism also dissented from Rush's specific therapeutic beliefs, they shared his concern that too much faith in nature would injure both patient and profession.

Defensive animosity toward the healing power of nature escalated during the second quarter of the century as critics became convinced that American skepticism had taken a decidedly new and invidious turn. According to the increasingly rigid model that began to emerge, from the late 1820s some American physicians had carried their faith in nature's beneficial actions in disease to its extreme: they had renounced traditional remedies in their writings and shunned them at the bedside. These skeptics had severed the link between intervention and identity, debasing their standing as regular physicians and, by their example and teachings, endangering the integrity of the regular *profession* itself. This model was a vastly distorted version of reality; nevertheless, it provided a remarkably resilient image and formed the basis for most of the arguments of physicians who feared the implications of an excessive reliance on nature.

Before the 1830s most critics saw an enfeebled application of art as the primary danger to be feared from a dependence upon nature. Nathaniel Chapman, a successor of Rush at the University of Pennsylvania who vehemently disagreed with many of the elder physician's beliefs, was typical in the thrust of his objections to the concept of the healing power of nature. The notion "that fever will run its course and that all the practitioner can do is to abate its force," he told his students in 1816, "is a dangerous one and should be combatted . . . It begets a feeble practice and suffers the disease to go on til it is beyond our power."[21] Later in the century this type of criticism became more widely and vigorously voiced. It was imperative that the practitioner at least make an effort to interrupt the course of a disease. As an Ohio physician asserted, "I do not believe it is our duty to stand by and do nothing: we ought to study every disease, and interfere."[22]

From the early 1830s on, the range of concerns of those who found fault with a dependence upon nature expanded. Critics became increasingly troubled by the implications of skepticism for the profession's position and for professional identity. Some practitioners responded by staving off the assaults against therapeutic tradition they perceived in the turn to nature. Skeptics were branded with "infidelity to the healing art."[23] Excessive faith in nature, critics charged, violated the physician's profession of his ability to heal and, in the assessment of one practitioner, "virtually proclaims the existing medical profession worse than useless."[24] Further, it indicted the practices of physicians who retained their confidence in drugs and used them aggressively.

In the eyes of his assailants, the skeptic's doubts about his own effectiveness negated his "profession" of therapeutic competence, correspondingly dissipating the confidence of his patients. "Skepticism and distrust," a Boston physician argued, were "inconsistent with proper activity and perseverance in the use of means of cure[.] Surely faith and confidence are essential to the successful prosecution of our art, and we cannot inspire our patients with what we have not ourselves."[25] A New York physician who wrote in 1859 to vindicate "the character and honor of the profession" expressed the opinion of many physicians when he charged that the skeptic's notion "that all the physician does is to amuse the patient whilst nature cures the disease" was "a labored effort to destroy public confidence in the medical profession."[26]

In the perception of critics the most extreme implication of the belief that nature healed was that the physician became superfluous; his professional role was annulled. As early as 1830 Chapman had commented in a tone of dismay on the idea that the course of diseases could not be curtailed by art: "Could I believe this opinion to be correct, I would at once without hesitation strike the flag of my profession, and cease to pilfer a generous public of their money by such a fraud and impostance."[27] New Orleans medical editor Bennet Dowler echoed this view thirty years later, asking, "Can an honest man hold such opinions, and at the same time continue to practice his profession?" If the physician believed "that Nature only, not the doctor, is competent either to relieve or cure the sick," he replied, it would be unethical to continue to practice medicine.[28] By implication, those practitioners who did persist in seeing patients while at the same time extolling nature were behaving unethically.

The notion that too great a faith in nature unfitted a man for the regular profession was due in part to the tacit association between nature trusting and sectarianism. Many physicians maintained that the rising emphasis on nature's role in healing was an injudicious response to sectarian therapeutics, and especially to homeopathic infinitesimals. One version of this argument held that some physicians were capitulating to sectarian rhetoric that denounced regular drugging to the public. Such physicians were guilty of giving in to ill-informed public demand in order to make themselves more competitive against sectarian rivals, and thereby of responding to an illegitimate source of therapeutic change. Another version of this argument began with the premise, widely shared among regular physicians, that homeopathic treatment was physiologically equivalent to therapeutic abstinence, and therefore was tantamount to relying entirely on nature for cure. Some physicians, this argument continued, believed that clinical statistics purportedly showing homeopathic successes both illustrated the power of the *vis medicatrix naturae* and suggested that regulars had been attributing to art much of what was due to nature. "Absurdity and heresy can go no farther," scoffed one Cincinnati critic.[29]

This connection between an allegiance to nature and what regulars regarded as quackery had another, more threatening dimension. Whether or not the emphasis by some regular physicians on the healing power of nature was actually caused by homeopathic example and propaganda, many practitioners believed that it would inevitably be taken by sectarians as an endorsement of their creed. Regarded in this way, skepticism directly harmed the regular profession by sustaining its enemies.

It is telling that religious metaphor was among the most common devices for expressing criticism of skepticism. Physicians were well aware of the theological resonance of the terms *skepticism* and *nihilism* and exploited it in their polemics. Skeptics were guilty of disbelief in the efficacy of medical art, and of proclaiming their heretical faith in nature. "The worshippers of this faith look upon drugs as meddlesome, if not profane interferences, downright polypharmacy and 'damnable heresy,' " one practitioner charged.[30] The apostasy of those who followed nature threatened to corrupt not only their individual standing (and the salvation of their patients) but also that of the professional community. By renouncing his profession of faith in the redemptive power of medical art, the skeptic weakened the collective faith and confidence of orthodox physicians.

Growing faith in the *vis medicatrix naturae* coincided with the perception of many physicians that the standing of their profession was declining in American society. A leading cause to which they attributed this deterioration was an overreliance on theories and speculative systems of practice. Critics who questioned the very existence of the *vis medicatrix* saw it as yet another theory that had to be overturned in order to free the profession from dogmatic rationalism and uplift its place in society. This theory, according to one writer, was an "enthusiastic superstition that gives to nature a *personality* altogether unreal or imaginary"; another practitioner who shared his view argued that those who confided in the curative power of nature were suffering from "a blind idolatry of a false principle."[31] Many practitioners heeded the call to rebuff the "attack upon those who prefer to follow the light of experience and common sense rather than the delusive guidance of mere speculation and theory."[32]

Given the widely prevalent caricature of skepticism as a therapeutic posture that directed nonintervention, the charges critics brought against it were largely cogent. Yet if the skeptics did in fact preserve professional legitimacy in their own eyes (and they did), a problem emerges. If they were able to endorse a noninterventionist stance at the lectern and carry through with it at the bedside, then the postulated link between therapeutic activity and professional identity either was breaking apart during the middle third of the century or was nonessential in the first place. Neither of these was the case. The skeptics did not propose or practice inactivity. The portrait painted by their many critics was not true to life; instead, the artists projected their own anxieties and professional insecurities onto the canvas. In reality the connection between intervention and identity remained intact. To show that skepticism did not and could not mean inactivity in American medicine, it is first necessary to ask: Who were the American skeptics and nihilists?

Physicians who stressed the healing power of nature and questioned the prudence of aggressive drugging were not all cast in a single mold. In matters of restoring health the relative weight practitioners accorded to nature and art varied widely. Although representatives of both extremes practiced in virtually all parts of the United States, those who emphasized nature's beneficial actions were most concentrated in New England, while a relatively large proportion of its detractors practiced in the South and West. Advocacy of nature also changed over time, becoming increasingly common from the 1820s. Early in this period especially, a large proportion of the physicians who drew attention to nature's ability to cure were distinguishably elite—socially prominent, often European trained, and institutionally eminent. So too, though, were many of their harshest opponents, and elite status is not a reliable predictor of physicians' attitudes toward nature and art.

Nevertheless, there can be no doubt that if any physicians in America during this period truly deserved the title "skeptics," their leadership was centered in New England. Boston was the chief American shrine to the faith of nature in medicine. The most prominent spokesmen for the movement taught at Harvard Medical School, and a large number of proselytizers studied there. Furthermore, many of these physicians were associated with the Massachusetts General Hospital, either as visiting physicians or as resident students. If during the four decades preceding the Civil War skepticism ever meant noninterventionism, it surely would be evident in the thought and practice of this cluster of Boston physicians. Showing that the link between identity and interventionism remained intact in this stronghold of American skepticism illustrates the distortion of reality in the critics' caricature. At the same time, it suggests the worth of investigating the origins of this caricature, which was so prevalent among American physicians and which they took so seriously.

Harvard medical professor Jacob Bigelow's 1835 address to the Massachusetts Medical Society on "Self-Limited Diseases" was widely hailed and condemned as the opening proclamation in the nature-trusting movement. But in fact the ideas Bigelow presented were by no means novel in the Boston vicinity when he gave his address. Moreover, while there can be no doubt that both homeopathy and the teachings of the Paris clinical school strengthened the movement, the self-conscious faith in therapeutic moderation that Bigelow expressed thrived in Boston before either of these two forces could have given birth to it. Bigelow's address, and the movement as a whole, had roots deeply embedded in the native soil of New England.

The therapeutic teachings of Boston physician James Jackson, Sr., for example, well illustrate the advocacy of therapeutic moderation and respect for nature that was evident in New England by the early decades of the nineteenth century. In part, Jackson's therapeutic posture was encouraged by his preceptorship in the mid-1790s under Edward A. Holyoke, an eminent Salem physician known for teaching moderation in treatment. Jackson's study in London at the turn of the century reinforced this position. Because Bostonians who traveled abroad to study medicine during the middle and late eighteenth century tended to study in the large hospitals of London, where they were imbued with the emphasis on practical clinical teaching, they returned to America with a different attitude toward healing than did students from other regions of the country (such as Philadelphia and Charleston) who preferred to attend lectures in Edinburgh, where the more theoretical precepts of William Cullen were taught. This Bostonian medical emphasis on experience over theory, in the appraisal of one historian, translated into a less aggressive therapeutic stance than that adopted by, say, the Philadelphian Benjamin Rush.[33] In any event Jackson's institutional position in Boston medicine—physician to the Boston Dispensary, leader of the Massachusetts Medical Society, long-term professor and reorganizer at Harvard Medical School, and cofounder of the Massachusetts General Hospital—made his therapeutic teachings singularly influential in the vicinity.

Jackson self-consciously urged on his students an undoctrinaire approach to therapeutics, enjoining them to treat according to the peculiar indications of the patient rather than by fixed rules. There were two general modes of healing diseases, he maintained, active and expectant, and each was adapted to certain diseases at different stages. Jackson shared with Rush the belief that some diseases could be actively broken up by treatment. "If we see the patient early," Jackson told his students, the "active mode is employed with the intention of either checking or rendering the disease safer, or of arresting it at once."[34] But contrary to Rush's creed, Jackson believed that active treatment often did more harm than good, and the physician's wisest management was in "leaving the cure to Nature."[35] Certain diseases that had to run their natural course and could not be curtailed by art, such as smallpox and measles, called for the expectant method of care.

Jackson made it clear in his lectures, however, that in employing this method the physician did not become inactive. "Even in the expectante method we are obliged to make use of the active method, with regard to certain symptoms, wh if left to themselves, would interrupt or render the disease more violent."[36] He explained that the "expectante waits for nature but still attends to nonnaturals [such as diet, exercise, and excreta]. If any thing happens bad [we] must remove; i.e., don't try to shorten disease but prevent aggravation."[37] It was the physician's task in the expectant approach to "guard against the obstacles which may hinder the method of Nature."[38] As Bigelow would later do in his address on self-limited diseases, Jackson stressed the importance of knowing a disease's natural course and its natural tendency to cure.

Jackson spoke for a much more humble therapeutic position than did Rush, one that placed great reliance on nature. Yet he did not turn away from art, even when using the expectant method, nor did he question the usefulness of the physician. By both medicinal and hygienic prescriptions the physician could prolong life, prevent the aggravation of disease, and mitigate suffering.[39] Jackson both reiterated his therapeutic reserve and acknowledged his use of active drugs in an

1833 letter to his physician son, adding, "But I hear you say, how then have you *so much* faith in medicine. *So much!—how much?*" Answering his own question, he continued, "[I] never fall into the error of believing that I cure (in the common sense of this word) any larger proportion of my patients." He explained, "I do not like this use of the word cure—this prejudiced sense of it. For it is a very good word in its proper sense & I do not know any substitute—accordingly in my lects I always state that it is derived from *cura*—the physician shd take care of the sick—he is or should be more capable of this than other persons—but he s[hould] not undertake by drugs to overcome all their dis[ease]s."[40]

The New England vein of therapeutic moderation that Jackson's thought represents was both reinforced and reshaped by the precepts of the Paris clinical school. Many of the physicians who were to become the leaders of Boston medicine traveled to the Paris hospitals for study from the 1820s on, especially from the early 1830s through the 1850s. In therapeutics the leading features of Parisian medicine included an emphasis on the healing power of nature, a doubting attitude toward the efficacy of medical treatments until they had been proven of value by rigid observation and analysis, and the numerical evaluation of the worth of therapeutic practices based on empirical clinical observations.[41] Although therapeutics was the dimmest part of the new vision of medicine the Bostonians brought back with them, their French experience nevertheless encouraged them to question the efficacy of medical art and influenced both their practices and their teaching.

Partly because Boston had a tradition of therapeutic reserve dating back to the eighteenth century, its physicians were particularly receptive to the outlook of the Paris school. Perhaps, too, the Unitarian sensualism and allegiance to Locke prevalent among Boston's upper classes made them especially open to French medical sensualism in the tradition of Condillac and Cabanis. Bigelow expressed a very widely shared opinion when, late in his life, he explained that it was Pierre Louis—French clinician, proselytizer of the numerical method, and mentor to an influential congeries of Boston physicians abroad in the 1830s—who was principally responsible for the turn away from aggressive drugging. "Before Louis came, a great many believed implicitly in the power of medicine to cure diseases, and it would have been deemed a heinous dereliction of duty not to prescribe a certain round of medicine in every disease," Bigelow explained. "Louis's works checked all this; taught us the importance and necessity of a closer study of nature and of each fact in medicine."[42]

The Parisian experience of Jackson's son, James Jackson, Jr., illustrates the kind of shift in therapeutic outlook that French teachings could bring about in a young American. He attended medical lectures at Harvard, then departed for Paris in 1831. Having studied with his father, he was well acquainted with the elder physician's therapeutic inclinations.[43] Soon after his arrrival in Paris, young Jackson expressed his impatience with the feebleness of the practice he witnessed there. Enthusiastically writing to his father about the large number of patients with bronchitis he had observed and the overwhelming opportunities he found for studying the natural history of the disease, he digressed: "I cannot help stopping a moment to speak of the impotent and of course inefficient efforts to save the lives of those thus affected." Venesection was rarely used, he noted, and "instead of trying the effects of emetics and extensive blisters—as we shd do, they wait till death is just at hand and then, order a blister of 3 inches square to the legs or thighs—it is really aggravating to see the corpses upon the table stained by the marks of this useless painful practice. I had read of French practice and heard of it, but I had not the slightest conceptn how little they are acquainted with the science of Therapeut[ics]."[44]

At first the young Jackson criticized the therapeutic apathy of the two clinicians he worked with most closely, Gabriel Andral and Pierre Louis. In one letter that his father later published, he highly praised Louis's clinical teaching and skill in arriving at a diagnosis. But the elder Jackson edited out his son's additional comment on Louis—that after making his diagnosis, "he finishes there—he is very weak at therapeut, and is perfectly satisfied c[um] a correct diagn."[45] Yet as what a family medical friend called "his hearts idolatry of Louis" grew stronger, young Jackson wholly gave himself over to being Louis's disciple in "the *exact study of disease.*"[46] Andral and Louis, he wrote to his father, "have taught me the danger of admitg anything wh is not deduced fr *well-observed* facts,"[47] and this included therapeutics. When he had left Boston, he explained to his father early in 1833, he had wanted above all to become "a good physician," but that objective had changed. "Now my much more ardent desire is to do my part in clearing away some of the clouds wh hide the truth in our difficult medical science. I am beginning to regard myself as one of those whose education has been such that it is in his power & whose disposition is such that it wld be his delight to seek and find *truth*, pathological & therapeutic. You & I do not look upon this subject c[um] exactly the same eyes."[48]

In several of his letters the younger Jackson tried to describe the clarity of the French way of seeing to his father without accusing him of therapeutic myopia. Through Louis's plan of clinical observation and the numerical method, the younger Jackson believed, therapeutic truth could be discovered, but it was not yet known. "This is to me a painful subject, for I would fain believe in all the therapeutics which you believe in; and yet the evidence that it is true must be derived from your and my general impressions. Now, when I have had such ample opportunity to see the futility of such evidence . . . I ask myself, honestly, how far I can trust all this?"[49] He closed cautiously, saying, "I trust you will not misunderstand the early part of my letter: it is not that I disbelieve in the effect of Med[icine]; . . . but that I do not think *proof* has been given of what is believed."[50] In another letter he exclaimed, "Our poor pathology and yet worse therapeutics; shall we never get to a solid bottom: shall we never have fixed laws? shall we never *know*, or must we be ever doomed to suspect, to presume? Is *perhaps* to be our qualifying word forever and for aye?"[51] His father published these remarks but deleted the last part of his son's letter, which said: "On readg over these pages, I am almost tempted to burn them. For I fear . . . that you will imagine me more sceptical than I am as to the science of Therapeutics . . . Let me say in one word then; That as a *Doctor* (if I were one) I believe in the *use* of many remedies wh as a *scientific man* I am not entirely persuaded to be useful . . . You see I'm half afraid of yr answer."[52]

In the senior Jackson's assessment, he and his son shared a common therapeutic outlook; the only difference was that his view had been tempered by the practical exigencies of clinical experience. "You seem quite sober on the subject of your scepticism on the subject of therapeutics—& evidently fear that you & I much differ much [*sic*] in that respect," he replied to his son. "I would not have you troubled on that score . . . This is a matter I have thought of & looked at in all the respects in wh you seem to regard it. You suppose me to have more faith in the power of remedies than I have. Yet in many points I have no doubt a practical faith wh I could not at once impart to you."[53] Time and experience at the bedside, the elder Jackson confidently believed, would teach his son that he *must do something*, however uncertain or unsustained by proof the therapy might be. Skepticism in principle could not mean noninterventionism in practice. "Do not believe that in practice you need wait for mathematical certainty. There is a propitious incredulity as well as the opposite.—However I have no fear that you will ultimately fall into the practical error of extreme skepticism. Meanwhile be as rigid as you will in your scientific inquiries & conclusions." He closed by assuring his son that he would find others in Boston on his return who shared his uneasiness. "If you do not find me ready to doubt with you as much as you wish," he wrote, "you will find others—Dr Bigelow & Dr Ware are excellent doubters."[54]

Jacob Bigelow, one of Jackson's "excellent doubters," soon had the chance to witness Parisian medicine for himself. He and Oliver Wendell Holmes sailed together to France early in 1833, and the younger Jackson introduced them to the medical life in Paris. He wrote to his father of Bigelow, "I carried him to see Louis & his [numerical] Tables—they delighted him—he told Louis we might now hope to see Medicine a Science, that he had done for it what Cuvier did for Comp[arative] Anat[omy] &c."[55] The philosophy of the Paris school was surely one topic of conversation on the return passage, when young Jackson and Bigelow were traveling companions. The former had scant opportunity to proselytize the skepticism he had acquired in Paris, however, for in 1834, at the age of twenty-four, he died of typhoid fever. Aptly, his father took charge of his case, and Bigelow, reverently observing the French zeal for pathoanatomical correlation that James had so admired, performed his autopsy.[56]

Whatever influence Bigelow's own brief visit to Paris may have exercised in forming his address on "Self-Limited Diseases" in 1835, the ideas about treatment he encountered in Paris were not new to him. His inclination toward therapeutic moderation had been evident for the preceding two decades. As a student Bigelow, in a step unconventional for a New Englander, had elected to attend medical lectures at the University of Pennsylvania. There he heard Rush, but was more influenced by the therapeutically moderate professor of materia medica, Benjamin Smith Barton. Still, Bigelow later recalled that when he first started practice and a patient died under his mild therapy, he felt guilty at the possibility that Rush may have been right, and that he should have been more aggressive in his treatment.[57] On his return to Boston from Philadelphia he became associated in practice with the elder Jackson and clearly was influenced by his views on therapy. Even in 1817 when Bigelow wrote the preface to his *Medical Botany*, he made clear his desire to reduce rather than extend the therapeutic armamentarium, a penchant for simplicity in materia medica that he also applied to his work on the *Pharmacopoeia of the United States* (1820).[58]

For the quarter century before he gave his address, Bigelow had functioned within a Boston medical environment in which a favorable attitude toward the healing power of nature, an emphasis on recognizing the natural course of diseases, and a humble appraisal of the physician's ability to cure were all common. What made Bigelow's essay important and influential was not its originality but its clarity and force. He sought to convey a single important point, and he did so with straightforward language and single-minded direction. His prominent position in Boston medicine strengthened the power of his remarks: when he gave his address he had been a Harvard Medical School professor for two decades, was attending physician at the Massachusetts General Hospital, and was nationally prominent for his role in preparing the *Pharmacopoeia*. The context in which his paper was presented, as the annual address to the Massachusetts Medical Society, gave it special visibility. As one physician commented, "Its publication by the Society placed it on the table of every regular physician of the Commonwealth, and within the reach of most educated men."[59]

Bigelow did not question the physician's ability to actively cure with drugs in many diseases, but only in those he designated as "self-limited." By such a disease Bigelow meant "one which receives limits from its own nature, and not from foreign influences; one which, after it has obtained foothold in the system, cannot, in the present state of our knowledge, be eradicated, or abridged, by art,—but to which there is due a certain succession of processes, to be completed in a certain time." These processes, he proposed, "may tend to death, or to recovery, but are not known to be shortened, or greatly changed, by medical treatment."[60] Even in such "self-limited" diseases, Bigelow did not advocate a passive course. "The question will naturally arise," he acknowledged, "whether the practitioner is called on to do nothing for the benefit of his patient; whether he shall fold his hands, and look passively on the progress of a disease, which he cannot interrupt. To this I would answer,—by no means." The physician could save the patient from "the ill-judged activity of others"; palliate the patient and sustain the family with clear prognostication; and manipulate sleep, diet, and environment to produce an atmosphere conducive to nature's most favorable operation.[61] Often this approach demanded the timely interposition of the same active drugs that were the mainstays of Rush's practice. Nonetheless, such a position was humble. To recognize the value of drugs, Bigelow asserted, the physician must be prepared to acknowledge the limitations of art.

In the literature in support of nature trusting that proliferated in Boston during the decades following Bigelow's address, the relative roles he had ascribed to nature and art in healing were reanalyzed and redefined, but not fundamentally changed. Oliver Wendell Holmes said little new when in 1860 he promoted the healing power of nature in his widely known annual address to the Massachusetts Medical Society, "Currents and Counter Currents in Medical Science." Holmes had studied medicine in the early 1830s at Harvard with James Jackson, after which he spent three years in Europe following especially Louis's instruction in Paris. Returning to Boston he was appointed physician at the Massachusetts General Hospital for several years, and from 1847 held a medical professorship at Harvard. Holmes unambiguously placed his address in the tradition of Bigelow's talk of 1835, which, he observed, "has given the key-note to the prevailing medical tendency of this neighborhood, at least, for the quarter of a century since it was delivered."[62] He also recognized the singular strength of this intellectual tradition in Boston. "If there is any State or city which might claim to be the American head-quarters of the nature-trusting heresy," he asserted, "that State is Massachusetts, and that city is its capital."[63]

Since the time of Bigelow's address, Holmes maintained, the one important new element in medical discourse was the growing popularity of homeopathy, a movement against which he had led the New England crusade from the early 1840s. With that movement's rise, Holmes noted, "the old question between 'Nature' so called, and 'Art,' or professional tradition, has re-appeared with new interest."[64] Holmes represented in new language the importance of striking a balance between nature and art, and the dangers of excessive drugging. The physician should not abandon drugs, but his task was much broader than merely administering them. He should be a "Naturalist" who studies and explains the operations of nature in disease and creates an atmosphere conducive to healing.[65]

It is clear, then, that critics were wrong in saying that the Boston nature trusters were rejecting active drugs in *principle*. But what about in *practice?* Were critics correct in their charge that the expectant practitioner stood at the bedside with folded arms while nature did all the work? Simply put, they were not. The therapeutic activism of the Boston skeptics can be displayed by an analysis not only of their normative rhetoric, but also of what they actually did in the sickroom. In the records of medical practice kept by such physicians as Jackson, Sr., Bigelow, and Holmes, it is unmistakably clear that these men used all of the leading therapies that Rush employed—such bleeding techniques as venesection, leeching, and wet cupping; mercurial purgatives such as calomel; strong emetics such as tartrate of antimony; blisters, setons, and sinapisms; and opiates such as Dover's powder and laudanum. At the end of the 1840s, for example, when both Bigelow and Holmes were physicians at the Massachusetts General Hospital, each of them prescribed all of these therapies, including venesection, in treating the hospital's inmates. Their practice was milder than that of some more assertively heroic physicians, and at times their self-conscious attentiveness to diet, rest, and exercise was apparent. But they were not inactive.[66]

The fact that skepticism in Boston did not mean noninterventionism or the rejection of drugs is clearly displayed by the practice at the Massachusetts General Hospital. As a group the hospital's medical staff represented as strong a body of nature trusters as was to be found anywhere in America, including among its ranks such "skeptics" as Jackson, Bigelow, Walter Channing, John Ware, and Holmes. Furthermore, medical theory held that the kinds of patients recruited by the hospital required less aggressive therapy than the same physicians might prescribe for their private-practice patients.

If skeptics rejected traditional, active remedies anywhere, then they would be expected to have done so at the Massachusetts General Hospital. They decidedly did not. The agents of heroic depletion declined dramatically in use there as elsewhere from the 1820s through the 1850s, but were widely prescribed nonetheless. Their commonness is illustrated by the frequency of the three practices most emblematic of heroic depletion—mercurials, antimonial emetics, and bloodletting. In the male medical wards, the percentages of patients for whom these practices were used in the 1830s, 1840s, and 1850s were, respectively, for mercurials 50.8, 41.4, and 28.7; for antimonial emetics 22.0, 12.1, and 6.8; and for bloodletting 34.8, 22.1, and 14.3. Opiate use in the hospital became increasingly common, being prescribed during these decades in, respectively, 45.1, 54.2, and 62.5 percent of the cases. The employment of tonics and stimulants such as alcohol, quinine, and iron compounds also progressively increased. All of these practices, including venesection, were occasionally applied at the hospital through the 1860s. Plainly drugging had not been vanquished and expelled from the hospital's wards. Indeed, although the mean duration of stay declined over this period, the mean number of treatments given per case increased from 7.4 in the 1830s to 7.9 in the 1840s and to 8.7 in the 1850s.[67]

Even when physicians in the hospital explicitly allowed nature to take its course, they were not therapeutically inactive. In 1832 a student attending Jackson's clinical lectures on a febrile patient in the hospital copied into his notebook, "General plan of expectant treatment & consistently with this an emetic or a cathartic."[68] In the same year Walter Channing directed that his prescription of "Medicine expectante" be written into the case record of a male domestic afflicted with fever; without violating this order, the house physician, the young Holmes, gave the patient both ipecac and opium that night for pain. Leeching, cupping, and calomel were all administered to another patient for whom Channing ordered the same prescription.[69]

Leaving disease to its course did not mean leaving the patient alone. Lecturing in the hospital to students on the case of a nineteen-year-old female domestic admitted in 1830 with fever, for example, John Ware, one of Jackson's "excellent doubters," noted, "In this case, [it is] manifest that disease made great inroads in organs of Head and abdomen. Object to relieve these & nothing else." Accordingly, he told them, he had determined to "leave disease to [its] course . . . Where effect of remedies is doubtful—not as some do, do anything[,] rather do nothing—nothing rather than anything wh [will] exhaust & may do hurt—When we are doubtful about our way in a muddy path by twilight, throw the horse the reins & trust to sagacity—So in disease—rely on nature—give her the reins—whenever come to a stand—In conformity was practice in this case." The patient's case history reveals that the practice corresponding to the normative statements "do nothing," "rely on nature," and "leave disease to course" included administering within seven days thirteen different treatments, among them calomel, mustard plasters, laudanum (tincture of opium), and thirty-seven leeches applied to the head and epigastrum.[70]

For the Boston skeptics, the bond between professional identity and therapeutic intervention clearly was not broken either in principle or in practice. They regarded prudent action as an essential part of their professional task and never doubted that the physician had an active role in the healing process. The caricature of them as noninterventionist was untrue, but it is nonetheless revealing. In part critics constructed a model of the "skeptics" that embodied what they were afraid might come to pass rather than expressing the way things were. This endeavor reflected the sensibilities of a profession very much on the lookout for heterodoxy in its ranks and fearful of the consequences if the corruption of medical orthodoxy went unchecked. Even though homeopathists believed themselves to be therapeutically active, in the eyes of regulars they gave no active remedies and thereby provided an example of true noninterventionism. Nature trusting, to some regulars, represented yet another sect whose adherents should be denounced and expelled. Furthermore, while the Americans who studied in Europe did not return as therapeutic nihilists, the development of genuine nihilism in the Vienna school of the 1840s, most vividly expressed in the extremism of clinician Joseph Dietl, seemed to substantiate fears that it was possible for an eminent regular physician to renounce medical art.[71]

The caricature of therapeutic skeptics also reflected the fear of any internal criticism that could diminish the profession's claims to efficacy. While those physicians who stressed nature did not reject drugs, they did say that physicians were less able to cure by art than either the public or regular practitioners had previously thought. This more humble attitude threatened an insecure profession anxious to hold fast to all its disputed claims to power. By opening established dogma to critical questioning, skeptics placed professional tradition, and the reassurance it gave the practitioner, in a precarious position.

The rhetoric of younger physicians who avowedly located themselves in the newer tradition of Parisian medicine was particularly well calculated to elicit resentment from older practitioners who perceived in it a threat to *their* tradition. Youth and Parisian training often characterized those who first advocated the healing power of nature and questioned the efficacy of art. Assaults on therapeutic skepticism were consequently fueled by resentment against the pretensions of French knowledge and the young practitioner's insufficient deference to established tradition. More fundamentally, resentment was directed against physicians who critics believed did not adequately appreciate or share the insecurities of their professional brethren. The particular locus of the Boston nature trusters is revealing in this regard. As the leaders of the regular medical profession in Boston, they were unusually well entrenched. For men such as Jackson, Bigelow, and Holmes, this security came only in part from the esteem of other physicians and derived substantially from their social position, institutional power, and family and community ties. Security was, to be sure, a permissive rather than a determining factor: some other medical Bostonians who shared this security, such as George Cheyne Shattuck, Sr., retained a stauncher faith in the physician's ability to cure with drugs. Nevertheless, those who spoke for a more humble assessment of the power of medical art were often among those least fearful of the consequences for their own position and power.

More than elite professional status was involved here. Whereas there were striking numbers of nature's advocates in some of the older cities outside the Northeast, such as Charleston and New Orleans, where connections between medical institutions and long-functioning patterns of familial power and social deference were established, it was in the newer regions of the South and the West that condemnation of the healing power of nature was most robust. Frontier hardiness may have sustained arguments for heroic drugging, but it hardly explains them. In Cincinnati, for example, where even the elite of the regular profession actively felt threatened by sectarian competitors throughout the antebellum period, denunciation of skeptics was fierce. These regular physicians, in contrast to Boston's elite, felt an urgent need to assert their regularity. At the same time they battled with powerful sectarian groups for control of the city's medical institutions, such as hospitals and boards of health, and not infrequently lost.

Much of the animosity directed against the Boston nature trusters reflected the perception that medical members of a smug Boston establishment were irresponsibly making statements about the relative merits of nature and art that involved little danger to themselves but substantial risk for the regular profession as a whole. The majority of the profession did not enjoy their security, but it suffered from their indiscretions. This resentment was especially evident in the reaction to Holmes, whose identity was not grounded entirely in his position as a medical practitioner. Indeed, he had given up private practice in 1849 and resigned from the Massachusetts General Hospital two years later to become a full-time author and lecturer. By the time he gave his Medical Society address in 1860, he was becoming better known as a literary than a medical figure. His speech received a hostile reception from many physicians—in part, as the New York physician Austin Flint observed in a letter to Jackson—because "Dr Holmes was misapprehended by many, who imagined that he was willing to bring the art of medicine into discredit. Their suspicions were formed by knowing that he did not engage in practice. They feared that he was disposed to give encouragement to the homeopathists." While Flint believed that "time & reflection will make it all right," others did not shrug off so easily the perceived affront to the regular profession.[72]

Holmes's lack of caution in selecting his words was partially to blame for the tumult that followed his address. His carelessness was displayed by his endlessly quoted remark, "I firmly believe that if the whole materia medica, *as now used,* could be sunk to the bottom of the sea, it would be all the better for mankind, and all the worse for the fishes."[73] Henry Jacob Bigelow, Jacob's son, aptly described the character of this comment's reception when he recalled a decade later, "A distinguished friend of mine once stated, that, if all the medicines in the world were thrown into the sea, it would be better for the world and worse for the fishes. Unfortunately, we all thought he said *physicians,* and very properly rose in a body to hurl back the startling insinuation."[74]

The membership of the Massachusetts Medical Society resolved that it "disclaims all responsibility for the sentiments contained in this Annual Address" and directed that this resolution be published with Holmes's essay. One southern editor commented that no resolution could restore Holmes "in the estimation of *real* medical men."[75] The distinction he implied was significant. Holmes did not fully share the anxieties and insecurities felt by many physicians whose identities derived largely from practice. In that sense he was not, in their appraisal, a *real* medical man, which in America meant one who treated patients. A Kentucky medical society had written into its "Code of Etiquette" the direction that physicians should avoid "indulgence of any affected or, jocular scepticism concerning the efficacy and utility of the healing art."[76] Holmes's flippant remark clearly violated this rule.

A letter written by Samuel D. Gross to a lay friend in 1862 is typical of the response of moderate physicians who thought Holmes had gone too far. Gross, an eminent surgeon and Philadelphia medical professor, began by stating his support for the move in therapeutics toward "conservative medicine," by which he meant a plan that supported nature's operations, was expectant when appropriate, and used strong drugs when they were called for. He then turned to Holmes's recent address. "As to Dr. Oliver Wendel Holmes," Gross wrote, "he belongs to a class of nampy pampy men who, if they are not a positive disgrace to medicine, are certainly a great hindrance to it. They are pseudo-philosophers, who in their conceit & vanity, never hesitate to deride legitimate medicine whenever an opportunity offers." He added wryly, "You need not wonder at the singular, semi-apologetical 'Letter' of Dr. Jackson, now close on the borders of 90 years, when you are told that he is the father-in-law of Holmes. It is evident that he wrote his little brochure with the desire of shielding the poet-doctor from the just indignation of an offended profession."[77]

Gross was mistaken about the relation between the two men (they were cousins, and Holmes married Jackson's niece), but he was perceptive in discerning the embarrassment about Holmes's language felt by those who shared his medical views, and their fear that their own therapeutic position had been presented in a fashion that would attract ridicule. Jackson did write to the Massachusetts Medical Society asking it to withdraw its resolution disclaiming responsibility for Holmes's essay; but even though the resolution was reconsidered, it was not retracted.[78] And as Gross observed, Jackson published in 1861 a treatise entitled *Another Letter to a Young Physician*, which was explicitly an explanation of what Holmes had and had not intended to say, as well as a statement of Jackson's own therapeutic faith.

"Within the last year [since Holmes's talk in May 1860] a grave question has been agitated among us," Jackson began, namely, "whether there is any good to be derived from the practice of medicine."[79] He noted that "an impression has been received, in and out of our profession, that Dr. Holmes meant to represent the medical art as useless, and even as productive of evil, at least so far as the administration of medicine is concerned. Somewhat similar opinions have been formed, by some persons, in respect to the faith of my learned friend, Dr. Jacob Bigelow, in the utility of our art. I do not understand that either of these gentlemen is thus sceptical."[80] Holmes had been misunderstood. "His great object was to inculcate caution in the practice of medicine," Jackson proposed.[81] He proceeded to explain that nature trusting did not mean loss of faith in drugs. "It must not be understood that in pursuing the expectant course, we necessarily avoid the use of all medicines; still less, that we leave the patient without any directions as to the treatment in other respects. By leaving a case to nature, it is not meant, that we must leave it to chance."[82] Potent therapies such as mercury, antimony, and bleeding remained valued parts of his own armamentarium; no practice was to be used or eschewed routinely. His therapeutic faith, Jackson affirmed, was entirely compatible with that of Holmes and Bigelow.

Holmes's difficulty had much to do with his desire to entertain and perhaps startle his audience. In his quip about scuttling the regular medicine chest, and elsewhere in his address, he sacrificed direct expression and the possibility of persuasion for the sake of displaying wit. But the underlying problem of relating language to meaning in therapeutic discourse was a serious one even for physicians more sober than Holmes in their choice of words. The Boston practitioner Henry Ingersoll Bowditch, for example, was one of many physicians seeking a middle therapeutic path who found existing caricatures and labels inadequate to precisely express their therapeutic ideal. After graduating from Harvard Medical School and serving as a house physician at the Massachusetts General Hospital, Bowditch left Boston in 1832 to spend two years studying in Europe. Along with Holmes and his close friend Jackson, Jr., he studied with Louis, whose commitment to exact observation became a central theme in Bowditch's medical work.[83] He entered practice when he returned to Boston and in 1859 was appointed professor of clinical medicine at Harvard. In his clinical lectures Bowditch denounced the therapeutic nihilism, which he called "Pure Naturalism," represented by the Viennese clinician Joseph Dietl. "Thank God! I am not one [of] these—Nearly 30 yrs [ago] I returned as a young man from the wards of my Master the great Louis teeming with scepticism in regard to the beneficial effects of all remedial measures whatsoever."[84] From that time onward, he continued, he progressively gained greater faith in drugs. Still, according to his son's later appraisal, "In his practice my father was not what might be called a 'therapeutist' in the common acceptation of the word, and he was always rather a skeptic in the use of drugs."[85]

Condemning the heroic practitioner and the skeptic alike, Bowditch urged upon his students a plan of practice that ordinarily avoided the extremes of heroic and expectant practice while occasionally adopting each of them, what he called "the middle course" or "the golden mean." Lecturing to students at the Massachusetts General Hospital six months after Holmes had delivered his famous address, he asserted that while some physicians "are fools and knaves and use drugs unbecomingly," the "lovers of Nature" were overreacting. "I fear we are becoming carried too far and in attempting to make a good step forward we shall fall beyond the mark & as it happens always by driving a good principle to an extreme we actually produce evil." He recognized, however, that it was in rhetoric and not in practice that the American "Naturalists" appeared to be abandoning interventionism. "So far as I have had an opportunity of seeing the practice of many of the Naturalists—they really do use some of the most powerful of the drugs." The practices of the skeptics and of "their opponents or for want of a better term the common every day practitioner," he observed, "differ only in the degree and the amount of remedies used."[86]

Bowditch's relation to those whom he called skeptics reflects a persistent theme in the nineteenth-century American medical profession's management of therapeutic change, the problem of extremism. How was it possible to correct the errors of the past—in this instance the overreliance on drugging and utter distrust of nature epitomized by Rush—without overreacting against it? Physicians found it much easier to resolve this problem in their therapeutic activities than to put their solutions into words—easier, that is, to alter gradually their own practices than to find a satisfactory balance in telling their colleagues how they should change theirs. The normative statements of physicians were at times therefore far more radical in their departure from tradition than their practices ever were. Despite rhetoric that occasionally implied noninterventionism, the fact is clear that those physicians most strongly identified as therapeutic skeptics did not reject traditional therapies in principle or in practice. Their calls for attention to the healing power of nature may have been voiced with a stridency that belied their real goal of moderation; such proclamations certainly disturbed, threatened, and perhaps frightened some of their counterparts. But even Holmes never meant to endorse passivity. For antebellum regular physicians, therapeutic activity remained an inseparable part of proper professional identity.

— 2 —

Epistemology, Social Change, and the Reorganization of Knowledge

B<small>ETWEEN THE</small> 1820s and the 1850s American physicians held steadfast to their belief in the necessity of therapeutic activism and in the value in principle of traditional remedies. Yet far from being static, this was a period of signal change in therapeutics. Although they retained their faith in such established therapies as bloodletting, alcohol, and opium, practitioners began to use these treatments with frequencies and intensities that deviated sharply from earlier conventions. More fundamentally they increasingly questioned the sources and character of their therapeutic knowledge. How could the practitioner assess the worth of therapeutic practices, and how was therapeutic progress to be effected and judged? The answers rationalistic systems of practice provided made physicians more and more uneasy. Their mounting attack on such systems and their concomitant celebration of empiricism pervaded the medical literature. This transition in epistemological thinking was among the most important and revealing transformations of medical therapeutics in nineteenth-century America.

From the 1820s on, many American physicians began to see a reorientation from rationalism to empiricism in therapeutic knowledge as crucial to the clinical and social success of their profession. It is in some respects surprising that epistemological issues mattered so much to them. After all, American physicians saw themselves as preeminently practical men who valued practice over theory, as active therapeutists more than as truth-seeking scientists. Their intense concern with the epistemological foundations of therapeutic knowledge suggests that more was at stake than the underpinnings of theories. The production of epistemological rhetoric becomes more understandable if it is viewed as a form of behavior elicited by professional anxieties. The vigor with which American physicians assailed rationalistic systems and the praise they lavished on therapeutic empiricism were among their varied reactions to perceived shifts in the profession's social standing. The vehemence that typified epistemological criticism stemmed in large measure from the desperation of a profession that believed itself to be in decline.

Members of all professions in America during the second quarter of the nineteenth century shared the complaint of declining power and status. In medicine, even though many individual practitioners maintained prestigious positions in their communities, regular physicians believed that their profession as a whole had been debased in the public view. Populistic medical sects such as Thomsonianism, as well as sects like homeopathy that appealed to a more affluent clientele, challenged both the orthodox profession's claims to intellectual and therapeutic superiority and its economic well-being. The rescinding of medical licensing laws by the states in the 1830s and the 1840s institutionalized the stripping of professional privilege. Such laws had been principally honorific but had nonetheless distinguished regular physicians as singularly legitimate.[1]

Beyond these external indicators of deterioration, physicians detected ample evidence of decline within the regular profession itself. The proliferation of proprietary medical schools, many with low standards and purposes, greatly increased the number of poorly trained practitioners holding M.D. degrees. This erosion of standards confirmed charges of unmerited pretensions. The overabundance of regular physicians increased the difficulty of earning a living by practice, a circumstance that heightened competition, discordant rivalry, and professional disunity. Tensions were aggravated by the fact that while the lowest levels of the profession were growing, so too was the topmost layer. More American physicians than ever before were acquiring rigorous medical training, particularly in Paris. These men often held inflated aspirations for the profession's knowledge, practice, and institutions and were well prepared to believe the worst of the large masses of meagerly educated regular practitioners. "Our own profession, what with its ignorance, its heresies, and its moral sense, has lost the respect of the community and sunk to the level of a trade less honest & less useful than that of the rudest mechanic," one prominent Philadelphia physician lamented in 1857. "Alas! it should be so when every year is adding to the learning & science, & skill of our leading men & those around them."[2] This growth at the extremes created a group of ambitious, thinking physicians anxious to improve the standing of their profession by uplifting their backward brethren.[3]

The desire to shore up the profession was expressed in a variety of ways. State and local medical societies multiplied, and the national American Medical Association was formed in 1847 to promote unity among physicians, distance regulars from sectarians, and reform medical education. Societies attempted to arbitrate difficult interactions among physicians with formalized codes for professional etiquette, to reinstate licensing laws, and to elevate the standards of education while curtailing the number of new graduates. The profusion of new medical journals in the 1840s and 1850s represented one effort to increase the level of intellectual activity within the profession. The fact that physicians played visible roles in a variety of civic and cultural activities— including public health work from the 1840s on—can be regarded at least in part as another aspect of the same endeavor to improve their profession's standing.[4]

The adjustments physicians made in response to the debased position of the profession extended to its cognitive structures as well. The energies that drove efforts to elevate the profession by promoting social harmony, theoretical accord, and intellectual vitality also fostered a change in the character of therapeutic knowledge. It is not difficult to locate the principal intellectual origin of the epistemological shifts that characterized this period in French clinical empiricism, but the energy with which physicians scrutinized and assailed the very foundations of their therapeutic knowledge is best understood in terms of the social and intellectual functions epistemological reorientation served for a profession seeking to consolidate its legitimacy, prestige, and authority.[5] Rationalistic systems of practice came to represent the causes of degradation, and physicians turned to empiricism and to an attack on rationalistic systems in particular as a way of vindicating the regular profession. By denouncing the internal sources of the profession's problems, by dismantling systems, and by substituting empiricism for an ostensibly rigid rationalism, they sought to use therapeutic epistemology as a vehicle for professional uplift.

Rhetoric about therapeutic rationalism and empiricism was produced for several audiences. Orthodox writers, drawn largely from a well-educated elite, believed that they were speaking primarily to the poorly trained masses who purportedly followed a more extreme and mechanical therapeutic course than themselves. These practitioners needed to be forcibly roused from their ignorance and lethargy; in particular, their betters sought to wrench them away from their dependence upon rationalistic systems in practice. In this way thinking physicians sought to elevate the profession's collective standing and improve their own situation in the process.

Implicitly at least, many proclamations of allegiance to empiricism and denunciations of rationalistic systems were also directed to the public. The simple message was that although misplaced trust in systems had led orthodox physicians to commit therapeutic errors in the past, the public should not lose faith in the regular profession since physicians had recognized their earlier mistakes and corrected them through the empirical observation of nature. Contrasts between homeopathic and Thomsonian reliance on exclusive dogmas and regular adherence to empirical fact became commonplace. By confessing their past epistemological crimes while pointing to their present good behavior, regular physicians sought to distinguish themselves from sectarians and at the same time to defend their profession against accusations of therapeutic abuse.

Above all, though, the physicians who were most preoccupied with reforming therapeutic epistemology were talking to themselves. They were confident that their thinking was enlightened, and improvement in their own activity was not the end they sought: it was the thinking and actions of others that required change. Beyond catalyzing the uplift of the profession by educating its inferior practitioners, epistemological criticism served an important symbolic function for these men by affirming that they had identified a key source of and remedy for the profession's ills. By denouncing the evils of rationalistic systems and pointing to empiricism as the path to redemption, they could reassure themselves that they were doing what was necessary to bring about professional salvation. From their oratory they also derived the self-satisfaction of proclaiming their own sanctity while exhorting sinners to see the error of their ways.

The systems of medical practice most familiar to early-nineteenth-century Americans, such as those of Rush and of Scots William Cullen and John Brown, embodied the remnants of the Enlightenment hope that some unifying medical principle would be found, a law of disease and treatment that would prove as fertile for medicine as the law of gravity had for the physical sciences. A unified, rationalistic explanation of pathology characterized such systems, which often distilled the apparent diversity of disease phenomena into a single pathogenic process. Consistent with the notion that all diseases represented essentially the same morbid alterations, systems of practice tended to reduce treatment to the few operations needed to rectify these derangements. The simplified approach to disease and treatment such unitary systems posited inclined their adherents to literally systematic, routine practice. This assumption by American physicians that many followers of systems prescribed by rote was reflected in the common use of the term *system* to refer not only to a particular explanatory schema but also to more general therapeutic preferences, as in the heroic, drugging, or expectant systems. All systems claimed to have been validated by experience, but their most striking feature was the rationalism that underlay their erection and operation.[6]

By 1820 most American physicians had become ambivalent about rationalistic systems. Although practitioners were attracted by their comprehensiveness, sanction of traditional authority, and reassuring guidance to therapeutic activity, they tended to regard the therapeutic certainty systems seemed to offer as a seductive illusion belied by the complexity of bedside experience. A growing, often fervently hostile reaction against systems characterized therapeutic thought during the remainder of the antebellum period.

Three principal elements comprised the assault upon systems. The first was an empiricist reaction against their rationalism, an attitude that embodied both a new faith in the primacy of experience and a changing concept of what constituted science in medicine. The second was a particularist reaction against their universalism, propelled by the objection that systematic rules were inapplicable to individual patients. The third was the perception, driven in part by the ongoing popular critique of regular therapeutics, that systems bore an inherent tendency to extremes and thereby encouraged practices that injured patients and the profession alike.

A key to comprehending the professional meaning of talk about therapeutic epistemology is the recognition of the multiple connotations rationalism and empiricism held for American physicians. Discussions about the proper nature of therapeutic knowledge—its generation and organization—turned upon the opposition of rationalism to empiricism, and it was along the rationalism-empiricism axis that the leading shift in therapeutic epistemology proceeded. Nevertheless, in medical writings both terms had ambiguous meanings that did not bear any necessary relation to either their etymological or their intuitive meanings. Either word could take on directly opposite senses in different contexts.

Four groups of meaning for *rational* and *empirical* convey the principal significations of these terms in regular therapeutic discourse between about 1820 and 1860. In their *methodological* senses, they referred to the ways physicians acquired, assessed, and applied knowledge, as well as to the epistemological character of the knowledge upon which therapeutic explanation and practice were based. In their *professional* meanings, the terms characterized groups of medical practitioners according to their professional legitimacy, ideological allegiances, and therapeutic inclinations. Methodological and professional meanings took on both positive and negative connotations, resulting in four different usages for each term. Although confessedly arbitrary and overlapping, these categories of meaning are adequately precise to permit the tracing of the principal thrusts of physicians' arguments in a singularly confusing body of rhetoric.

When used in its methodological sense with a positive connotation, the term *rational* meant, at its simplest, prudent or judicious. "By Rational Medicine, in its proper meaning," a North Carolina physician asserted, "we understand simply, *common sense* in the practice of physic; prescribing according to the indications, relying upon no exclusive system in the treatment of disease, but invoking all reasonable plans."[7] At times *rational* referred to rules of practice deduced from general principles,[8] but by 1820 this usage was not common. More usual was the contrast of rational medicine to systems of practice. Medicine, a Richmond practitioner argued, should be based upon a rational method of induction from facts that would free it from "the trammels of authority" and "the arbitrary dictum of the master," and would at the same time avoid a "blind empiricism."[9]

Rational was also given the opposite methodological meaning by critics who linked it firmly with exclusive systems and condemned it with them. In this negative connotation, it meant separated from experience and overly devoted rules that led to practice by rote. Typically, a medical student in Nashville concluded in an 1860 essay that "science, in its whole extent and compass, is necessarily Empirical, and that the means and methods of Rationalism are not available for purposes of scientific inquiry."[10]

Rational in its positive professional sense meant grounded in medical knowledge and traditional wisdom and was a term applied to a regularly educated physician. It was sometimes very nearly synonymous with "regular," for both terms denoted the qualities that set the proper member of the medical profession apart from all other practitioners. It was with an eye to this sense of the word that Jacob Bigelow elected to name his professional plan "Rational Medicine."

In his essay bearing this title, Bigelow reviewed the other methods of practice (artificial, expectant, homeopathic, and exclusive) and judged them all to be systematic and professionally degrading, concluding, "If no alternative were left to the physician and patient but the extreme and frequently irrational methods which have now been briefly described, practical medicine might well take its rank as a pseudo-science by the side of astrology and spiritualism."[11] However, if regular physicians would but take up an enlightened attitude and eschew the unwarranted therapeutic confidence characteristic of exclusive systems—that is, adopt a rational professional stance—professional elevation would be inevitable.[12] This positive professional use of *rational* was far more common than its negative counterpart, which referred to a professional ethos characterized by rigid allegiance to authority, dogmatic obedience to tradition, and doctrinaire practice supported by the excessive therapeutic confidence that faith in exclusive systems granted.

Empirical, used in its positive methodological meaning, denoted knowledge and practice firmly grounded in experience and observation; it was discriminating and unclouded by theory. As the explanatory support of rationalistic systems was dismantled, the operations of many regular therapeutic agents were left unaccounted for, and both such remedies and their use were termed empirical. "An Empirical remedy," a Virginia medical student recorded in his class notebook in 1860, "is one where the modus operandi is not understood. The[y] become *rational* as soon as enough data are gathered, to understand their action."[13] Especially from the 1840s onward, physicians acknowledged that much of their practice was not fully explained and was unavoidably empirical. An M.D. degree candidate in Charleston argued that because so much in medical teaching was unsettled, the *"practitioner can not be controlled by any settled principal [sic] but must 'discriminate,'* and of course *his* treatment must often become empyrical, to a considerable extent."[14]

The negative methodological meaning of *empirical* was more complex. While it always referred to mechanical, indiscriminate practice, the supposed cause of that routine could be either insufficient or too much reasoning. The blundering habit of an ignorant practitioner was empirical, but so was the practice of the formally educated physician who trusted too completely in speculative systems. "Medical practice," one physician asserted, "should always be relative; it must be proportioned" to conditions rather than to names of diseases; "all else is empiricism."[15] Such unthinking application of rules of practice was what Samuel Cartwright had in mind when he claimed that therapeutics suited to the particular needs of northern climates "becomes rank empiricism when applied to the rest of the world."[16]

Reflecting the prevailing semantic muddle, *empiricism* in its negative methodological sense most often referred to an excessive reliance on rationalistic systems of practice. Physicians frequently used the term this way in decrying the abuse of a specific therapeutic agent, as when a New Orleans practitioner charged that the prominence of mercury in the systems constructed by Rush and John Esten Cooke had "led to a degree of empirical administration of that drug."[17] A student at Transylvania in the early 1840s who wrote a thesis denouncing the systems of Brown, Cooke, and François J. V. Broussais used the terms "systematic empiricism," "systematic course," and "systematic routinism" as synonyms. "It can but be mortifying to every true admirer of his profession," he wrote, "to see his own noble science quaking under the galling chains of Empiricism . . . But we think the day is rapidly advancing, when medical men will be guided in their therapeutic ministrations; by the facts as presented, irrespective of predilections for this or that system."[18]

Empirical was seldom used with a positive connotation in its professional meaning, although occasionally a practitioner was deemed judicious for his discriminating, empirical practice based upon bedside experience. Nineteenth-century American physicians had inherited a long-established equation of the empiric and the quack, and it was ordinarily in this sense that professional postures were judged empirical. The term *empiric* had acquired this condemnatory meaning in England by the seventeenth century, when medical practitioners whose knowledge of practice avowedly came from experience were scorned by Oxbridge-educated fellows of the Royal College of Physicians who flaunted their cultivated rationalism. The self-conscious turn to methodological empiricism by some physicians associated with the Royal College, such as licentiate Thomas Sydenham, complicated the word's medical meaning but did not dispel its association with quackish behavior.[19]

Therefore when a western practitioner wrote in 1847 of "the senseless empiricism of homoeopathy," he implied nothing about that sect's epistemological foundations, but merely condemned it as quackery.[20] Breaches of professional etiquette by regular physicians were also termed empirical. For example, an Ohio medical society wrote into the rules of ethics it adopted in 1829 that improper consultation behavior was "empirical in the extreme" and cause for public censure.[21] Three decades later, this was the sense in which a local medical society's committee on ethics judged medical advertising and public boasting to be empirical, "derogatory to the dignity of the Profession." The committee reported that "these are the ordinary practices of empirics and are highly reprehensible in a regular physician."[22]

The disparity between *empirical*'s persistently negative professional meaning and its increasingly positive methodological meaning created a tension that inevitably disturbed physicians. It was as an explicit plea for the resolution of this confusion that a student at the University of Pennsylvania submitted "An Essay on Empiricism" as his medical thesis. The word *empiric*, he began, was "used as synonymous with Quack, Charlatan, Imposter &c, to point out those whose practice does not meet the requirements of the profession to which they pretend to belong." He wrote "to protest against the use of a word whose definition comprehends so much that is useful, and which defines the very foundation of true Medical Knowledge." Empiricism, he argued, was essential to the "Scientific Physician."All medical theories were founded upon empirical practice, and without this basis would be useless to the practitioner. Through this semantic paradox, "we are placing the regular Physician, in an anomalous position, for adopt[ing] Empiricism as a title to designate Imperfect practice, founded upon false principles, as we now do, we must compel him to disavow all treatment based upon the results of his own experience and which are not yet explained by theory . . . This presupposes and in fact asserts that medicine is not a progressive science; but is now at a stand still, having years ago attained its highest culmination of perfection. And who of its votaries, will admit that?" In order for physicians to avoid perpetual contradiction in discussing the nature of their medical knowledge, he urged, the misused term *empiric* to mean charlatan should be abolished. "Call him an ignoramus," he pleaded, "but not an Empiric."[23]

The sociopolitical connotations of the regular profession's epistemological rhetoric had destroyed the integrity of its vocabulary. By the second quarter of the nineteenth century the terms *rational* and *empirical* taken by themselves were all but meaningless in medical discourse and had only what concrete significance context conferred. Both could mean discriminating or mechanical, professional or quackish, scientific or ignorant; they were synonyms and antonyms of each other and of themselves. This multiplicity of meanings for the two words most central to the ongoing reassessment of therapeutic knowledge confused programmatic statements and greatly clouded discussion.

Categorizing the ways these terms were used makes it possible to identify several general characteristics of the deliberation about therapeutic knowledge. For example, although all of the usages described above were current throughout the period between 1820 and the Civil War, in their professional meanings *rational* retained a generally positive connotation while *empirical* remained predominately negative. In part this can be attributed to the common-sense meaning of rational as reasonable and not irrational. These continued language patterns are also explained by the fear among regular physicians that any softening of their condemnation of "empirics" might compromise their position.

The terms' methodological meanings did not have the same stability, however. *Rational* acquired an increasingly negative connotation as physicians reacted against the rationalism of systems, which became methodologically suspect as one source of the imagined indiscriminate drugging for which the regular profession was incessantly rebuked. Concurrently, the methodological meaning of *empirical* became steadily more positive as physicians deliberately turned to clinical experience and questioning of theory as a way to reform medical knowledge. This dual transformation in methodological usages clearly reflects the predominant shift in therapeutic epistemology from rationalism to empiricism.

This analysis of word usage further explains certain difficult expressions in the nineteenth-century therapeutic vocabulary in a way that does not assume that physicians were characteristically illogical. For example, the widely used term *rational empiricism* is best read to mean prudent, discriminating methodological empiricism—that is, professionally respectable empiricism explicitly dissociated from the equation of empiric with quack. The term had a wholly positive connotation, combining the positive methodological meaning of *empiricism* and the positive professional meaning of *rational*. Similarly, this analysis of meanings explains how Bigelow's "Rational Medicine" could have become a rallying point for American therapeutic empiricists. Bigelow was openly sympathetic with French-inspired medical empiricism,[24] but because of empiricism's overwhelmingly negative professional meaning, he did not have the option of adopting the label Empirical Medicine. Yet there was no real contradiction between his empiricist commitments and the term he selected, for his plan for medicine was rational in the professional meaning of the word though staunchly empirical in methodology.

While the trend of therapeutic thought during the second quarter of the nineteenth century clearly was away from rationalistic systems and toward empiricism, the revolt against system was by no means monolithic. By the 1820s the systems of Cullen and Rush were seldom taught as unified bodies of knowledge and practice, but elements of their ideas remained ubiquitous. Cautioning against dogmatic adherence to systems and at the same time presenting one's own tenets as the tested products of clinical experience was a convention in medical teaching. Thus Charles Caldwell warned students in Lexington that "blind devotion to authority [is] . . . an obstacle to acquisition of knowledge," and David Hosack advised his classes in New York to "avoid an attachment to any particular theory—Treasure up your knowledge from the sick room," while both men proceeded to proselytize their own theories.[25]

Two new systems of practice, those of John Esten Cooke and François J. V. Broussais, rose to vogue among some American physicians during the 1820s and 1830s, the very time when the reaction against systems was mounting. An allegiance to observed fact tempered by a dogged attachment to theory—the substantive core of the physician's epistemological dilemma—was apparent in the sympathy and revulsion that practitioners displayed toward the ideas of Cooke and Broussais. Assessments of these, the last rationalistic systems to attain major influence, illustrate the increasing antagonism yet underlying ambivalence American physicians felt toward system.

Cooke's theories gained little support before the late 1820s, when he was appointed professor of the theory and practice of medicine at Transylvania University in Lexington, Kentucky, published his *Treatise on Pathology and Therapeutics*, and cofounded the *Transylvania Journal of Medicine and the Associated Sciences*. These were influential forums for disseminating his ideas, especially in the South and West. Although Cooke's treatise was massive, the essence of the pathological and therapeutic system it presented was simple. Miasmata, which he held to be the remote cause of fever (and virtually all diseases), weakened the action of the heart; cardiac dysfunction in turn diminished the pulse, enfeebled capillary circulation, and led to the accumulation of blood in the vena cava. Congestion of the vena cava constituted the essential phenomenon of disease and deranged the body's functions, especially suppressing the secretion of bile. By stimulating biliary secretion and arousing weakened organs, the practitioner relieved congestion and restored health. To this end the leading remedy was calomel (compounded with rhubarb and aloes) in the cathartic Cooke's Pills.[26]

Despite the manifest rationalism of this unitary theory, Cooke asserted that his ideas were grounded in observation alone. In the tradition of invoking Newton's name for self-legitimation, Cooke, as John Brown had done, prefaced his treatise by stating that he was applying "the method of philosophizing of the great Newton" to medicine. He rejected the theories of Cullen, Brown, and Rush as based on assertions and not evidence, hypotheses rather than observations.[27] Cooke conveyed his allegiance to fact in his classroom teaching as well. "We should evidently be guided, in our practice, by . . . fact alone," a Transylvania student wrote in his medical thesis, which he dedicated to "John Esten Cooke, . . . My esteemed Preceptor," in 1833. "It is this which should distinguish the physician from the Empiric, & this alone should determine his superior claims upon an enlightened & liberal public," he continued. Denouncing deductive systems of practice, he perceived professional salvation in Cooke's "Theory of Congestion"; through it, "we are not forced to resort to idle hypothesis, or vain speculation, to explain the phenomena observed in disease; but rest our explanation upon the facts observed, & their concurrent testimony, with the general plan of treatment."[28]

The timing of his system's demise had as much to do with Cooke's own career as with his medical doctrines. Along with two other Transylvania faculty members, Cooke left Lexington to found the Medical Institute of Louisville in 1837. At the same time he redirected his energies to religion, taking up as his own the welfare of the Protestant Episcopal Church.[29] Bereft of his active support, Cooke's system was assailed in all parts of the United States with only scant defense.

Reaction against Cooke's system was strongest in Cincinnati and Lexington, homes of the medical schools in greatest competition with the new Louisville school and the medical centers of the region in which Cooke's teaching had been most influential. The vehemence of the western denunciation of Cooke is largely attributable to proprietary rivalry, but the specific charges brought against him are nonetheless revealing of the prevailing antisystem animus. "The *bilious pathology*," a lecturer in Cincinnati typically asserted in 1843, "which hangs like an incubus about the profession, rests upon vague assumptions; that is, the explanation of nearly all diseases upon a supposition of deranged or vitiated biliary secretion, rests alone upon hypothesis, is the offspring of erroneous observation, and in its results is destructive in practice."[30] One of the many Transylvania students to write his thesis in the early 1840s as a brief against Cooke was more personal in his attack. "The Vena-Cavism of Cooke, we thank God, has, like its originator, one foot in the grave," he wrote. "It has (as I candidly believe) set back medicine in the Valley of the Miss[issippi] at least twenty years."[31] Cooke's influence on American therapeutics was dramatic but transient. Only on the practices of physicians who had come directly under his tutelage was the imprint of Cooke's doctrines generally deep.

The influence of Parisian clinician F. J. V. Broussais, though less direct, was more extensive and lasting. Broussais's formulation of an assertively antiontological "physiological" conception of disease in the 1810s and 1820s had given him a scientific prominence that Cooke never approached. "*Broussais* is a genius," one American studying medicine in Paris wrote to his sister in 1836. "He seized the Science of Medicine like a good old Doctor would a bottle of lotion, and shook it manfully: France, Germany, all Europe, parts of Asia and America have felt the agitation."[32] Broussais's eminent position in the Paris school lent authority to his publications, a number of which were translated and published in the United States during the late 1820s and the 1830s, and gave him a means of reaching socially powerful and intellectually ambitious American medical men.

Broussais's model of pathogenesis and treatment, like Cooke's, was reducible to a simple plan. He denied the existence of specific diseases and held that overstimulated bodily functioning leading to anatomical lesions (almost always expressed as inflammation of the gastrointestinal tract) was the process held in common by most diseased conditions. Because the central feature of disease was overstimulation or pathological irritation, the indication for treatment was to physiologically lower the patient. Therapy was therefore selectively antiphlogistic, consisting in most cases of a low, debilitating diet and local depletion by leeches. In sharp antithesis to Cooke's advocacy of mercurial purgatives, Broussais eschewed cathartic drugs, which he maintained would further irritate the already inflamed gastrointestinal tract.

These ideas especially attracted Americans who hoped to combat the influence of rationalistic systems, countering undue speculation by attending to facts. Broussais had decried earlier systems and their builders, "those obscure & purely speculative logicians, who follow in the treatment of human infirmities, the chimeras of their imaginations, rather than the real disorders which are presented to their senses."[33] Edward Hall Barton, a Louisiana proselytizer of Broussaisism in the early 1830s, saw its founder as a staunch Baconian and his "physiological medicine" as a therapeutic counterweight to the mercurial drugging of the "purgo-maniacs."[34] Barton ridiculed the disciples of Cooke who saw "nothing but congestion of the *vena portae*"; "Here is 'unity of disease,' with a vengeance; *uno morbo; uno remedio.* Here is simplicity without truth, and uniformity without principles."[35] He was aware of no inconsistency between assigning Cookeism to "the borders of empiricism" and embracing Broussais's philosophy of therapeutics.[36]

But other physicians challenged Broussaisian theories as "highly-wrought but unfortunately unfounded opinions."[37] Pierre Louis was a vicious opponent of his countryman's theories, and his American students formed a major nucleus of opposition to Broussais's ideas.[38] Criticism grew progressively stronger until by the 1850s Broussais had become a standing symbol of rationalism's dangerous seductiveness. Summing up the prevailing assessment in 1857, a Nashville medical student stated that with Broussais's theories, "a new era sprang forth in the History of medicine, and his doctrines were made resplendent by the honor of his name. But it was reserved for later Philosophers to expose his premises, refute his theories, and bring medicine back to the light of truth by the test of experience." He concluded, "The day of personal authority and universal sway in our science has passed and the great American principles of free thought and free speach, prevails."[39]

Despite dissimilarities in the constituency, cultural locus, and intellectual origins of the therapeutic ideas propounded by Cooke and Broussais, the criticisms brought against their theories followed remarkably similar tacks. A student of Cooke at Transylvania who wrote his thesis in 1833 on "The Theory of Broussais" decried it as a "delusive phantom, wrapped in mist & physiological enigmas, & obscured in the depths of sophistry." Plainly mimicking his preceptor's teaching, he stated that "to establish principles by fine spun theories, & bold assertions, is a phantom, no longer to be imposed on the medical world . . . All correct theory must have for its basis alone, matters of fact, from which all our principles are to be deduced: short of this, we will be involved in uncertainty & error."[40] These words could as well have been composed by a Broussaisian critic of Cooke's theory, or indeed by any American physician of the period assailing systems generically. Regardless of the particular theory, the elements of its denunciation were the same: rationalistic medical systems fostered practice by rote and therapeutic extremism, which in turn undermined the public's faith in regular medicine, drove patients to quacks, and degraded the profession. The vocabulary, logic, and accusations that went into criticism of therapeutic knowledge had all become parts of a formalized convention that turned upon the perceived evils of rationalism.

The assault on system became even more strident in the 1840s, when it was epitomized by Elisha Bartlett's empiricist manifesto *An Essay on the Philosophy of Medical Science* (1844). In this treatise the Paris-trained New Englander decried medical rationalists in untempered words and bitterly implicated rationalistic systems in "the abominable atrocities of wholesale and indiscriminate drugging." He explicated only to denounce the tenets of Cullenism, Brownism, Rushism, Cookeism, Broussaisism, "and all the host of other so called rational *isms.*"[41] Pathological systems were "*a priori* abstractions, under the misnomer of laws, or principles," and it was not merely deluded but dangerous to deduce therapeutics from them. "I hope," Bartlett concluded, "that the true character of all these pretended medical doctrines is now sufficiently obvious to the reader. I hope he is prepared to judge them according to their deserts, and to assign them their appropriate position *without* the pale of legitimate science."[42]

By the 1840s and 1850s the very term *system* had become an epithet of derision. It functioned in medical rhetoric as a discrediting modifier that implied treatment in which theoretical commitments hobbled therapeutic discrimination. Those who pledged their loyalty to the healing power of nature, for example, were decried for taking up "the *expectant* system," "the *system of nature*," or "the do-nothing system."[43] Even Bartlett's therapeutic empiricism was disparaged as a system: it was a pity, a Cincinnati physician commented, "that one so calm, reflecting, and philosophical as Dr. Bartlett evidently is, should be led into a position, or medical *system*, . . . and thereby greatly impair his standing as a *teacher*, and his usefulness as a practitioner."[44] To call a therapeutic position a "system" was to damn it as unprofessional and ultimately dangerous to both the profession and the patient.

What accounts for the vehemence of the assault American physicians mounted on systems of medical practice and their purported rationalism? In part, of course, the empiricist impulse must be ascribed to new attitudes toward medical knowledge brought back from France by the Americans who studied there in increasing numbers. Pierre Louis correctly described the task his American students had set for themselves when he wrote to Henry I. Bowditch that they were constructing "a barrier against the spirit of system."[45] The clinical empiricism of the Paris school often took the radical, unyielding stand Bartlett espoused; indeed, Bartlett's empiricist treatise was the most coherent single statement of the French medical ethos, leading historian Erwin Ackerknecht to label him "the philosopher of the Paris clinical school."[46] French medicine contributed fundamentally to the empiricist revolt against rationalistic systems. Yet the French philosophical impulse fails to account adequately for the stridency with which system was besieged. It is that stridency, that sense of urgency tending at times to desperation, that must be explained.

"System" became an objectification of the profession's social, economic, and intellectual ills. Rationalistic systems of practice were identified as a major cause of the profession's degradation, and therefore the countering empiricist critique of medical knowledge included a program of concrete changes through which specific problems could be alleviated. Attacking medical systems was also a symbolic action against the sources of professional despair, and the vehemence of the attack reflected the intensity of the anxiety that drove it. A crusade against rationalistic systems, declared under the banner of empiricism, gave regular physicians a rallying point and a project for reform. American therapeutic rhetoric underwent a self-conscious reorientation toward empiricism that in part took on the form and role of a medical jeremiad, a lamentation of decline that explained the profession's shortcomings and called on physicians to repent and thereby reclaim for it its proper place.

Regular physicians held systems accountable for the degradation of their profession in a variety of ways. One pernicious tendency of rationalistic systems was to generate overconfidence in drugs. Blind adherence to a theory, critics charged, fostered dangerously aggressive use of venesection by Rushites, mercury by Cookeites, and leeches by Broussaisists, and it also fostered inert practice by the followers of Bigelow and Holmes. The therapeutic monism typical of systems also excluded many useful therapeutic agents and discredited others by encouraging their overzealous use. "I reject all systems of medicine believing them to be highly pernicious," a Kentucky professor disturbed by this fact began his lectures in 1843. "The most powerful sanative agents in the materia medica are expurged from use in consequence of such systems."[47] By corrupting the use of the regular armamentarium, systems inevitably diminished the physician's power to heal.

The recognized tendency of systems to encourage therapeutic extremism further injured the regular profession by delivering weapons into the hands of sectarians. Patients who were overtreated with orthodox therapies would lose confidence in the regular profession and seek relief elsewhere. "So inveterate, with some, has become the *habit* of administering mercury—so common its use in all cases, without distinction of age, sex, habits, or constitution, and, we had nearly said, disease—," a Cincinnati physician claimed in 1842, that it had the effect of "driving the community from regular physicians."[48] Persistent sectarian attacks on excessive drugging by orthodox practitioners did much to erode the regular profession's image. Most often these accusations focused on the routinism that blind allegiance to theory and rationalism purportedly generated. A professor at the Cleveland Institute of Homoeopathy denounced allopathic excesses to his classes with examples of cases "treated by the murderous systems."[49] The link in popular imagery between regular physicians and drugging by rote, which sectarian rhetoric helped forge, was welded by the equation of the orthodox practitioner with the "mineral doctor" or "calomel doctor."[50]

In fact, underlying most regular considerations of the role that systems played in determining the socioeconomic standing of the profession were the examples of Thomsonianism and especially homeopathy. By challenging the regular profession's intellectual hegemony, denouncing its practices to the public, and competing with it for patients, these sects were a leading source of its experience of decline. Furthermore, regular physicians clearly saw both sects as themselves rooted in rationalistic systems of practice. After all, Hahnemann had cast homeopathy in substantially the same eighteenth-century mold that had given shape to the systems of Cullen, Brown, and Rush; as regular physicians assessed it, homeopathy offered an unambiguous example of extreme rationalism informing a dogmatic system of practice with dire consequences. The rise of this explicitly heterodox system of medicine at the very time that orthodox physicians were embracing the ideal of empiricism led those regular practitioners who did not adopt homeopathy to dissociate themselves from its adherents and from its intellectual misdirection, including its grounding in rationalism.[51]

Physicians attributed much of the profession's social dislocation to the disunity of its members, which they held to be another result of dogmatic commitments to rationalistic systems. The strife among them was notorious. "When we see Faculties in particular, and the whole fraternity of Physicians in general," a Maryland student observed in 1846, "we see acrimony, sarcasm, criticism, and ire, towards each other."[52] The bitter disagreements that faith in different systems produced inevitably debased the public's assessment of the profession. As one practitioner explained, "Opposing views in practice, among regular physicians, induces the belief that one of the parties is in error, and weakens public confidence in the whole."[53]

Systems further damaged the regular profession's standing by rigidifying the medical mind and thereby hindering therapeutic progress, physicians held. Blind devotion to authority fostered complacent practice in which the chief criterion of therapeutic propriety was conformity to systematic rules. "This formality," a Washington City physician asserted, "this routinism, is the bane of improvement in our science."[54] The most pernicious effect of a rationalistic system was to determine what its adherent saw and what he ignored at the bedside. "When once a particular set of doctrines have been imbibed," a Transylvania medical student wrote in his 1841 thesis, "they exert a secret but powerful influence over all our habits of thought and principles of reasoning; and, unknown to ourselves, perhaps, give their peculiar hue to every subject of investigation and reflection . . . The mind rejects as improbable, unsatisfactory or anomalous, all those facts and principles opposed to, and 'grapples with hooks of steel' such as seem to chime in with preconceived opinions and impressions."[55] Faith in systems both sustained inferior practice and blocked the profession's escape from its degraded position by checking therapeutic improvements.

This explication of how systematic medical practice had contributed to the profession's decline was not just a lament; it also provided a concrete plan for action, a project by which professional salvation could be attained through epistemological change. In a turn away from systems and in a deliberate reorientation from rationalism to empiricism, physicians perceived a means of actually improving both the practice and the status of the orthodox profession. They hoped to better regular practice by altering the knowledge that directed it, substituting a moderate, discriminating approach carefully grounded in experience for the mechanical practice and extremism associated with rationalistic systems. Professional disharmony would be alleviated through a shared allegiance to facts, minimizing the divisive influence of commitments to conflicting systems of practice. By providing better practice and by presenting a unified professional front, regular physicians would scotch sectarian competition and criticism and elevate the profession in the public regard.

The very act of attacking rationalistic systems played an important role in allaying physicians' anxieties. The energy that informed the attack went well beyond that necessary to expound their shortcomings and develop a program for reform. Moreover, physicians recognized that not all of the profession's problems could logically be attributed to systems: not only had systems dominated medical thought before the chief signs of professional decline began to be evident in the 1820s, but physicians also acknowledged other sources of professional debasement, such as the condition of medical education. Nevertheless, they repeatedly affirmed their faith in the transcendent power of epistemological reorientation to catalyze professional redemption.

Systems became an identifiable target onto which a degraded profession could project the causes of its anxieties and that it could blame for its woes. By denouncing this symbolic villain, physicians could reassure themselves that the medical profession would not stay in the anomalous position it temporarily occupied. An assertive proclamation of allegiance to empiricism and aggressive attack on rationalistic systems meant that the profession was actively doing what was necessary in order to redeem itself. It had seen the light and was renouncing its past epistemological sins, confident that salvation would ensue. Analyzing systems of practice in order to condemn them gave physicians a medium through which they could express, understand, and act on the sources of strain in the profession.

The emerging emphasis on therapeutic empiricism was expressed predominantly through a self-consciously critical attitude toward existing therapeutic knowledge. Especially from the 1830s onward, American physicians placed growing stress on the role of clinical medicine in disseminating therapeutic wisdom and gaining new knowledge. Clinical education in particular offered a medium for institutionalizing commitments to empiricism, allowing medical students both to, as one New Orleans school's announcement put it, "familiarly look disease in the face"[56] and to think critically about established knowledge.

"Clinical Medicine," a committee on that professorship at the Medical College of Ohio reported to the faculty in 1831, "does not . . . occupy itself on *Systems* of Pathology and therapeutics."[57] A report to the Baltimore Almshouse on the prospects of clinical instruction reflected a similar attitude three years later. The aims of clinical teaching, the report noted, "ought to be somewhat superior to the imposition of carrying out into practice some favorite abstract system: something elevated far beyond the servile drudgery of enforcing dogmatic routine . . . We should not only test the validity of former opinions & practice but institute researches for the discovery of new facts from which to trace new & more satisfactory inductions." By experience at the bedside, the student would be freed from the faith in systems that had tethered the profession.[58]

The stress on a critical, undoctrinaire attitude toward therapeutic knowledge that made clinical medicine the pivot of ascendant empiricism was formally expressed in therapeutic stances such as Bigelow's "Rational Medicine." As one Boston reviewer noted, Bigelow explicitly formulated his therapeutic philosophy to counter all exclusive systems of practice.[59] Calling for a doubting posture toward all therapeutic rules and practices that had not received rigorous clinical validation, this position was one extreme statement of a questioning attitude that became increasingly common after the 1820s and especially the 1830s. Bigelow's therapeutic views, a Charleston reviewer claimed, had done "more, we believe, toward establishing something like a rational method—negatively at least—in the treatment of . . . maladies, than any other single effort."[60]

The qualification "negatively at least" was crucial. Even those physicians who most ardently supported the movement toward empiricism in medical therapeutics recognized that it would be primarily destructive in its initial thrusts. After all, the first step in therapeutic reformation was to be the leveling of rationalistic systems. Some critics of "Rational Medicine" loosely equated the assault on systems with an attack on the medical principles that gave the regular profession its identity. "*Rational Medicine*," a North Carolina physician charged, "has become a sort of watchword, by which the enemies of the Regular Profession have been rallied into an organized opposition against principles that we honor and reverence."[61] Many more critics acknowledged that therapeutic empiricism was desirable in order to right the imbalance favoring rationalism and system, but held that reformers had tipped the scales too far in the opposite direction. "Systematic medicine is no more," Bennet Dowler could write in an 1859 review of Bigelow's *Brief Expositions of Rational Medicine.* "General theories of therapeutics are distrusted or repudiated." The systems of Cullen, Brown, Rush, Cooke, and Broussais were discredited, Dowler observed, and this was good. But, he cautioned, "on the other hand, extreme skepticism in therapeutic agents and a supreme devotion to, and belief in, the healing powers of Nature have followed. Skepticism continues. It increases. If extremes meet, here is an example: too much and too little faith."[62]

The empiricist program for therapeutics was principally one of tearing down. To be sure, empirical clinical observation promised in time to generate new therapeutic knowledge, not merely to test the old; but culling out error was the principal task undertaken during the four decades preceding the Civil War. "It was formerly supposed that the door to all human knowledge was only to be opened by the subtle casuistry and formal logic practiced by the schoolmen," a student of Elisha Bartlett wrote in his medical thesis. "Who of you has not seen some old physician, an advocate of the exploded theories of Hunter, Cullen, Brown, or Good, who would deny palpable facts, if detrimental to his theory; who would decry all therapeutical agents and modes of treatment that had not been so timely born as to receive the decisions of the good and great of ages past; who had rather fail by rule, than succeed by innovation; and plead the antiquity of their errors in bar of reason and common sense?" Undue reverence for the past, he held, had blocked the progress of medicine and debased the profession; American physicians could no longer indulge themselves in the false certainty of dogmas. "Ours is a sterner and less pleasing duty," he tellingly concluded. "It is the allotted task of our age to remove the crumbling relics of a false philosophy."[63]

Like their French mentors, many American advocates of empiricism interpreted the demolition of "crumbling relics" as a return to an older past, that of Hippocrates. The radicalism of the new departure in therapeutic epistemology was frequently blunted by historical allusions to the empiricism of classical Greece. As they interpreted it, the ongoing revolution in epistemology was to be a truly complete one, not merely overturning rationalism but continuing full circle to its starting point at empiricism. Having demolished the rigid structures erected by eighteenth-century system builders, physicians were once again free to apply Hippocratic methods of observation and to adjust their therapies to the specific characteristics of patient, place, and society. Empiricism was a comforting posture from which to confront the new ideas and changes that emerged during the nineteenth century. While it had reassuring roots in classical medical tradition, it simultaneously accommodated the expectation that practice would adjust to new circumstances, making therapeutic change less threatening.[64]

The revolt against system contributed to the rise of a self-consciously modest therapeutic outlook. Physicians lost their reassuring faith in rationalistic systems and the certainty they promised; empiricism provoked caution and a view of therapeutic truths as tentative. Many physicians' rhetoric sharply reflected their sense of working with a very temporary body of knowledge. "We do not know enough," James Jackson wrote in 1861 as part of his advice to young physicians, "to enable any one to offer a satisfactory *system of rational medicine*. In many instances, certainly, our practice is founded on experience alone. In the good sense of the word, our practice is *empirical*." Stressing particularly the profession's ignorance of physiology, he cautioned, "Before we can make a system of rational medicine, our stock of knowledge must be increased in all and each of the various departments of our science."[65]

Jackson's remarks were prudent as a statement of professional humility and also prescient in their stress upon physiology. In the 1870s a concerted attack would emerge against the sterility of clinical empiricism, coupled with a call for physicians "to develope a system in the treatment of disease which shall be founded on something more rational than tradition or empiricism" and produce a "rational system of therapeutics."[66] *Rationalism* would begin to reassume a positive methodological connotation and *system* to regain its legitimacy in therapeutic discourse. Empiricism had broken the rationalistic systems of an eighteenth-century mold; experimental laboratory physiology would be the foundation for a New Rationalism. "Physiology," one physician proclaimed in 1879, "leads the way to a *rational system of therapeutics.*"[67]

— 3 —

The Principle of Specificity

Underlying most of the criticisms regular physicians brought against rationalistic systems of practice was the objection that they fostered mechanical, indiscriminate treatment. That physicians actively regarded the specter of treatment by rote as such a menace to both therapeutic success and the profession's standing reflects the pivotal place the principle of specificity occupied in professional values. Specificity—an individualized match between medical therapy and the specific characteristics of a particular patient and of the social and physical environments—was an essential component of proper therapeutics. Treatment was to be sensitively gauged not to a disease entity but to such distinctive features of the patient as age, gender, ethnicity, socioeconomic position, and moral status, and to attributes of place like climate, topography, and population density.

The commitment of American physicians to therapeutic specificity was remarkably durable. Despite the dramatic upheavals that occurred in therapeutic theory, epistemology, and practice during the first two-thirds of the nineteenth century, the principle of specificity endured virtually uncontested as a central dogma in the regular therapeutic belief system. Not until the late 1860s did its primacy begin to weaken substantially.

Admonitions to heed the various elements encompassed by the principle of specificity permeated therapeutic instruction. A medical teacher in Ann Arbor in 1855, for example, itemized the "circumstances which modify indications" for correct treatment: "Age of the patient. The Sex . . . Constitution . . . The temperament. The disease going on in the organ. Idiosyncrasies, or personal peculiarities. Variation of the pulse. Habits of the patient. Tolerance of medicines. Climate. The prevailing epidemic influence. Race. Profession. Severity of the disease."[1] Professors routinely taught that such individuating factors as race, age, gender, diet, habit, occupation, climate, and season modified the character of disease and the operation of drugs, which last was also influenced by the form, dose, and combination of medicines administered.[2] Concrete directives for exercising specificity pervaded therapeutic discourse.

The commitment to the principle of specificity gave therapeutic knowledge an epistemological status fundamentally distinct from that of the basic medical sciences at least through the 1860s. In contrast to such branches of medicine as anatomy, physiology, and chemistry and to the mechanical manipulations of surgical and dental treatments,[3] which were universalized in their generation and validation, medical therapeutics was specific to patient and place. Constructing universally applicable rules of practice was a wrong-headed endeavor, for the validity of therapeutic knowledge was restricted to a type of patient and environment that closely approximated those from which it had been drawn in the first place. "Idiosyncrasy, or the peculiarities of the individual, are as anomalous and impossible to reduce to rule and measure, as the passage of the clouds," a Boston physician asserted. "What is true of one place may not be true of another."[4] By stressing the specificity, not universalism, of therapeutic (and to some extent diagnostic and prognostic) knowledge, physicians expressed their conviction that knowledge pertinent for certain places or individuals could be inappropriate for others, directing practice that was dangerous to the patient and to the physician's reputation.

In establishing the limitations specificity placed on generalizing therapeutic precepts, physicians took care to point out that this did not draw into question the universality of certain other categories of medical knowledge. The qualifying footnote a South Carolinian appended to his translation of Broussais was typical: "The Southern climate of the United States seems to require more bold and decisive practice, than the Northern climate of Paris and London: hence, to us, the therapeutics of Broussais . . . appear feeble; but the *principles*, founded on the physiology and pathology of the tissues, are undeniable and universally applicable."[5] The same distinction between the universal basic medical sciences and principles of medicine on the one hand and region-specific therapeutic knowledge on the other supported the notion that, as one medical editor put it, "while the principles of medicine are uniform, its practice must be learned in the locality in which these principles are to be applied."[6] Thus an Alabama physician arguing vigorously that southern students must learn at southern bedsides made it clear that he was pleading for the specificity only of therapeutics.

"As to the study of the *rudiments* of the science of medicine, (Anatomy, Physiology, and Chemistry,) they can be learned North, as well as South, for *they* are the same everywhere," he pointed out. "Again, there is no material difference in the practice of Surgery or Midwifery, North or South."[7]

The exercise of specificity was an essential part of proper professional identity and helped distinguish the physician who shared regular values from the quack. Responsible practice required not merely a mastery of medical principles, but also a cultivated ability to discriminate among patients' needs in selecting therapy. Regular physicians regarded nonspecific (or disease-specific) treatment—that is, treatment that was not individualized to each patient's needs—as a manifest stigma of charlatanry. They pointed to the failure of sectarian practitioners to discriminate among the therapeutic requirements of different places and patients as one of the most blatant signs of their routine, unethical, unprofessional practice. For example, as regular caricatures depicted them, Thomsonians regarded all disease as essentially a deficiency of heat, which treatment sought to restore. Guided by this simple theory, they ignored the differences among individual constitutions and treated all patients with assortments of six standardized therapies. Homeopathists were equally systematic: the homeopathic physician blithely prescribed a uniform therapy for all cases classified as the same ailment. Homeopathists no doubt would have regarded this criticism as unjust, holding with good reason that their treatment was sensitively matched to the patient's symptoms. Nevertheless, compared to the lecture notes of regular medical students, those of homeopathic and eclectic students more strikingly resemble cookbooks, cataloging a fixed recipe for each disease.[8]

A regular physician who disregarded the principle of specificity would be reduced to the ethical status of a quack. Referring to the debasement of practitioners who matched a disease with a drug "good for" it, a Kentucky physician wrote in 1822 to his brother studying medicine, "I do not wish to see you a mere *Blue Pill Pedlar* nor doctor who caries in his Pockets something that is *good for* this & that complaint."[9] A medical student in Nashville used similar language in describing the kind of recently graduated "regular M.D." whose ignorance degraded the profession. "They know precisely what is good for the colic, for the recipe is safely preserved which was never known to fail," he wrote in his own thesis in 1857. "They have also a host of others suited to any number of diseases which in foreign lands were successful in the hands of some prominent physician—thinking perhaps (if they think at all) that diseases having the same names at the north as at the south-pole have also the same characteristics, and pursue the same courses." In his appraisal, "such students are not entitled to the name, neither are they worthy ever to be classed among honorable Physicians." Such a routine practitioner would soon lose his patients to a more discriminating one, and be left with "the reputation only of a brainless quack, or at best, a respectable humbug."[10]

An image of practice that imprudently ignored therapeutic specificity was the leading target of the regular assault upon rationalistic systems. The rhetoric accompanying that attack decried systematic treatment while extolling specificity. At the same time, by stressing empirical observation, antirationalism further secured the central standing of specificity in regular thought. Discriminating observation took into account the great variety of factors that purportedly modified proper therapeutic activity, and many physicians found in ascendant empiricism support for the principle of specificity.

Yet rationalistic systems did not necessarily disregard therapeutic specificity in principle. Rush's critics feared the tendency of his system to produce uniformity in treatment and assailed him for undervaluing specificity, for example, but he did call for the variation of practice according to circumstances. In keeping with the characteristic beliefs of the Jeffersonian circle, of which he was the most prominent medical member, he held that political and social organization, the physical environment, and health were all linked, making disease and its treatment functions of both place and culture. "Diseases of warm & cold climates require different treatment," a student listening in 1809 to Rush's directives wrote in his notebook. "The season of the year should be attended to. Epidemics differ . . . The dress & moral habits should be attended to. The inhabitants of Egypt require stronger purges than other persons. The nation of which a person is a native should be attended to."[11]

The growing emphasis physicians placed on empirical observation and their allegiance to specificity encouraged them to question the validity of established therapeutic knowledge—not its validity for the particular circumstances under which it had been generated, but rather for the specific characteristics of their own patients and environments. Although the principle of specificity was by no means new, starting in the second quarter of the nineteenth century it was celebrated with a fresh vigor fueled by faith in therapeutic empiricism and by the reaction against systematic practice. Reinforcing each other, specificity and empiricism urged physicians to reassess therapeutic truth by looking to their own experiences.

Trust in inappropriate sources of authority came to be seen as a cause of ineffective practice and professional decline, as rationalistic systems were. An Indiana practitioner, for example, attributed the de-

graded condition of the profession in the West in large measure to the
continuing reliance of young physicians on knowledge acquired in New
England schools. "They do not discriminate between the diseases here
and what they have been accustomed to," he complained, "and so
treating, at first, our diseases according to the letter of the books, they
experience the sad mortification of losing a large number of their patients, and thereby obtain a bad reputation."[12]

It is important to stress that at least until the 1860s, disease-
specific treatment was in most instances professionally illegitimate.
Beginning in the 1820s physicians did increasingly recognize the existence of specific diseases characterized by distinctive congeries of
symptoms, but they believed that a host of environmental influences
could nudge one disease into another and that a single disease could
take on a variety of forms. Disease entities were not fixed but fluid,
and the actions of remedies were also inconstant. Moreover, two patients with identical diseases could require opposite treatments. This
was precisely the point Harvard medical professor John Ware made in
admonishing his students in the 1840s and 1850s to distinguish between "a pathological and a therapeutical diagnosis—the diagnosis
which determines the technical character of the disease, and that which
determines the principles upon which it is to be treated." The name
of a disease was not a trustworthy guide in treatment, he urged, for
"cases of which the pathological character is precisely the same may
require a treatment diametrically opposite."[13] In most instances, a name
could at most suggest therapeutic possibilities and point to likely courses
the disease might follow that could be anticipated therapeutically.

It was in the context of disease-specific treatment that a "specific"
was ethically suspect. "By this term," a Tennessee medical student
explained in his thesis, "is meant the indiscriminate administration
of certain medicines for the cure of Diseases which Diseases are treated
by name without reference to symptoms or accompanying complications."[14] A "specific" exerted an invariable curative action on the disease to which it was matched, regardless of the particular patient or
environment. Its mode of action was obscure; unlike most treatments,
which produced readily discernible physiological alterations (such as
catharsis, emesis, or stimulation), a specific acted by virtue of its mys-
terious antagonism to a single disease. Such assumptions ill fitted
within regular medical thought. "No scientific physician willingly admits the existence of specifics," one practitioner asserted. "Such an
admission is a germ of quackery."[15]

In denying the existence of specifics, physicians had hedged on
two possible exceptions, cinchona bark and especially its derivative
quinine for intermittent fever and mercury for syphilis, at least since

the time of Sydenham's writings in the seventeenth century. One medical student asserted of intermittent fever in 1857, "It is emphatically a specific disease dependent on a specific cause and requires a specific treatment, and that treatment is Quinine. As the Bible is *the Book*, so is *Quinine the remedy.*"[16] Physicians varyingly affirmed and denied the status as true specifics of these two remedies and a few others such as digitalis for dropsy, but before the 1860s nearly all regular physicians agreed that treatment-disease matches were exceptions to therapeutic canon, not models for progress.

Even in proposing that a remedy was nearly always indicated in a particular disease, physicians were often careful to point out that it did not constitute a specific. Bloodletting was "a sine qua non in treating yellow fever," Daniel Drake told his students at Louisville in 1847, but he cautioned that it "is not *a* specific but *a* remedy."[17] A Cincinnati practitioner perhaps best summed up the regular profession's appraisal of specifics in listing his reasons for pronouncing their use to be unprofessional "empiricism": "First, disease is not an entity, or real existence, but is only the organic and functional forces, or powers of life, modified by perversion of activity;—second, disease obeys certain laws, and these laws can only be controlled by a careful adaptation of exterior influences to the state of the patient; and third, all remedies are relative agents, that is, they only can act curatively by a *judicious* application to the *individual* case in hand. *Individualism*, not *universalism*, attaches therefore to all our therapeutic measures."[18]

The notion of specifics was connected not only with quackery but also with systems of practice. The therapeutic and pathological monism characteristic of systems, the reasoning that forged this link went, meant that there was in effect only one disease and one plan of treatment; therefore treatment was necessarily disease specific. Critics of Cooke's system, for example, charged that he used mercury as a specific in treating all fevers.[19] Attacking rationalistic systems for their advocacy of specifics was another way of saying that systems encouraged mechanical practice and ignored therapeutic specificity. Because of the association of specifics with charlatanry, such an attack doubly indicted systems as professionally disreputable. Neither the construction of systems nor the search for specifics, antebellum physicians increasingly argued, offered a promising avenue to therapeutic progress.

On one level treatment sought to adjust the overall physiological condition of the patient, elevating the debilitated body and lowering the overexcited one. It was also directed to individual symptoms as they arose. But the response to these indications the physician elected had to take into account other knowledge about the individual patient and environment, knowledge made up of an array of signs as significant as the symptoms themselves. "Scarcely any two cases of disease are to be treated exactly alike," the editors of a Boston journal declared. "The treatment in every case of disease is to be varied according to a thousand varying circumstances."[20]

In principle therapy was determined by the combination of disease and a host of specific factors that can be broken down into two broad categories, characteristics of the individual and characteristics of the place. No rigid rules defined the weight or meaning ascribed to each modifying influence. Variables were seldom demarcated sharply, for few measures of a person's therapeutic category were as discrete as gender and age, and most attributes of patients were intertwined with those of their environments. Nevertheless, a general consensus did exist about the therapeutic implications of the most significant factors.

The most inclusive term for those characteristics of the individual patient to which treatment was properly specific was *constitution*. "The 'constitution' of the patient," a Massachusetts physician wrote in 1861, is "the sum of all the influences of locality, station, hygiene, occupation, habit, diet, or accident, which have acted upon the individual from the time of his birth, until the period of the disease we are treating."[21] Heredity and life experiences created a constitution *sui generis* for each individual. "We cannot find two persons equally endowed with the same constitution," a medical student in Charleston observed in 1859, explaining that because of this, "in giving calomel to different persons with bilious fever; the dose that would produce an action from the liver in one case would not do it in another; & in giving quinine to different persons, some will take eight grains or more without any injurious effects and the same dose would almost deafen another."[22] The more knowledge the physician had about the patient's constitution, the better able he was to judge therapeutic tolerance and need.

A less idiosyncratic index that offered a general characterization of a patient's constitution was *temperament*. This concept had been established in medical thinking since the time of Hippocrates, though by the nineteenth century it had lost much of its earlier rigidity, preserving the terminology of classical humoral pathology but little of its explanatory significance. "The constitution of the human frame varies in different individuals, & this variety or difference exerts an influence on the mind & diseases of People. This peculiarity of organization is called Temperament," New York medical professor David Hosack explained in the 1820s, "and they are four in number": sanguineous, choleric, melancholic, and phlegmatic.[23] Each temperament was associated with its characteristic physiognomy, behavior, types of disease, and therapeutic needs. "Temperaments," a medical student in Philadelphia noted in 1844, "will each require its appropriate and peculiar treatment, even when labouring under the same character of disease, and in the same stage of the disorder."[24] Not only did persons have their own characteristic temperaments, but so too did climates, places, and nations; the kind and strength of temperament expressed in an individual patient were determined by a combination of heredity and environment. Habits, modes of living, and age could modify temperament. Because each temperament correlated with a general therapeutic approach (such as venesection for the sanguineous and cathartics for the choleric or bilious), this construct displayed one of the clearest interactions of place, climate, person, and treatment.

Another form of the same sort of categorization, the view that different races required different medical treatments because of racially defined constitutional peculiarities, grew necessarily out of the principle of specificity. Most antebellum physicians endorsed the proposition that blacks required distinctive treatment, though they were less agreed on whether they typically needed more or less aggressive therapy.[25] Therapeutic discrimination among races placed the greatest emphasis upon hereditary determinants of constitution, though monogenecists traced race itself back to environmental origins. "Race," of course, could refer to very broad ethnic divisions. "Race, has a very great modifying influence" on the actions of remedies, a Tennessee student in Philadelphia noted in 1855. "An amputation, would be much more dangerous, in the full plethoric beer drinking Englishman, than in the very active Frenchman or Italian. It is because the former, is much more liable than the latter, to inflammations, on account of his peculiar mode of life. And so it is with medicines. A medicine which in the usual dose would scarcely affect the one, would produce in the other, the most inordinate effects."[26]

The distinctive medical treatment of blacks was not predicated on biological inheritance alone but on socioeconomic and occupational status as well. Indeed, physicians saw many of the conditions of life that molded therapeutic discriminations as linked to class and occupation. "Among different classes of the inhabitants of the world," a student in Lexington noted in 1848, "inflamation, and inflamatory constitutions vary," requiring differing degrees of supportive or depletive treatment. Laborers, physicians generally maintained, were ordinarily possessed of robust constitutions and overstimulating maladies. "Diseases of a purely inflammatory character are more common among the peasantry, and the labouring class of the community, than among epicures, and those who occupy a higher station in life, and live in indolence and luxury," the student commented. "Just in proportion to the advance . . . [of] refinement, does the inflamatory disposition sub-side; and diseases of a more malignant character increase."[27]

The therapeutic implication of this association was that more aggressively lowering treatment was appropriate for sick laborers than for the more refined classes. In 1834 a New England physician portrayed a similar image of "the healthy, the vigorous and the robust, such as we know is the New England labourer" in arguing that "a great pro-portion of the diseases of New England are diseases of excited action, requiring the employment of the lancet and other depleting measures to an extent unknown and unparalleled in other countries." He sug-gested that "we may account in part for this notorious fact, by con-siderations of climate, but the constitutional peculiarity of temperament must be mainly ascribed to an over-nutritive and over-stimulative diet." This nourishing diet, he claimed, constituted a social basis for dis-tinctively American therapeutics.[28]

Social behavior and physical environment combined to distin-guish the therapeutic needs of the city from those of the country. One Boston physician who believed that more energetic lowering treatment was demanded by rural than urban inhabitants attributed this to the notion that the urban atmosphere was vitiated by human respiration.[29] Benjamin W. Dudley, lecturing in Kentucky in the 1830s, taught that the environment of a city such as London or Philadelphia enervated its inhabitants. "A particular mode of living in those large cities," he claimed, meant that "their diseases are of a nervous, rather than san-guineous character," requiring elevating therapy opposite to the de-bilitating treatment appropriate in the country. "The treatment of the same disease, Erysipelas for instance, in one of these large towns and here, would be totally different. In one you would stimulate, in the other deplete."[30]

Discussion about therapeutic specificity that considered the dif-ferences between city and country often centered on the applicability to country practice of therapeutic knowledge generated in cities and codified by urban physicians. The primary distinction was most often drawn between country private practice and urban public practice, that is, charity practice in hospitals, almshouses, and dispensaries. Dissim-ilarities in the environments in which practice was conducted and in the types of patients recruited suggested that urban hospital knowledge and that befitting rural practice were fundamentally distinct.

It was not obvious, given the prevalent faith in specificity, that the findings of therapeutic research in hospitals were applicable to anything other than practice in similar hospitals. This became a critical issue as the hospital came to be the leading locus for producing and testing therapeutic knowledge. Some physicians regarded such knowl-

edge as irrelevant to the needs of the majority of American practitioners. Even as late as 1882 a Michigan medical professor could assert that
the "descriptions of diseases and methods of treatment derived from
consultation, practice, or experience in large metropolitan hospitals
are not in all respects exact or applicable for cases occurring in an
ordinary American village or country situation, where well-housed,
well-fed, non-alcoholized people are seen in the beginning of their
diseases."[31] American respect for European knowledge in the medical
sciences notwithstanding, these same sorts of objections were brought
against *most* European therapeutic knowledge, coming as it did not
only from a different region of the world but also from such dubiously
valid analogues for American practice as the great hospitals of London
and Paris.[32]

By reinforcing the rising emphasis on empiricism, specificity urged
that students learn through clinical experience; but it suggested at the
same time that experience in hospitals might add little to the therapeutic acumen of most students, who were destined for private practice. In this respect it provided the basis for one of the most compelling
arguments against training students in hospitals. Motivated in addition
by proprietary interests, a professor at a country medical school in New
York State argued in 1846, "Let a student of medicine from the country
take a course of instruction in the hospitals of one of our large cities
and then let him go home and commence practice among the yeomanry
of his native town and he will soon find that he has a set of very
different patients a different class of diseases and that [they] require a
very different course of treatment from those he found in the hospitals."[33]

Especially during early attempts to establish hospital instruction
as an essential component of medical education, reformers felt constrained to defend the value of hospital experience by pleading its
therapeutic similarities to private practice. A report on clinical instruction at the Baltimore Almshouse in 1834, for example, endeavored to
scotch the prevailing beliefs "that the modes of treatment in Private
& Public practice are fundamentally different[, and] that the energetic
practice adapted to domestic cases could not be born by patients in
public infirmaries or hospitals." It acknowledged that hospital inmates
were rightly characterized by dissipated habits, listlessness, and constitutions broken down by poverty, but urged nonetheless that "la-
mentably accurate as this picture is, still the same lines & colourings
are discernible in private practice." Extolling the value of clinical study
to the student, the author concluded that "a mind trained to this kind
of investigation & practice, can readily adjust itself to any other."[34]

Just as variations in patients' social situations indicated different therapeutic courses, so too social changes modified diseases and people in ways that directed alterations in the prevailing therapeutic tack. One such change was expressed in the addition of a new temperament to the four known to the ancients: the "nervous" temperament, characteristic of modern civilization. "This temperament," David Hosack explained, "like the nervous affections which are the result of it, has never shewn itself, but among societies brought to that state of civilization in which man is farthest from nature."[35]

The dominant therapeutic tendency produced by social changes in America, physicians generally agreed, was a shift from depletive to supportive treatment occasioned by the increased refinement of living. Like the late-nineteenth-century neurasthenia, a characteristically urban, upper-middle-class nervous debility, maladies of the nervous temperament demanded supportive rather than depletive treatment. In this instance the anxieties of modern society were identified as the engines of therapeutic change. Dudley noted in his lectures at Transylvania in 1834 that the "genl predisposn to inflaman is declining." This could, he proposed, be attributed "to introdn of luxurious modes of living; for among labouring classes we find the inflam[mator]y predisposn as strong as ever[. They are] not as often ill as the luxurious but [their] inflamns more violent."[36]

Conversely, populations such as Indians and mountain men celebrated in popular imagery as especially rugged had characteristically overexcited illnesses. "Among the savage tribes of people," a student at Transylvania wrote in 1848, "scarcely any other diseases prevail, than those of an inflammatory nature, . . . and this circumstance may be referred to their mode of living."[37] The therapeutic implication of this belief was that while the "savage," like the hale laborer, was effectively treated with the antiphlogistic therapies that highly inflammatory conditions called for, the civilized American whose constitution was subjected to "that enervating influence of luxurious habits" could not withstand such treatment and demanded stimulation in its stead.[38] To this extent physicians regarded therapeutic change as socially determined.

People could alter their therapeutic requirements by changing their physical environments as well as themselves. The example of this physicians most often cited was the change brought about by the settlement and cultivation of a new region: the very acts of clearing the land, changing the vegetation, and turning the soil, physicians had maintained since the colonial period, altered the type of prevailing diseases. As settlement progressed, social changes were added to the remolding of the land to effect an overall environmental transformation, and change in the inhabitants' therapeutic requirements was the expected consequence.[39]

While people could substantially modify some of the attributes of a place that influenced therapeutic need, most attributes were less malleable. Apart from rural versus urban areas, large geographic regions, distinguished by their temperature, rainfall, topography, and vegetation, were the most conventional units for discussion about therapeutic specificity to place. The discriminations most fervently supported by American physicians were those between the Old World and the New, but the peculiarities of regions within the United States had a central place in discussion as well. "As surely as there is a distinction between foreign and American medicine," one New Orleans physician asserted, "so surely is there a distinction between Northern and Southern medicine."[40] When in 1834 John Leonard Riddell, attending lectures in Ohio, copied into his class notebook, "Says 10 grs. of calomel is as effectual in Pennsylvania, as 50. in the Valley of [the] Mississippi," he was recording the sort of assumption about therapeutic regionalism pervasive in antebellum America.[41] The North, South, and West were distinctive habitats, and accordingly differing treatment was required in meeting the specific needs of the inhabitants and unacclimated transients in each region.

The ubiquity of malaria in many parts of the South and West and its scarcity in the North in the early nineteenth century made the therapeutic distinction between malarial and nonmalarial regions a prominent one. Malaria was taken to be not a disease but a noxious miasm or effluvium arising from decaying organic matter that contributed to a variety of pathological conditions, especially periodic fevers. In addition, it purportedly altered the character of nearly all diseases in a region where it prevailed. Just as it was believed that during years of cholera or yellow fever epidemics the prevailing "epidemic constitution" altered the character of other maladies, so too the malarial environment continually redirected the course of local diseases.

The constitution of the person who lived in a malarial area was gradually transformed, many physicians believed, as was, in consequence, the type of management required when he or she fell ill. Physicians widely maintained that quinine (or cinchona bark or another of its derivatives), regarded as a stimulant, was indicated in treating most patients affected by the malarial taint. "Treat diseases of Rice plantations & low grounds upon the stimulant plan," Joseph Jones told his students at the University of Nashville in 1866. "Avoid all depletion as far as possible; and in the climate fevers, administer sulphate of quinia boldly . . . for this is the great remedy in the diseases of swamps and ricefields, even in the pleurisy & pneumonia of the winter season, for they are in such sections of the country motified by the slow action of malaria upon the system."[42] John K. Mitchell, lecturing to students at Jefferson Medical College in Philadelphia, similarly directed that in yellow fever, "Bleeding and Mercury in the first stage are the great means of cure, especially in northern constitutions," but for the same disease recommended "Sulphate of Quinia in malarious districts."[43]

Reflecting quinine's classification as a stimulant or tonic, physicians held that residents of malarial regions required more supportive treatment when sick than those of nonmalarious districts, and withstood heroic depletion only with difficulty. "In acute inflammatory affections," one practitioner asserted, "we would not think of treating with the same activity, a subject who had for years lived in a miasmatic district, and been subject to all its contaminating influences, as we would the hale mountaineer. In miasmatic districts, then, where the system is to a certain extent impressed with its peculiar influence, we should have great care in the use of active remedies."[44]

Some argued that the extensive use of quinine in the malarial districts of the South and West had led to a distinctively aggressive therapeutic confidence among practitioners in those regions. Quinine's striking efficacy, coupled with the fact that malaria engrafted itself into all diseases, Oliver Wendell Holmes suggested in 1848, "creates a natural tendency to 'heroic' practice, and accounts for an habitual boldness in the application of powerful agents which is reserved for exceptional cases in other latitudes. All these circumstances re-act upon the whole tone of thought; they modify the feelings, the style of talking and writing, the very bearing and physiognomy of the physician and the lecturer."[45] A professor at Indiana Medical College agreed. "In the West, the physician may in reality take to himself more credit— may with more propriety say I *cure* fever, than his eastern brother," he wrote in the following year. "A careful temporalizing course must mark the practice of the eastern man. [But] the western physician lays his hand on a potent agent, and without fear makes a dash at the disease and conquers it . . . Sins of ommission are more commendable in eastern than western practice."[46]

The *climate* of a place, like the *constitution* of a person, was a broadly inclusive term denoting a variety of factors that modified disease and treatment. "We understand by climate," one student wrote, "since Hypocrates, a country or region, which may differ from an other in respect to the season, qualities of the soil, heat or coldness of the temperature &c."[47] Among the variables of climate thought to fashion therapeutic behavior the most important was temperature, as reflected in the belief that heat and cold modified disease, the human constitution, and the action of remedies in ways that required different therapeutic strategies for different seasons. Mitchell, for example, told his students in Philadelphia that "bleeding is more successful in cold than in warm weather," while a student attending lectures in Boston copied into his notebook, "Dr. Jackson says the remedies we use in July and August begin to fail in September and October."[48]

The therapeutic differences physicians claimed existed between hot and cold regions were fully congruent with those between warm and cold seasons. In lectures delivered in New York during the first three decades of the century, Hosack repeatedly advised students, "Inhabitants of Hot climates will not bear the same mode of treatment as those of Cold."[49] He explained that "in warm countries or tropical climates the inhabitants are more subject to debility . . . Their diseases are of a low grade." To treat such persons, Hosack recommended "the early & free use of Tonics & stimulants; they do not bear evacuation."[50] In contrast, the inhabitants of cold regions tended to have robust, energetic constitutions. Their diseases were most often of an inflammatory character, Hosack claimed, which required not stimulation but depletion.[51]

These distinctions between hot and cold climates provided a clear differential between the North and the South and constituted the keystone around which arguments for the therapeutic particularity of the regions were constructed.[52] The notion that climate combined with other modifying influences to demand distinctively northern, southern, and western therapeutics was a cardinal corollary to the principle of specificity.

The judgments American physicians made upon the regional appropriateness of two mainstays of the antebellum armamentarium— venesection and mercurials—display the sort of differences in treatment therapeutic regionalism implied. Regular practitioners widely held that although mercury was on occasion valuable in treating patients in all regions of the country, it was demanded more frequently and in larger doses in the South than in the North. The premise was that mercury stimulated biliary secretion, which was often weakened in the South because of the climate. Heat from the sun, and often malaria as well, stimulated the liver, exhausting that organ and leaving it debilitated. A student attending medical lectures in Charleston typically explained in 1835 that to therapeutically arouse torpid southern livers, "we are compelled to resort to what would be considered by northern practitioners, enormous doses of calomel, without which, we would be continually foiled in our attempts to cure the biliary disorders of the South."[53]

On the other hand, many physicians held therapeutic depletion

by venesection to be suited to the constitutions and maladies of northern patients but badly borne by southerners. "Here," Chapman said in
a lecture on continued bilious fever in the region of Philadelphia, "it
is almost uniformly inflamatory, exacting for its management the very
constant and profuse use of the lancet, but in the Carolinas & Georgia
this must be wholly laid aside, or sparingly & discriminately employed."[54] Although the use of bloodletting diminished in all regions
of the United States during the first two-thirds of the century, faith in
its differential regional suitability persisted.

Through the late twentieth century, both prudent and invidious discriminations among patients on the basis of such factors as age, gender,
stamina, ethnicity, socioeconomic class, and residence remained a part
of what determined an individual's therapeutic management: treatment for a young, vigorous woman might be inappropriate for an enfeebled, elderly man, while a rural patient in the Third World might
receive substantially different care from that accorded a wealthy urban
resident of an industrialized nation. But it was a different type, and
not just degree, of medical reasoning that during the first two-thirds
of the nineteenth century bound relevant therapeutic knowledge by
the principle of specificity to typologies of patients and locales. Specificity not only defined in principle proper practice, professionally correct behavior, and a distinctive status for therapeutic knowledge, but
it also had important, practical institutional and epistemological implications. As long as specificity rather than universalism reigned, much
of the wisdom valued by the profession was necessarily tied to the
place where it was generated and used: it was in essence *local knowledge*. The self-conscious cultivation of the local and the particular by
physicians illustrates how deeply embedded specificity was in medical
institutions, thought, and activity.

One way of gaining knowledge about therapeutics that physicians
in the early and mid-nineteenth century regarded with an esteem comparable to that their descendants were to accord laboratory science was
the investigation of local meteorological conditions, in the tradition
of the Hippocratic treatise *On Airs, Waters, and Places*. Meteorological
observations, coupled with records of prevailing diseases and the success of various treatments, informed the physician about the pathological and therapeutic peculiarities of the district in which he practiced.
Much of the information gathered in this way was etiological. Lundsford P. Yandell, for example, recorded in his diary climatic changes
observed in his region of Kentucky and speculated on their pathological
influences. He also expected to derive therapeutic information from

his records, and entered detailed weather observations, descriptions of prevailing diseases, and the rationales and results of the therapies he used during the 1820s and 1830s.[55] Meteorological conditions, like patients' symptoms, constituted a therapeutic sign, and conceptually the two were so closely intermeshed that American practitioners often preserved meteorological observations and medical practice records in a common volume. They expected their observations to reveal patterns that would guide practice and indicate alterations in treatment as prevailing circumstances changed. Such observation was a particularly important source of knowledge for the neophyte practitioner or the newcomer to a region.

The records kept by Samuel Hildreth in Marietta, Ohio, between 1831 and 1854 display the stunning detail with which some physicians made and preserved their observations. Hildreth recorded daily the character of the weather, winds, and rainfall; thrice daily took thermometric and barometric readings; and included general remarks on clouds, frost, river conditions, and any unusual phenomena pertaining to weather, crops, or disease in his vicinity. At the end of each month and again at the end of the year, he discussed the relationships among these observations, the patients he had treated, changes in the region (such as cultivation, flooding, shifting population), the tendencies of disease, mortality (for which he tallied annual bills), and the shifting course of his therapeutic efforts. In this way Hildreth was able to correlate treatment and alterations in it with meteorological and sometimes social phenomena and to trace the changes in disease and treatment in his district over a period of decades.[56]

Private practitioners were not alone in gathering meteorological observations as an adjunct to practice. In 1838 the house physician at the Massachusetts General Hospital recorded his observations three times a day in the last few pages of the medical case history books. He observed the temperature and calculated a mean, noted the winds and precipitation, and commented on the general character of the atmosphere.[57] The records of the Baltimore Almshouse similarly noted, "We have now [a] Thermometer, a Barometer, Hygrometer & a Raingage, & have begun to keep meteorological tables," and at the Commercial Hospital of Cincinnati in the 1860s, the medical staff voted that a resident student "be directed to make & record thermometrical barometrical and hygrometrical observations three times a day."[58]

Medical societies were the most active sites for collecting local observations of weather, disease, and treatment. The South Carolina Medical Association solicited meteorological data from all parts of the state, and its constitution required the president to make a biennial report on weather and diseases. At a meeting of the Ohio State Medical

Society in 1853, members resolved "that this Society recommend, to each of its members, and Auxiliary Societies, to keep a record of the number of cases of each variety of disease, which may occur in their practice monthly, with brief accounts of the Topography of their particular locality, the State of the weather &c. &c. and report the same annually to this Society." The Baltimore Pathological Society resolved two years later that it was the duty of its members to record similar information on forms the society furnished.[59] Periodic reports on the character of diseases prevailing in a particular locality and the treatment they called for was a part of most societies' meetings.

By providing a forum for the collective pursuit of local knowledge, medical societies served an important therapeutic function. While it is true that most of them did little to contribute to the universalized basic medical sciences and that their meetings in this regard were thin in scientific content, they were the leading loci for the production and dissemination of knowledge about medical practice that was of considerable local import. This is not to deny that societies were animated principally by the desire to promote professional unity, mollify dissension among regulars, and distinguish them from their competitors. To reduce the meaning of the medical society for the individual practitioner to its socioeconomic dimensions alone, however, is to ignore the plain fact that local and even state societies served a practical intellectual function for the physician and were a source of knowledge that could be applied to practice. The energetic pursuit of locally oriented investigations of the relationships among environment, disease, and treatment that flourished especially from the 1830s through the 1850s in medical societies was at least in part an expression of the growing suspicion American physicians felt toward established sources of therapeutic authority. The development of local knowledge based on local observations reflected the burgeoning empiricist reaction against the universalism of rationalistic systems.

While the cultivation of local knowledge in medical societies was by no means restricted to the South and West, the hegemony of therapeutic teachings from the North and Europe made physicians in other regions particularly sensitive to their dependence upon precepts that might misdirect their practices. For example, Samuel Cartwright, addressing a medical convention in Mississippi in 1846, complained about the reliance of his state's practitioners on knowledge from other climates. "The diseases of the northern latitudes, and of the paupers of European hospitals, are delineated with the most minute accuracy, and the remedies, which the experience of all countries and ages has proved to be the most successful in their treatment, can be brought to bear upon them," he noted. But "in vain do we search medical books for an accurate description of those affections, as they occur in our practice, or for the most successful methods of treating them. Hence the necessity of a society, or some organization among ourselves, for learning the laws of those affections, and the remedies that each of us has found, by dear experience, to be most successful in their treatment."[60] Through the medical society, isolated observations could be elevated to practical regional knowledge, a commodity that only the physicians practicing in a region could produce.

It was in the mold of this sort of local investigation that a genre of medical literature common during the first two-thirds of the century was cast. Many medical students elected to write a thesis on the peculiarities of disease, meteorology, topography, and treatment of their home county, and in marked contrast to the majority of theses, which substantially echoed (and sometimes copied verbatim) the teachings of medical texts and professors, often these essays were impressively original. Commonly the student collected information for such a thesis by observing his preceptor's practice and talking with local physicians during the interval between his first and second courses of lectures. Because some candidates for the M.D. degree had practiced medicine for years or even decades prior to attending medical lectures, theses occasionally presented extensive observations from their authors' own practice. While most locally oriented theses were modest studies, Daniel Drake's massive treatise on *The Principal Diseases of the Interior Valley of North America* (1850–1854) was in its essence merely a singularly ambitious expression of the same kind of endeavor. Relying on his own observations and the private records of physicians such as Hildreth, Drake performed for a vast region some of the task many medical societies sought to perform for their own locales.[61]

Observation of the relations among local diseases, meteorology, and treatment offered one opportunity for research in an otherwise unencouraging environment. John Young Bassett's contributions on the topography, climate, and diseases of Huntsville and Madison counties, Alabama, to Erasmus Darwin Fenner's *Southern Medical Reports* in 1849 and 1850 are representative in this regard.[62] Bassett had studied during the early 1830s in France, where he had become solidly committed to the epistemological ideals of the Paris clinical school. Returning to Huntsville, he was painfully conscious of his isolation in an intellectually lethargic professional environment devoid of the clinical institutions necessary for research as pursued at the Parisian hospitals. In his essays Bassett traced the changes in his district's climate on the basis of his own meteorological journal (which Drake had already borrowed in preparing his treatise)[63] and correlated these changes with permutations in disease and treatment. Explicitly challenging

established therapeutic authority, he suggested that shifts in climate
had produced changes in the character of the region's diseases, which
in turn had demanded alterations in therapy. He claimed experience
with local practice as the sole basis for his therapeutic stance. Bassett's
work not only typifies investigations of local knowledge, but at the
same time lucidly illustrates the convergence in one man, working
within the constraining realities of the American environment, of commitments to the research ideal and empiricist epistemology of the Paris
clinical school, skepticism regarding the dominant sources of therapeutic authority, and focus on the local environment as an avenue to
therapeutic progress.

Many physicians held the practical instruction of northern textbooks and journals to be suspect for use in the South or West. What
was demanded was medical literature suited to each region's idiosyncratic requirements, which could be had only if practitioners would
observe local diseases for themselves and publish their pathological
and therapeutic discoveries. Because precepts applicable to medical
practice were necessarily region specific, unlike most scientific knowledge they could not be imported. "In the science of medicine," a Mississippi practitioner claimed, "there is no choice between a foreign
supply and home production. Our medical literature cannot be *man-
ufactured* for us abroad."[64]

The most forceful expression of calls for local knowledge was the
movement for regional medical education that was strongest between
the 1830s and the Civil War.[65] The movement was expressed most
stridently in the South and West, even though physicians in all parts
of the country endorsed its conceptual core, the principle of specificity
and the faith in regional therapeutic distinctiveness it sustained. This
reflected the self-conscious intellectual marginality of physicians in
these regions, a consequence in part of their dependence on northern
and eastern institutions and teachings, and their perception that this
reliance on external therapeutic authority fostered inferior practice.
One southern practitioner lucidly stated the premises of regional medical education in 1844, writing, "It is precisely because diseases are
not all entities, and do not preserve the same features, wherever met
with; and that remedies are *not all specifics*, or uniform and invariable
in their effects, that it becomes necessary to *study* them where they
prevail."[66]

Physicians in the South and West increasingly insisted that the
student trained in a northern school who moved to another region to
practice would be forced to either unlearn the practical precepts of his
northern teachers or face ruin. William W. Cozart, a medical student
from North Carolina, developed this theme in his thesis entitled "The

Place where Southern Students Should Acquire Their Medical Knowledge" (1856).

> The general principles of Medicine may be communicated by teachers that are competent without regard to locality. But the case is different in respect to particular ones, and their application to practice; those differing wherever the peculiarities of localities differ. And it is well known by the medical profession that diseases are modified by these places, and other circumstances; and in order that these indications should be met successfully, the adaptation of the treatment must be varied accordingly . . . As the northern diseases differ materially in their characters from the southern, the advantages therefore, southern students have by attending southern Colleges are no doubt considerable.

The southern graduate of a Philadelphia or New York medical school, Cozart claimed, "returns home in high spirits and with bright anticipations, 'sticks out his shingle,' ready and very willing to go to work." But however thorough his knowledge of medical science, he was destined to fail in practice, treating his first patients, in accordance with northern teachings, with general bloodletting and sedative medicines that produced dire results. "Now his bright anticipations are clouded; disappointments discourage him; and a sad experience teaches him that the instructive lessons of a northern institution will not answer, in the treatment of southern diseases. He cannot now under the circumstances establish an extensive practice," Cozart concluded; "the confidence of the people in him is shaken, he is neglected, despised, and soon forgotten."[67]

Education in southern and western schools, which proliferated after the 1820s, offered a sanative alternative. The potential strength of regional medical instruction rested in the opportunity for students to gain knowledge about disease and treatment appropriate to the environment within which they planned to practice. Advocates of regional medical education accordingly contrasted the universality of medical principles with the regional specificity of practice and stressed "observation at the bedside" of the types of diseases and patients students would later be called upon to treat as the hallmark of regional training. Incorporating those branches of medicine that *were* region specific—diagnosis, prognosis, and treatment—clinical training both gave regional medical education its identity and drew attention to the inadequacies of northern schools.

The fact that in the years before the Civil War hundreds of southern medical students annually elected to attend lectures at northern schools was in no sense a denial of the singularity of southern medical practice. As American physicians traveled to the hospitals of Europe in growing numbers during the antebellum period to gain knowledge about medical science despite their belief that European practice was doubtfully applicable to American patients, southern students similarly sought medical knowledge in northern schools while remaining wary of the practical precepts taught there. There were, to be sure, obvious political, social, and economic incentives for fashioning distinctively regional medicine with its own institutions. Much of the force that impelled the case for medical particularity in the South must be ascribed to the same engines that drove the rising defense of the southern way of life. It was patently not by happenstance that the growing preoccupation with regional distinctiveness in southern medicine coincided with the larger movement in the South toward economic, cultural, and political sectionalism and nationalism from the 1830s onward. Tensions engendered by the South's colonial agrarian economy, reliance upon slavery, and diminished political power, augmented by a regional sensibility piqued by external charges of immorality, intellectual sloth, and social retrogression, imbued all questions of the region's particularity with a strong emotional vibrancy. Furthermore, medical editors and educators, functioning within a medical marketplace in which competition for subscribers and students was acute, had a potent economic incentive for using southern medical distinctiveness as an argument for the advantages of regional literature and schools.

Nevertheless, implying that southern physicians promoted southern medical distinctiveness simply because they were southerners or because they were driven by invidious economic incentives explains away more than it explains. The movement for regional medical education was an affirmation of faith in the importance of local knowledge that was fully consistent with the principle of specificity. Erasmus Darwin Fenner, the leading defender of the South's medical singularity, had solid grounds for claiming a medical truth validated by national consensus as his authority when he denied a northern charge that the movement for southern medical education was politically motivated and represented "States Rights Medicine": "If this be *sectional medicine*," he retorted, "I cannot help it. It was not made so by me, but by Nature."[68]

Beyond its political and economic motivations, the argument for regional medical education and the commitment to local knowledge upon which it was premised represented to southern and western physicians one means of uplifting their profession. The inadequacy of the northern educational authority, on which many physicians depended, for practice in their area, southerners held, misdirected the southern practitioner, imperiled public confidence in the profession, and encouraged quackery. A distinctively southern medicine promised to remedy the low standing of the profession by raising public regard for the regular physician's ability to heal, thereby countering sectarian competition. It would also release southern practitioners from their dependence on the North and Europe, opening possibilities of scientific and institutional parity, and would galvanize the medical community, augmenting its intellectual stature and social power. The institutions of medical education offered physicians a concrete context in which to objectify their commitment to southern medical distinctiveness, thus becoming a vehicle for the vindication and vitalization of medicine in the South.[69]

What is especially striking about the movement for regional medical distinctiveness is its similarity to the concurrent campaign against rationalistic systems of practice. American physicians in both movements were attacking what they regarded as a routine, mechanical practice that ignored specificity, a practice they believed resulted from reliance on an inappropriate source of therapeutic authority. In the one case that authority was rationalistic systems; in the other it was the teachings of a different region or country applied without sufficient attention to modifying local influences. Both movements held that this adherence to inappropriate authority degraded the profession through the inferior practice it generated. It led to unsuccessful attempts to heal, undermining public confidence in the regular profession and giving sectarians legitimate grounds for charging the regulars with providing inadequate care. Faith in inappropriate authority, physicians held, also discouraged practitioners from questioning the cogency of therapeutic teachings for the needs of their own practices and so blocked progress.

Furthermore, in both movements physicians saw the key to professional upliftment in the rejection of established authority and substitution of something better. In one instance this consisted of dismantling rationalistic systems and constructing new therapeutic knowledge on the basis of experience at the bedside; in the other it involved a critical re-evaluation of established therapeutic knowledge, its revalidation (or invalidation) for use in contexts other than that in which it had been produced, and its augmentation or replacement by new knowledge developed by direct observation of practice and better suited to local conditions. In both cases this endeavor was informed by the growing allegiance to empiricism. The two movements were not in conflict with each other, and the individual physician could, and often did, embrace them both without disrupting the integrity of his commitments.

The commonality of these two movements underscores what antebellum physicians saw as the importance of the principle of specificity to therapeutic knowledge and to the status of the profession. In both the reaction against systems and the drive for regional medical knowledge, the sources, organization, and dissemination of therapeutic knowledge figured as crucial in anxieties about the profession's standing. By an active celebration of the principle of specificity—including a self-conscious eschewal of routine practice, whatever its source, and an emphasis on discriminating observation—physicians believed that they could elevate their profession. The growing commitment to empiricism reinforced specificity in fostering a doubting attitude toward existing therapeutic knowledge and practice, and it also encouraged physicians to look for themselves in order to determine what practices best answered the needs of their patients. In this way, physicians regarded the reformation of therapeutic knowledge, predicated on a due regard for specificity, as a vehicle through which professional redemption would be realized.

Yet allegiance to specificity as a tool for professional improvement was a two-edged sword. By the third quarter of the century, concern would begin to arise that the specificity of therapeutic knowledge, contrasted with the universalism of some other kinds of medical knowledge, meant that there was a widening gap between the perceived progress and growing certainty in the universal "basic sciences" and the stagnancy and inevitable uncertainty of therapeutics. Because of the seemingly limitless variability over place and time of what constituted valid therapeutic knowledge, there could be no fixed, universally applicable rules of therapeutic practice, no hope for therapeutic certainty. Some physicians would come to regard an emphasis on the principle of specificity as a humiliating affirmation of professional limitations and as ample grounds for therapeutic pessimism.

Only in the late 1860s and 1870s did a new therapeutic epistemology, coupled with a new ideology of professional identity, appear to some physicians to offer an alternative to despair. Those physicians who proselytized this new view unambiguously identified the constraining overemphasis on the principle of specificity and the empiricism to which it was bound as causes of the retardation of therapeutic progress. The alternative they proposed was the creation of a fundamentally new epistemological status for therapeutics, grounded in the universalism of experimental laboratory science. The advocates of this posture sought to replace sterile clinical empiricism with a New Rationalism based on experimental science, while at the same time substituting a new optimism premised on the possibility of universality for the pessimism generated by the specificity of therapeutic knowledge. The principle of specificity, however, was so deeply embedded in the profession's values that such open violence to it could not be done without producing considerable anguish.

PART II

The Process
of Change

— 4 —

Therapeutic Change

To be fully exploited as a probe into the mind of nineteenth-century American physicians, therapeutic rhetoric must be interpreted against the backdrop of behavior. Only by knowing what physicians actually *did* is it possible to assess the significance of what they said they did and ought to be doing. The kinds of sources historians most often rely on are indispensable for describing how physicians portrayed their activities and for understanding the purposes and justifications of their therapeutic procedures, but they do not reveal their actions. Although some insights into therapeutic activity can be gleaned from such narrative sources as diaries, published case histories, clinical lectures, and letters advising patients, such sources are often only anecdotal, and sometimes are more normative than descriptive.

The most revealing sources of information about the therapeutic behavior of private practitioners are practice records made for personal use. A small minority of physicians kept case history books in which they logged their patients' signs and symptoms, their own therapeutic efforts, and the consequences of treatment. All too often, though, physicians recorded only exceptional cases in such volumes.[1] Furthermore, many tired of the labor after a couple of years (or even days), so the duration of case history books is often brief.[2] Underlying the making of these volumes was the physician's belief that by writing down his experiences he could improve his practice and perhaps contribute to collective knowledge as well; but the kinds of information recorded were often idiosyncratic. While such documents do lay open the bedside activities of a few physicians, they lack the uniformity requisite to support meaningful comparisons.[3]

Most practitioners kept patient records solely for financial purposes. In the account books and financial ledgers that survive in abundance, they listed their services and the corresponding charges.

83

Sometimes individual drugs dispensed directly to the patient are specified in such records; far more often physicians recorded only the
general type of drug administered, such as cathartic or emetic, or the
even less enlightening term *medicine* or *prescription*. While it is sometimes possible on the basis of these records to tell that a physician was
prescribing a certain drug frequently, it is seldom certain that he was
not using other, unrecorded treatments even more regularly. However,
most physicians did routinely itemize certain services, including vac-
cination, tooth extraction, and attendance at childbirth. Venesection,
as a surgical procedure, was among the services that were ordinarily
specified for billing purposes, and therefore more can be learned about
its relative frequency than can be known about any other therapy.

Pharmacy prescription books are also valuable indexes of prescribing habits in communities where drugs were not dispensed primarily
by physicians themselves. The prescriptions pasted or copied into such
registers itemize all of the drugs ordered for the patient and specify
dosages, and therefore drug usage revealed by pharmacy prescription
books from different places and times can be compared statistically.
Yet the usefulness of these records is limited by their scarcity for the
first half of the century, the paucity of patient information they provide,
the restriction of information to drugs (excluding diet, other regimen
instructions, and procedures such as venesection and cupping), and the
frequent failure to identify the prescribing physician.

Virtually the only detailed, systematic information about nineteenth-century therapeutic activity over an extensive period of time
that can be meaningfully quantified is that obtained through hospital
records. The rigor with which hospitals recorded case histories varied
widely, but the records of the two American hospitals analyzed here
are sufficiently detailed and complete to illuminate the complexity of
therapeutic change over the long duration. With a richness private
practice documents do not offer, these records disclose the marked
variability in therapeutic orientation and actual treatment that typified
medical practice in different contexts; show that even within a single
institution such categories as heroic depletants, palliatives, and heroic
stimulants were not monolithic, and that the individual treatments
within a single category rose and fell on diverse schedules; and forcefully reveal the absence of outright rejection of established therapies
and the continuity of therapeutic practice over time.

Therapeutic change is described here on three progressively nar-
rower and more detailed levels. On the first the shifting objectives of
treatment between the 1820s and 1880s are sketched. This brief account, based more on narrative sources than on practice records, analyzes how physicians thought about the end point of their therapeutic

actions—that is, what they thought it meant to heal. Second, the broad trends in therapeutic activity during this period are described. This overview of therapeutic trends is generalized primarily from records of private pratice but draws on narrative and hospital sources as well. Third, and much more extensively, the fine structure of therapeutic change as it occurred in the limited contexts of two large hospitals is delineated on the basis of patient records.

From Natural to Normal: The Changing Therapeutic Perspective

The transformation of therapeutic practice between the 1820s and the 1880s is best understood against the backdrop of a simultaneously shifting conception of what it meant to restore health. A fundamental albeit subtle permutation in medical thinking was embodied in a change in medical language. Throughout the first half of the century the term *natural* was commonly used to describe the model state of well-being that was the desired end point of therapeutic activity; by the mid-1870s *normal* had almost completely replaced *natural* used in this way.

During the first two-thirds of the nineteenth century physicians viewed disease as essentially a systemic imbalance. The many, often conflicting theories of pathogenesis shared the underlying assumption that for therapeutic purposes the primary characteristic of sickness was excessive excitement or enfeeblement. Treatment was premised on a model of the body as an interconnected whole, and therapy that responded to individual symptoms, which indicated deviations from the natural condition, also modified the system's imbalance. The fundamental objective was to restore the natural balance, which was accomplished by depleting or lowering the overexcited patient and by stimulating or elevating the patient enfeebled by disease.[4]

The notion of what constituted a natural state was closely connected to the principle of specificity. The natural condition was defined not for a population but for the individual and was molded by such individuating factors as ethnicity, gender, family background, and moral status. Moreover, what was natural for a person during one season, in one physical or social environment, and at one age changed as that person grew older, altered his or her social position, or moved to a different part of the country. The physician best able to know what was natural for the patient and most capable of restoring the system to a natural balance when it was disrupted was a practitioner well acquainted with the patient's personal history and with the peculiarities of the locality and its diseases.

The idea that therapeutic efforts should seek to restore the diseased system to a natural condition did not imply that nature was capable of accomplishing the task. Physicians who barred nature from the sickroom agreed with those openly devoted to the healing power of nature in viewing the natural state as the objective of medical care. Relying principally on the body's natural healing powers to restore balance and aggressively drugging the patient to force his or her system back to a natural condition were merely two strategies for attaining the same end. Nature's spontaneous operations in disease did, however, give hints as to how treatment could restore systemic balance. Hemorrhaging, for example, might indicate a plethora of blood in the body, which could recommend therapeutic bloodletting to equilibrate bodily fluids. In epidemics of unknown character attention to nature's inclinations was particularly important, for nature provided the physician faced with an unfamiliar disease an indication of possible therapeutic tacks.

Etiological theory sustained this way of thinking about disease and cure. With only a few exceptions (smallpox and syphilis being the most notable), etiology in the early nineteenth century was nonspecific. Diseases were thought to be generated not by discrete causative agents— one invariably producing pneumonia and another typhoid fever—but rather by a variety of destabilizing factors acting singly or more often as an ensemble to unbalance the system. Cold, anxiety, and miasmas could all produce analogous impressions on the human body, and the character of the predisposing epidemic constitution prevailing at a certain time could have as much power as these exciting causes in determining the form disease assumed. Just as illness itself was regarded as an imbalance, its genesis was often attributed to excesses or deficiencies in the way a patient lived. The conjunction of natural equilibrium and health fitted easily within a moral context, for unbalancing immoderation could follow not only from improper behavior regarding heat, fresh air, exercise, and food, but also from drinking, piety, and venery.[5]

Beginning in the mid-nineteenth century, the way physicians looked at the objectives of treatment began to change. They came to think of disorders less as systemic imbalances in the body's natural harmony, and more as complexes of discrete signs and symptoms that could be analyzed, separated and measured in isolation. The Paris school's emphasis on the anatomical localization of diseases introduced some measure of such analysis, but the conceptual shift in the third quarter of the century went much further. The hallmark of the new way of thinking about the goals of treatment was the reduction of signs of bodily order and disorder to objectively measured, quantified norms.

In the 1850s the "normal" began to replace the "natural" as the paradigm of order and health. Physicians looking for guides to therapeutic intervention gradually turned away from judging a patient's well-being by comparison with the natural state of health for that individual. They began instead to weigh specific indicators in the patient against criteria of health expressed as norms for a population and as the universalized norms defined by laboratory science.

Therapeutic attention from the 1860s onward focused increasingly on individual physiological processes as meaningful in themselves, not merely as indicators of systemic disarray. In practice physicians became preoccupied with bringing disordered processes back into line with fixed norms. During the 1860s and 1870s quantification and graphical representation of such variables as temperature, pulse rate, and respiration rate, together with the quantitative assay of, for example, the chemical composition of urine, became common methods of tracking the course of disease. Treatment was in turn explicitly aimed at making these measurements match figures that represented normal standards.

Changes in etiological theory reflected and supported these shifts. Physicians began to think more in terms of discrete disease entities and disease-specific causation and less in terms of general destabilizing forces that unbalanced the body's natural equilibrium. This change was expressed most clearly in bacterial etiology but did not result from it. Myriad specific chemical, fungal, and animalcular causes of disease had been proposed from the 1840s onward, and especially since the 1860s. Accompanying a more rigid ontology of diseases—in which disease was held to be something abnormal but discrete and identifiable—was the idea that treatment could restore health not merely by righting imbalance but by specifically manipulating abnormal processes or even etiological agents. With the crystallizing concepts of specific diseases and specific causes, specific therapy also gained a growing legitimacy, and diagnosis in turn attained a new therapeutic importance.

The replacement of the term *natural* by *normal* in clinical discourse between the 1820s and the 1880s mirrors this shift in the way physicians thought about disorder and hence in what they believed was to be modified by treatment. This alteration, evident in all the conventional records of medical language, is perhaps most vividly exhibited in the changing use of the two words in hospital medical case histories. These records have the advantages of offering a sustained documentation of clinical language over an extensive span of time and of having been produced with a reasonably consistent purpose and format.

Figure 1 shows the changing frequencies with which the words *natural* and *normal* appeared in a sample of about four thousand cases taken from the male medical wards of the Massachusetts General Hospital in Boston and the Commercial Hospital of Cincinnati.[6] The crude frequencies of use show that the words were extensively employed in case histories at both hospitals. Moreover, while the use of *natural* declined over time (from 38.9 percent to 2.3 percent of the case histories at the Massachusetts General Hospital between the 1820s and 1880s, and from 24.1 percent to 1.8 percent at the Commercial Hospital between the 1830s and 1880s), the use of *normal* increased (during the same period from 0 percent to 64.0 percent at the Massachusetts General Hospital, and 0 percent to 57.8 percent at the Commercial Hospital).

Figure 1 leaves no doubt that after midcentury physicians in these two hospitals used *natural* less often and *normal* more often. The changing usage of these words vis-à-vis each other is more clearly seen in Figures 2 and 3, which show by decade the percentages of cases in which *natural* and *normal* individually were used out of all of the case histories in which one or both terms appeared, normalized to a total of 100 percent. Between the 1830s and the 1880s, *normal* virtually replaced *natural* in clinical case records. The most marked period of change in clinical vocabulary occurred between about 1860 and the

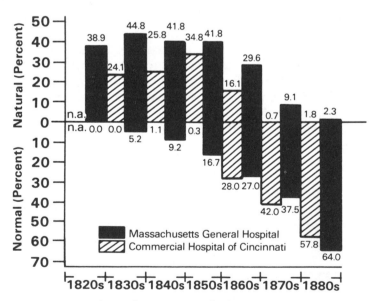

Figure 1 Percentage of case histories in which terms *natural* and *normal* appear.

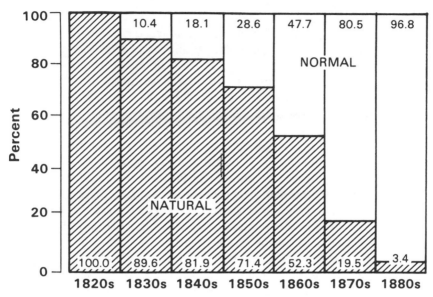

Figure 2 Massachusetts General Hospital. Percentage of case histories in which terms *natural* and *normal* appear (out of all cases in which one or both terms appear, normalized to 100 percent).

mid-1870s, precisely the years during which the shift in medical thinking postulated above was progressing most rapidly.

A contextual analysis of the ways these words were employed makes it clear that the changes indicated by the quantitative evidence are not merely coincidental. Early in the century physicians writing case histories at the two hospitals used *natural* to describe virtually all of the various signs and symptoms they observed, often recording the condition of an organ or a structure such as the skin, tongue, pupils, or abdomen in terms of its variance from the natural state. Functions or inclinations such as respiration, appetite, sleep, mind, urination, voice, or the way a patient answered questions were also appraised in terms of their naturalness, as were the color and character of urine, sputa, and dejections, and of blood expelled spontaneously or drawn therapeutically. *Natural* and *unnatural* further referred to the patient's physiognomy, called countenance, aspect, or expression. The physician directly observed and judged most of these factors, but because the patient was best acquainted with his or her natural condition, often the patient's assessment was solicited and heeded. Thus common entries in the case records took the form: "[The patient] thinks he passes more urine than natural"; "Says his breathing has been much shorter than natural"; "Urine, he thinks, is unnaturally yellow"; "Says appetite unnaturally good."[7] All of these characteristics are described in later case records as "normal" rather than "natural."

This substitution was marked soonest in the descriptions of two types of patient characteristics. The first was stethoscopic discernment of heart and lung sounds. At the Massachusetts General Hospital particularly, where the transition in terminology was more gradual and was apparent earlier than at the Commercial Hospital, many early uses of *normal* occurred in stethoscopic reports. A second common category in which the semantic change appeared early was quantified temperature, respiration, and pulse. Before the 1850s these patient characteristics were noted principally in qualitative language assessing their naturalness, and even early quantifications were often followed by comments on the natural or unnatural character of the pulse or respiration. As their description came to hinge more on a number than on character, physicians increasingly used the word *normal* rather than *natural.* These two kinds of signs had in common the intervention of some intermediary tool such as a stethoscope, thermometer, or timepiece into the physician's direct observation; the patient was unable to convey information about his or her condition without instrumental

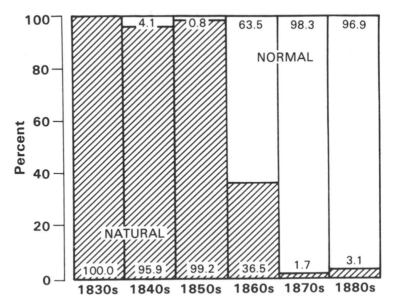

Figure 3 Commercial Hospital of Cincinnati. Percentage of case histories in which terms *natural* and *normal* appear (out of all cases in which one or both terms appear, normalized to 100 percent).

aid. This removed an element of patient subjectivity, and rendered the patient without special training incapable of interpreting the meaning of these signs in relation to his or her natural condition.

The eclipse of the term *natural* in clinical language was closely associated with the growing quantification of clinical observations from the 1860s onward. As temperature and pulse charts became common in clinical records beginning in the 1870s, qualitative references to the charts were almost invariably phrased in terms of conformity to or deviation from the normal. Similarly, in describing the results of quantitative laboratory analysis of urine, for example, physicians almost always spoke of normal and abnormal (rather than natural) urea, chlorides, or uroxanthin. While the use of the word *normal* went beyond the description of quantifiable patient signs and symptoms, its application was most solidly linked to recording variables that could be compared with quantified norms.

To the extent that words reflect and mold thinking, this alteration in clinical language marked an important change in cognition.[8] The shift in the way physicians thought about disease—from a disruption of natural balance to a deviation from fixed norms—had fundamental implications for medical theory, epistemology, and professional identity. What is important here is the associated shift in the way physicians thought about the objectives of therapeutics.

The Changing Course of Therapeutic Practice

Therapeutics in early-nineteenth-century America has conventionally been characterized by its bold or heroic practice. More precisely, the heroic practice of this period should be termed heroic depletive or heroic antiphlogistic therapeutics to differentiate it from the heroic stimulative therapeutics that emerged later in the century. Reliance on heroic depletive therapy was premised on the belief that most prevailing diseases were overstimulating; while in principle diseases could be either sthenic (*sthénos* = strength) or asthenic, nearly all those the physician encountered were sthenic, tipping the patient's vital balance to a dangerously overexcited condition.

The task of treatment was to lower the morbidly animated patient to a healthy, natural state. Sthenic conditions were associated with an inflammatory or phlogistic (*phlogós* = flame, *phlogistós* = inflammable) state; therefore therapy that sought to quench morbid elevation was commonly called antiphlogistic treatment. The term *heroic* reflected the belief that aggressive intervention was often called for to effect the therapeutic lowering. Ordinarily the system was first cleansed of matter that might impede its functioning. Draining off excess excitement from the body was not entirely metaphorical, for it was often accomplished by draining fluids thought to stimulate the internal structures. Heroic depletion was brought about by such drugs as cathartics (calomel, corrosive sublimate, jalap), emetics (tartar emetic, ipecacuanha), and counterirritants (blisters), by low diet, and by drawing blood.

Heroic depletive practices gave clear evidence that they worked. The physician knew within limits the likely changes in symptoms a certain treatment would elicit, and frequently shared these expectations with patients and their families. No one could doubt that the violent purging that followed a large dose of calomel or such blatant signs of mercury poisoning as loose teeth and bleeding gums were the sequelae of treatment. Similarly, when a patient with a hard, fast pulse, high temperature, and delirium became calmer—physiologically lower— after a large volume of blood had been let, the treatment's effect was undeniable. Sleep promoted by opiates further testified to the ability of the physician to alter his patient's physiology at will. Confirmation of the treatment's efficacy was generally rapid, and the physician, patient, and patient's family could all witness and appreciate the simple fact that it was working. This was important, for it not only reaffirmed the validity of the treatment and the therapeutic system of which it was a part, but also demonstrated that the physician was in control. Occasional failure to cure did not necessarily negate the usefulness of a therapy but only emphasized its limitations. Death, after all, was a part of Nature's (or God's) order.[9]

Diagnosis was of only secondary importance in determining appropriate treatment. To the extent to which the physician asserted control over a disease by naming and explaining it, diagnosis was of course an important part of managing a patient. Furthermore, it was a useful aid to prognosis, for it indicated a range of the most likely patterns and outcomes a particular case might take. Yet treatment was essentially symptomatic.

There was no paradox in the emphasis on symptomatic treatment and the concurrently held belief that most diseased conditions required lowering. Therapeutic depletion could be produced in a variety of ways, and it was an important exercise of the physician's judgment to determine the best means of accomplishing it on the basis of what he knew about the patient's background, the environment, and the symptoms he observed. He also matched dosage to symptoms and their severity. Dosage determined the type and not merely the degree of a drug's action; many physicians regarded calomel, for example, as a stimulant in a small dose but a depletant in a large one. Often the extent of treatment was gauged only by what was required to bring about a desired physiological result. Ordering that bleeding be continued to syncope or swooning was a common way of indicating the amount of blood that should be taken by venesection, for a few ounces taken from one patient might have the same effect as many ounces taken from another.[10]

The public shared many of the most fundamental assumptions underlying this way of thinking about illness and therapy, though not the specific dogmas of the rationalistic systems of practice. It would be an oversimplification to say that regular physicians and lay Americans held in common a single medical belief system: not only was there a wide gap between professional and popular culture in etiological and pathological ideas, a gap that grew wider as the century progressed, but some laypeople baldly rejected regular therapeutics in favor of alternative belief systems such as homeopathy. Nevertheless, most lay Americans adhered to the beliefs that restoring health meant returning the system to its natural balance and that this was to be done principally by cleansing the body with drugs like cathartics and emetics, lowering or elevating the vital energy, and responding to individual symptoms. The letters lay men and women wrote to each other and to their physicians strongly mirrored regular medical thought in the basic expectations they expressed about healing.[11] Even patients who elected to use an unorthodox materia medica, turning either to a sectarian practitioner or to sectarian self-help, largely shared popular assumptions about the objectives and means of cure. Thomsonianism, for example, sought to restore the natural balance by the heroic use of botanical purgatives and internal and external stimulants.

The heroic antiphlogistic therapeutics of the early nineteenth century was to a large extent informed by medical systems. Even though a reaction against systems characterized American medical thought from the 1820s onward, the organization of knowledge into systems continued to mold the ways physicians thought about pathology and treatment. A practitioner trained in the tradition of Rush and sensitive to the dangers of capillary congestion was more likely to resort to venesection than, for example, a Cookcian preoccupied with hepatic pathology and inclined to prescribe massive doses of calomel. Regional variation in medical training was in itself sufficient to forestall any single system from gaining hegemony over American therapeutics as a whole: Rushian influences spread from Philadelphia mainly through the mid-Atlantic region and the South; Cooke's system was taken up principally in the South and West; in New England, no rigid system prevailed, and practice was distinguished principally by the preference for milder treatments and the inclination to trust nature. Moreover, mobility was high among physicians, especially young practitioners searching for a place to establish practice. Within each section of the country the diversity among the prescribing habits of individual physicians was sufficiently striking to belie any notion that medical systems engendered uniformity in treatment. The practice even of those physicians whom existing secondary literature would predict to be mechanical and doctrinaire was remarkably complex and varied.[12]

This diversity emphasizes that in its application heroic antiphlogistic therapeutics was not monolithic. All regular American physicians drew their treatments from roughly the same armamentarium, but they employed various therapeutic agents to different degrees and with their own idiosyncratic modifications. What united their practices was not that they all routinely venesected and purged (which they did not), but that they sought to attain a shared therapeutic objective by exploiting a common arsenal.

Bleeding and purging, and particularly the use of venesection, mercurials, and tartar emetic, have symbolized heroic depletion both to later nineteenth-century physicians and to historians, and with sound reason. Yet the heroic therapeutics of the early nineteenth century is better characterized by the attitude it embodied toward treatment, and especially by its faith in the cardinal need for depletion, than by its reliance on certain practices. Bleeding and purging persisted in practice after the inclination to heroic depletion that informed their earlier use had been reversed in favor of stimulation. Nor were there any necessary links among the depletive therapies other than their usefulness in effecting the ends of the underlying therapeutic philosophy. While there were resemblances among the usage patterns of the various heroic remedies, each individual treatment waxed and waned rather independently of the others.

Taken as a whole, heroic depletion was not as drastic as the image of it that has been perpetuated would suggest. Historians have commonly cited with horror or relish instances of treatment murderous in its effects—patients bled virtually to death, poisoned with mercury to the point of disfigurement, or purged to exhaustion beyond recovery. Such extreme incidents occurred, but this was not the ordinary course of things. Historians' image of such practice as typical results largely from a reliance on retrospective evidence, the recollections of physicians in the middle or late nineteenth century about how bad practice had been in earlier years. Such stories must be read for what they were, namely, self-satisfied statements about how much medicine had improved, frequently uttered with the intent of horrifying the faint-hearted among younger physicians. To base an image of medical therapeutics in early-nineteenth-century America upon such caricatures is to accept selective, sometimes lavishly embellished reminiscences as valid descriptions of everyday practice.

The decline in the severity of heroic depletive treatment was the most dramatic change in practice during the second quarter of the nineteenth century. Already evident in the 1820s, it became clearly pronounced during the 1830s, a decade that witnessed the sharp delineation in the medical literature and at the bedside of an explicitly antiheroic therapeutic stance. This antiheroic philosophy was more distinctive in the attitude it embodied toward therapeutics than in the practice it informed. The physicians who took it up used virtually all the same therapies as did those committed to heroic depletion, modifying only the purpose and extent of these remedies' use. Moreover, they questioned neither the assumption that the objective was to restore the patient's natural balance nor the belief that treatment should be symptomatic. They did, however, challenge the notion that the task of treatment was to break up disease with whatever imposition of force was necessary. Instead, they emphasized the self-limited character of many diseases and the alleviation of symptoms, leaving nature to restore the body to health. Through the second half of the century this antiheroic impulse constituted a parallel movement to heroic therapeutics. In practice few physicians stood at either pole, and those who proselytized one position differed from advocates of the other more in rhetoric than in bedside activity.

The use of venesection in private practice illustrates several of the broader characteristics of therapeutic activity and change. A wide diversity in the application of the lancet is evident from a quantitative analysis of the relative frequency with which charges for services recorded in daybooks and practice ledgers included venesection. In the 1820s, for example, John Hyde of Freeport, Massachusetts, venesected on 64 out of a sample of 2,384—2.7 percent—of his professional visits. During the same decade the corresponding figure for George Parker in New Market, Maryland, was 21.0 percent, while that for James Foster in Simpson County, Kentucky, was only 0.7 percent. The lack of uniformity is also clear among contemporaneous practitioners in a single region. In the 1820s in Ohio Edward Kemper of Cincinnati used his lancet on 3.8 percent of his professional visits; during the same years Isaac Parker of Mount Pleasant used his on 7.5 percent. In Maryland in the 1830s a Hagerstown practitioner bled on 5.3 percent of his visits, but William Rowland of Rowlandsville employed his lancet on 16.9 percent of his.[13]

These assorted figures exemplify the fact that in their employment of venesection all regular physicians did not practice in the same way.

Some patterns do emerge, however, that permit generalization. From the 1810s through the 1850s the incidence of venesection for the larger part of the American profession clustered between two percent and nine percent of recorded visits.[14] During the first half of the nineteenth century few orthodox physicians systematically bled the majority of their patients, yet before midcentury nearly all used the lancet to open a vein at least occasionally.

Regional patterns are also discernible. To be sure, at any given time the diversity in therapeutic bleeding within a single region was far greater than any systematic differences among the regions; therefore the relative frequencies in individual private practices do not exhibit sharp regional difference. But regarded in the aggregate the use of bleeding tends to cluster in ways that point to geographic variations. Venesection was used more aggressively in the mid-Atlantic region than it was in either New England or the Midwest, in both of which, however, regular practitioners resorted to the lancet more often than did their counterparts in the South. Even though region is not a reliable predictor of how an individual physician practiced, it is at least suggestive of the therapeutic behavior likely to characterize any group of physicians practicing in the same region.

It is evident from private practice records that venesection was already declining in use by 1820 and that its demise was a gradual process played out over the ensuing half-century. Venesection was not abruptly abandoned. The diversity among practitioners in its use at any given time was far greater than the overall change over any period of a few years or even a decade, so any single line drawn to describe its decline is specious. Nevertheless, the trend of relative frequencies of its use was progressively downward. In the 1820s and 1830s, the percentages of visits in which venesection was practiced tended to cluster between four and eight; in the 1840s, between three and five; and in the 1850s and thereafter, between a few percentage points and none.[15] Some few practitioners continued to venesect patients, albeit rarely, at least into the 1880s.[16]

In part the overall decline of venesection was due to the entrance into the profession beginning in the late 1840s of young physicians who rarely or never venesected, but practice records unambiguously indicate that not all of the aggregate decline in bleeding can be ascribed to this source. Some physicians who liberally bled their patients when they first began practicing used the lancet with diminishing frequency over the course of decades.[17] In certain instances this decline marked a complete loss of faith in the practice. For example, when Edwin Cowles was practicing in Cleveland in 1832 to 1833 he recorded venesecting patients on 7.2 percent of his visits; a sample of his practice for 1838 shows that he was bleeding significantly fewer patients. By 1848 to 1851 Cowles was no longer venesecting at all. In his case this represented a true rejection of regular medicine, for a certificate among his papers testifies that he had become a member of the American Institute of Homoeopathy.[18]

For most physicians the declining use of bleeding was less dramatic and less absolute and did not entail renunciation of the orthodox profession. A regular practitioner in a small Massachusetts town, for example, venesected on 8.9 percent of his visits in 1804 but only on 2.7 percent in 1822 to 1825.[19] Similarly, Henry Turner of Montgomery County, North Carolina, used his lancet on 4.3 percent of the visits he made between 1825 and 1829 and on 2.9 percent between 1848 and 1852. A more subtle change underlying this slight diminution is also apparent in Turner's practice records: during the later period bleeding tended to run only in the accounts of certain individual patients and families. Turner never bled the vast majority of his patients, but he venesected certain patients repeatedly over the years, indicating perhaps his perception of patient need or possibly that some patients especially insisted that they be venesected when sick.[20]

The example of William Rowland, a regular physician in Maryland, is especially revealing. Rowland unquestionably bled a much greater proportion of his patients than did most of his contemporaries, but during the years for which he kept records of his practice, 1835 to 1883, his use of the lancet steadily diminished. In a sample of his practice drawn from his account book for 1835 to 1838, he venesected on 16.9 percent of his visits; in 1841 to 1847, 11.6 percent; in 1853 to 1855, 13.3 percent; in 1863 to 1867, 10.4 percent; and in 1866 to 1883 (mainly the 1870s), 6.1 percent. The unusual detail and uniformity of Rowland's records make it possible to estimate the relative frequency of bleeding in his practice by case as well as by visit. At the start of his practice he was venesecting 38.2 percent of his patients at some time during their illness, while at the close of his career he was using the lancet in only 10.9 percent of his cases.[21]

Although the trends evident in the previous decades continued, in some respects the 1840s was a doldrum period in therapeutics. One notable development in the antiheroic posture was a more self-conscious emphasis on palliation. If the physician could not aggressively cut short the course of many diseases, he could create a healing environment enhanced by the alleviation of pain in which the natural healing processes could proceed. The relief of suffering rather than the active cure of disease, some physicians argued, was their principal task. In practice this meant the more frequent prescription of opiates, a tendency that became much stronger in the 1850s.[22]

The other important therapeutic development in the 1840s was the use of large doses of quinine in the West and especially in the South. Physicians advocated massive doses not only for periodic fevers but for all febrile conditions.[23] The use of quinine for typhoid fever, a practice that engendered much debate but nevertheless grew common, was singularly important. Typhoid was becoming one of the most common fevers in the South and West during the 1840s, physicians believed, and most regarded it as the model of a debilitating, asthenic disease that called for stimulants. The growing use of quinine certainly fostered and was encouraged by the notion that disease from the 1830s onward was shifting from an overexciting to an enfeebling type.

By the late 1850s stimulants, often given in large, frequent doses, had become the mainstay of many physicians' practices. This change turned on its head the model of disease and treatment assumed in earlier heroic antiphlogistic therapeutics: instead of being sthenic and requiring depletive treatment, disease was asthenic and called for stimulating therapy. Among the stimulants in common use were quinine, cinchona bark, iron compounds, and a high, strengthening diet, but by the 1860s the most aggressively used stimulant was beverage alcohol. Although they were by no means new to the armamentarium, whiskey, wine, and brandy attained a heightened prominence as the stimulants of choice in treating many acute diseases.

Stimulating treatments by no means fully replaced depleting ones. Various physicians defended in principle the extremes of heroic stimulation, heroic depletion, and antiheroic restraint. Most, however, did not stimulate, deplete, or trust in nature by rote. Even the most enthusiastic advocates of stimulant treatments did not abruptly reject the older drugs but gradually moderated their use.

The fullest fruition of heroic stimulation coincided with the Civil War and was lucidly expressed in the therapies given at military hospitals. Prescription books from such hospitals, requisition lists for medical supplies, and narrative accounts of medical treatment all testify to the fact that alcohol used as a stimulant and opiates as palliatives were the mainstays of military medical treatment during the war. For example, the prescription book of the Second North Carolina Military Hospital in Petersburg, Virginia, for 1864 shows that whiskey (or occasionally brandy) was a major or the sole ingredient in 61.8 percent of the prescriptions. The mean amount of whiskey prescribed for each patient was 4.9 ounces per day, a therapy often repeated for many days. Other tonics were given less frequently: quinine in 8.6 percent of the prescriptions and iron compounds in 4.3 percent. While alcohol use at this hospital may have been high, it was not aberrantly so.[24] The prescription book of another Confederate hospital at an unnamed place in Virginia for 1864 to 1865 shows that alcohol (usually whiskey but sometimes brandy) was given to 40.2 percent of the patients, typically in small doses such as one ounce three times a day. Iron was prescribed for 9.8 percent of the patients and quinine for 29.5 percent, though the second figure in part reflects the high proportion of patients diagnosed as having either intermittent or remittent fever (24.7 percent).[25]

While stimulation dominated military therapy, other treatments were not ignored.[26] Reflecting the fact that many of the patients suffering from disease had also been wounded, palliation held a central place in the practice of both hospitals; in Petersburg, 40.1 percent of the prescriptions contained an opiate.[27] Still, treatment was varied and sought to do more than stimulate and palliate. The 511 new prescriptions written in the record book contained sixty-one different ingredients, among them all of the cardinal drugs of heroic depletion. Mercurial prescriptions were common at both hospitals.[28]

Although a small proportion of the alcohol given at the Petersburg hospital may have been used as an anesthetic, ordinarily alcohol was prescribed to stimulate in diseases such as pneumonia, typhoid fever, and dysentery. Similarly, quinine, often used as an antiperiodic, was also given in nonperiodic fevers. Physicians commonly held camp diseases to be almost uniformly debilitating, and while this in part simply mirrored the view predominant in the 1860s that most illnesses were of an enfeebling type, the kinds treated in the military hospitals represented an extreme case. But even though the extent of therapeutic stimulation in Civil War hospitals went beyond that in ordinary private practice, the same approach to cure was evident at the civilian bedside as well. Physicians certainly transferred some of the experience and expectations they had acquired during the war to their private practices after its close. Nevertheless, while Civil War practice reflected and fostered the vogue for heroic stimulation in American medicine during the 1860s, it did not cause it: alcoholic stimulation simultaneously rose to therapeutic fashion in both Britain and France.

In certain respects the shift from depleting to stimulating treatment marked a complete reversal in American practice, but what was preserved in this transformation was every bit as important as what changed. Heroic stimulation, like heroic depletion, involved an aggressively active intervention in the course of disease. Both approaches used remedies that produced dramatic physiological changes: a patient and his or her family could not avoid noticing the effects of an ounce and a half of brandy given every hour any less than they could overlook the consequences of a large dose of tartar emetic. Moreover, a single objective guided the use of both stimulants and depletants, namely, to restore the patient's system to a natural harmony, the one by elevating and the other by lowering the vital balance. The shift was not accompanied by any fundamental alteration in the underlying assumptions about pathology and treatment that comprised the therapeutic framework.

Permutations between the 1820s and the 1860s in the dosages and frequencies of use of remedies do not fully indicate the extent to which therapeutic change took place. For example, the fact that patients were treated with calomel and venesection in both the 1820s and the 1850s does not establish that these treatments were employed for the same reasons at both times; they were not. In the 1820s calomel was used not simply to clean out the system but also for its alterative and systemic lowering effects; by the 1860s it was usually prescribed as a reliable purgative. Venesection offers an even more striking example of change. In the 1820s its objective was often to actively cure the patient, but by the 1850s it was frequently used principally to control pain.[29] A chronicle of the declining application of the lancet to let blood therefore masks what was in some ways the more significant shift, from an emphasis on cure to one on palliation, that was evident by the 1840s.

Although herioc stimulation peaked in the 1860s, the same decade also witnessed the general eclipse of heroic therapy.[30] To be sure, some older practitioners retained a heroic posture. And just as an Ohio practitioner could refer in 1881 to the "heroic uses of morphia and chloral" for the control of suffering, chemotherapy for cancer and surgical procedures such as the implantation of an artificial heart used in the late twentieth century could be regarded as heroic by merit of the aggressive interventionism that informs them.[31] But these two manifestations of therapeutic heroism were not based on the same assumptions about disease and the objectives of treatment as those that underlay both heroic depletion and heroic stimulation.

It was in the late 1860s and the 1870s that medical therapeutics in America in some respects began to look more like the practice of the early twentieth century than that of the early nineteenth. This gradual transformation involved no sharp break with past practices. Such new remedies as chloral hydrate, the bromides, and the salicylates came into common use, as did hypodermic injections and a revived enthusiasm for the therapeutic uses of electricity, but new drugs and techniques seldom fully replaced older ones.

A more dramatic shift occurred in the way that some physicians regarded the nature of therapeutic knowledge and the sources of progress. In the thinking of certain American physicians, therapeutic knowledge was accorded a new status characterized by a commitment to universalism rather than specificity. In daily practice the new orientation involved a gradual reshaping of physicians' conception of what they sought to accomplish by their therapeutic ministrations.

As physiological normality (often gauged by quantified norms) began to be regarded as the paradigm of health, patient management increasingly centered on the close monitoring of certain signs and symptoms in relation to these objective standards. A portion of the physician's exhibition of activity in controlling disease was transferred from therapeutic intervention to a self-consciously active vigilance. Treatment was gradually redirected toward altering specific physiological processes rather than changing the general equilibrium of the body. Equilibrium of course remained a common model of health, and in practice stimulants and supportive remedies continued to dominate treatment. But physicians began to turn away from a primary concern with systemic balance to instead break down the body into more discrete units or systems each of whose functioning could then be assessed and therapeutically addressed. In general, physicians used fewer drugs but aimed them more narrowly at manipulating specific physiological processes.

For example, during the 1870s and 1880s many physicians became preoccupied with temperature. The development of medical thermometry from the late 1860s on presented the possibility of quantifying temperature, precisely chronicling its changing course, and displaying this fluctuation graphically to give the physician a portrait of disease. Beyond merely substituting quantitative for qualitative terms, physicians began to think more in terms of temperature than of fever. This reordering of clinical cognition had important consequences for therapeutics, for whereas fever was a systemic phenomenon that could be altered only by changing the general condition of the body, temperature was a discrete entity representable as a single number so that physicians could think of and manipulate it independently from the patient's other signs and symptoms. Many physicians became absorbed with normalizing high temperature. The use of alcohol and quinine, already in vogue as stimulants, was given renewed sanction by the emergence of the notion that they reduced temperature as well. Physicians also brought into their practices new antipyretics such as salicylic acid, salicylate of soda, and antipyrine, and they experimented with a host of other temperature-lowering agents.

The therapies commonly employed in the 1870s and 1880s gave physicians more sensitive control of many physiological processes than they had possessed early in the century. Salicylic acid and subcutaneous injections of morphia mitigated pain; chloral hydrate and the bromides produced sleep; and aconite slowed the pulse. Furthermore, the physician could monitor bodily processes and identify deviations from the norm not only by measurements of temperature, respiration, and pulse and by such techniques as sphygmographic tracings, but also by quantifying, for example, chemical constituents of urine.[32] Beyond this focused manipulation of physiological processes, physicians increasingly emphasized hygiene, managing the patient's diet and physical environment in such a way that the process of healing could proceed unimpeded while the most deviant of the body's functions were corrected.

At the same time physicians became less concerned with the variety of patient and environmental characteristics encompassed by the principle of specificity. An emerging rationale for the use of various remedies matched a treatment to a specific disease or even to its cause. As microorganisms were identified as the purported causes of assorted diseases, for example, some physicians sought germicides that would provide disease-specific therapy. The belief that quinine, regarded as an antiseptic, could effectively cure intermittent fever caused by the *bacillus malariae* (an apocryphal but nonetheless revealing bacterium) was typical of a form of thinking common in the 1880s. Such reasoning did not directly alter bedside practice but rationalized it in new ways and fostered disease-specific treatment, thereby also increasing the therapeutic importance of diagnosis.

Although practice was in many respects transformed between the 1820s and the 1880s, several important elements of medical therapeutics persisted. Most of the drugs and practices common in heroic antiphlogistic treatment were still used in the 1880s, albeit less frequently and in smaller doses. Moreover, even though the immediacy of physiological impression that characterized the treatments of the 1820s had slackened by the 1880s, most of the practices used in the later decade still produced palpable changes in the patient's symptoms. In the 1880s the monitoring of deviations from normality and the management of a hygienic environment superseded to some extent the heroic intervention of the 1820s, but it remained clear that the physician actively controlled the patient.

The Massachusetts General Hospital and the Commercial Hospital of Cincinnati: Two Profiles

The medical case history records of hospitals provide the materials for sketching a finer-grained portrait of the changing use of medical therapies. Yet these records too have their peculiar limitations. The type of patient and environment found in a hospital and the distinctive

status the principle of specificity accorded to the therapeutic requirements of such an institution's inmates combine to make hospital treatment by itself untrustworthy as a mirror of private practice. Moreover,
medical prescriptions at a hospital represent a collective endeavor. The
medical staff changed over time, often more than one physician prescribed for a patient during his or her stay, and frequently it is impossible to determine which physician was responsible for a particular
therapeutic choice. While these circumstances tend to compensate for
personal idiosyncrasies, they also mask individual decision making.
Furthermore, even though in some ways hospital patients were a remarkably uniform lot, that does not warrant the assumption that the
therapeutic experience at a small voluntary hospital in one region of
the country closely resembled that at a large state-supported institution
in another. And while groups of patients within a single institution
could be endlessly subdivided according to their diseases, symptoms,
and backgrounds, this would vitiate the singular advantages of analyzing hospital records; yet the alternative, treating a changing and
heterogeneous patient population as analytically uniform, is not entirely satisfying either. Patterns of practice and change discerned at
one hospital offer but a single specimen of therapeutic reality; as they
illustrate practice in a limited context, they can suggest generalizations
but cannot establish them.

However restricting these caveats may be, the fact remains that
hospital case records offer the only systematic access to detailed patient
histories collected over a period of decades in a context that offers at
least institutional continuity. The quantitative description of changing
therapeutic practice over the long duration that is not possible for
private practice can be developed for some hospitals. The focus here
is on two exceptionally complete sets of hospital case records, those
of the Massachusetts General Hospital in Boston from 1823 to 1885
and those of the Commercial Hospital of Cincinnati from 1838 to
1881.[33] The limited purpose of this study is to identify some of the
possible courses of therapeutic change over more than six decades by
presenting two concrete examples, not to give a comprehensive account
of patient care in these institutions and much less to relate the histories
of the hospitals themselves. Still, some knowledge of the differing
environments within which medicaments were prescribed and records
kept is necessary to appreciate the contexts for therapeutic changes.

When the Massachusetts General Hospital (hereafter in this book referred to as the MGH) opened in 1821, it was a small, private, voluntary
hospital established expressly to accommodate the worthy poor.[34] Sov-

ereignty over the institution, including admissions, was held by the lay board of trustees, but once patients were in the house therapeutic decisions were controlled by the visiting physicians. James Jackson occupied this post at the hospital's opening, and was soon joined by Walter Channing, with John Ware as their assistant. There were generally three visiting physicians in any given year until 1847, when two new wings opened and the number doubled. These men, often medical professors at Harvard, were professionally and socially prominent, sharing the backgrounds more of the trustees than of the patients. Ordinarily they retained their association with the hospital for a number of years, providing one source of medical continuity. They visited the hospital to inspect and prescribe for patients and give clinical instruction to students, but, as Charles Rosenberg has explained, they played only a small part in the everyday internal life of the wards.[35]

The resident physician lived in the hospital and was more intimately involved with the patients' experience in the institution. Prior to 1850 he was a recent medical graduate, but thereafter this position was filled by a final-year medical student who was termed a house pupil. He recorded each patient's history at admission, wrote down the visiting physician's instructions, and chronicled notable changes in patient condition in the case record book for the visiting physician's inspection.[36] Experience as a resident pupil was a recognized portal to professional advancement, and both medical ability and social influence played parts in securing the post. Ordinarily a resident physician remained at the hospital in this capacity only for about one year.

The sample of patients analyzed here is drawn entirely from the hospital's male medical wards, enhancing the uniformity of the sample population over time by excluding both nonmedical patients and women. The 1,762 cases included in the MGH sample represent about a tenth of the male medical patients admitted between 1823 and 1885. (Unless otherwise specified, all subsequent statistics concerning the MGH patient population refer to this sample.[37])

Initially, admission to the MGH required the written application of the prospective patient, approval by a physician who visited him, and endorsement by the visiting committee of the lay Board of Trustees. In practice admission soon came to depend ordinarily on the inspection of the applicant by the resident physician, whose judgment was directed by criteria of fitness the board laid down. Another determinant of admission was the patient's ability to pay his own board, something that a third to a half of the patients did for much of this period. Free beds were in the greatest demand, and the likelihood of being admitted was higher if the patient could pay some of his own expenses. It was the hospital's rule to deny admission to incurables unless they could pay and to discharge patients when they were found to be incurable. The rationale was to prevent the hospital from becoming an almshouse or a permanent home for the sick poor. The hospital also sought to exclude patients with highly contagious diseases such as smallpox and erysipelas and to isolate them if they were admitted. Throughout this period the MGH refused admission to a significant proportion of its applicants.[38]

Once admitted, the male medical patient ordinarily remained in the hospital for several weeks and not infrequently for some months. The mean duration of stay among the patients sampled ranged, by decade, betwen 24.9 and 31.2 days, and did not present the steady diminution over time that the trustees persistently urged. In the hospital as a whole, free patients tended to remain a third to a half again longer than paying patients throughout this period. This phenomenon, a persistent cause for complaint in the annual reports, was interpreted as reflecting paupers' desire for a "comfortable home" rather than reasons of medical need. The MGH grew considerably between the 1820s and the 1880s, admitting 124 medical patients in 1823 and 918 in 1885, with the sharpest increase occurring in 1847 when two new wings were opened. The mean patient population in the hospital at any given time, including male and female medical and surgical patients, grew from 39 in 1839 to 112 in 1850, 131 in 1860, 120 in 1870, and 167 in 1885. Compared with other major American hospitals, its size remained modest and its accommodations unusually fine.[39]

While there was substantial physical and social diversity among the patients admitted to the male medical wards, a composite sketch of the typical inmate can nonetheless be drawn. He was most likely to be in his twenties. The mean age of patients (skewed above the median by a sizable number of elderly patients) grew progressively greater over the decades, increasing from 29.9 years in the 1820s to 34.2 years in the 1880s. Throughout this period the male medical patient at the MGH was most commonly a skilled or semiskilled worker, not an unskilled laborer; and the MGH blue-collar patient was at least twice as likely to be skilled as he was semiskilled. It was next most likely that the patient would be an unskilled laborer or a sailor, two occupational groups that together comprised just under a third of the patient population (somewhat lower in the 1880s). Finally, nearly a tenth to a fifth of the patients were (generally low) white-collar workers.[40]

It is difficult to document but easy to see that the occupational profile of the MGH's patients was lower than that of the general Boston population. In 1880, a year for which the city's occupational structure has been analyzed, 32 percent of Boston's male labor force held white-

collar jobs, while only 17 percent of the male medical patients admitted
to the MGH between 1880 and 1885 had attained this occupational
level.[41] Yet compared with the inmates of other large hospitals in the
United States, MGH patients had a strikingly high occupational standing. From the 1820s through the 1870s, better than half to two-thirds
were at or above the level of semiskilled blue-collar worker (with a
peak in the 1880s of 77.9 percent). This set the MGH patient population
apart in socioeconomic status from its counterparts in most contemporaneous hospitals, where patients were more likely to be unskilled
laborers or mariners.

During the 1820s the patient admitted to the MGH's male medical
wards was likely to be native born, with under one-fifth of the patients
identified as foreign born. This changed in the 1830s, and while native-
born patients predominated through the 1840s, during these two decades the division was nearly even. In the 1850s two-thirds of the patients were foreign born, a proportion that steadily diminished through
the 1880s but never fell under one half. During this period the individual admitted to the MGH's male medical wards was more likely to
be foreign born than was the randomly chosen member of Boston's
male labor force.[42] In any given decade better than half of the foreign-
born patients claimed Irish nativity, but the proportion was not overwhelming. Like the representation of foreign-born patients as a whole,
that of Irish-born patients peaked in the 1850s when it reached 42.4
percent. In that same decade 25.2 percent of the patients had been born
in neither the United States nor Ireland; but whereas the proportion
of non-Irish foreign-born patients thereafter remained steady at about
a quarter of the population, the proportion of Irish-born patients gradually declined through the 1880s to just above a quarter. From the
1830s, when the Irish-born population first became prominent, through
the 1880s, Irish patients tended to be somewhat older than their native-
born counterparts, and after the 1840s they tended to be discharged
sooner. Beginning in the 1850s, when the Irish presence peaked, resident physicians were consistently more inclined to comment on the
drinking habits of Irish than those of native-born patients.

Over the period as a whole, physicians assigned 208 different diagnoses to cases in the sample. No single complaint was dominant.
Pulmonary diseases, especially phthisis, were common throughout this
period, ordinarily accounting for better than a tenth of the admissions.
Typhoid fever was always prominent but was more variable, becoming
most common in the 1840s when it was the diagnosis given nearly a
fifth of the patients. Rheumatism was also often given as the diagnosis,
appearing with widely varying frequencies that ranged from a low of
7.4 percent in the 1840s to a high of 16.7 percent in the 1880s. Gas-

trointestinal complaints, including typhoid fever, were noticeably common in the 1820s and 1830s, when they accounted for about a fifth of the diagnoses; this tapered down to well under a tenth in the 1850s and thereafter. Although they were common at hospitals with different clientele and in other regions of the country, delirium tremens and malaria were rare at the MGH. Very few (usually only a couple of percent) of the MGH patients were identified as having been drinking when they entered the hospital. The proportion of those drinking patients identified as heavy drinkers did increase somewhat from the 1850s onward, reaching its height in the 1880s at about 10 percent.[43]

No clear trend characterizes the recorded outcome of hospital stay. Only in the 1880s were as many as half of the patients discharged as "cured," a tenth more than in the 1820s; but the proportion of patients "cured" always remained well over a third. The mortality rate among male medical patients rose steadily each decade from the 1820s, when it was 6.9 percent, to a zenith of 20.0 percent in the 1850s. Thereafter it declined again, reaching a level of 10.8 percent by the 1880s.[44] From the 1850s through the 1880s the mortality among native-born was somewhat higher than that among foreign-born patients, suggesting that native-born men may perhaps have been more reluctant to go to the hospital when sick and hence were more seriously ill when they actually reached the wards.[45]

The resident physician recorded each patient's history in a large ledger that was used for all the medical wards, male and female. During the hospital's early decades case histories often covered ten or more pages, but recordkeeping became abbreviated as the kinds of information recorded changed and became more quantified, and as the number of patients grew. By the 1870s, histories ordinarily consisted of only a few pages. When the patient was first admitted, the resident physician recorded his age, occupation, nativity, symptoms and physical signs, and the patient's own report of the inception and progress of his illness. Some of the information routinely garnered at one period of time was ignored at others; the appearance of the tongue, for example, was invariably noted before midcentury, but thereafter began to be ignored. Similarly, in the late 1850s and early 1860s the resident physicians were very much on the lookout for environmental sources of lead poisoning, and between 1843 and 1850 they recorded in great detail the replies to their questions about masturbatory habits. The resident physician also wrote down the names of the regular or sectarian medical practitioners a patient had consulted and of the drugs with which he had dosed himself, offering a unique record of working-class medical self-help practice. Occasionally the resident would also record the words in which the patient described his disease and the patient's speculations as to its cause. The diagnosis pronounced by the visiting physician was entered into a separate index at the end of the ledger.

Subsequently during the patient's stay the resident physician ordinarily recorded his changing condition daily. Through the 1850s this might encompass notations on the bowel movements, pulse, and appearance of the urine; later it often included quantified pulse and respiration rates and temperature, and perhaps the chemist's report on the urine's composition. When the visiting physician made his rounds he inspected the patient, was informed of phenomena observed since his last visit, and directed the treatment to be followed. The resident physician entered these instructions into the case history, changing the course of treatment himself only if the exigencies of the case urgently demanded it. He also noted the consequences of the treatments the visiting physician had prescribed on his last visit, such as sleep produced by opium, the alleviation of pain by salicylate, and quieting after venesection, as well as the condition of the blood that had been let.

Contrasted with the sort of institution the large hospital had become by the early twentieth century, the Massachusetts General Hospital and the Commercial Hospital in Cincinnati in the period from the 1820s to the 1880s appear remarkably similar.[46] Yet in some important ways that shaped the experiences of both physicians and patients, they were very different institutions. Unlike the private, voluntary MGH, the Commercial Hospital was a public institution, supported largely by the state and later the city. The Ohio legislature chartered the institution in 1821 as the Commercial Hospital and Lunatic Asylum of Ohio, and it was erected in part with state money in 1823. The need to care for the sick boatmen who landed in the Ohio River port of Cincinnati was a major justification for its founding, which was instigated in large measure by Daniel Drake. For most of the period from its early years through the end of the 1860s, the hospital held a contract with the United States Government to provide medical care for sick boatmen at fixed fees.[47]

The Ohio legislature retained ultimate control of the hospital until 1861, when it transferred governance to the city of Cincinnati. Thereafter financial support came chiefly from the city council, which levied a property tax to support the institution, renamed the Commercial Hospital of Cincinnati. Aside from boatmen, whose expenses the federal government still paid, the hospital as a municipal institution was designed primarily to care for the sick poor of Cincinnati and a few adjoining townships; if an ill transient could not pay for his own care, the hospital billed the city of his permanent residence. A reorganization of the hospital changed its name again in 1868 to the Cincinnati Hospital (and hereafter in this book CHC will designate the institution).[48]

From the outset, the Medical College of Ohio controlled the hospital's medical administration. The faculty contracted to visit and prescribe for patients in the hospital without pay in return for the privilege of bringing students into the house for clinical teaching. The Medical College also chose from among its graduates the men who would become resident physicians at the CHC, where, as at the MGH, hospital service was an important springboard to professional distinction.

This contractual arrangement was a persistent source of contention between the Medical College of Ohio and the other medical schools that abounded in Cincinnati. Those whom this arrangement excluded charged that as a public institution the hospital should open its clinical facilities to all medical teachers and students. Sectarians further challenged orthodox hegemony over the care of patients, and during the late 1840s and the 1850s faculty members of sectarian schools in Cincinnati demanded that the legislature divide the control of patient care among the major sects, including regulars. The faculties of other regular medical schools did not favor this plan, but throughout the remainder of the 1850s the regular Miami Medical College led a campaign against the Medical College of Ohio's "monopoly" on clinical access. Sectarians never gained the representation at the hospital they wanted, but the Miami Medical College did. In 1861, when the hospital was transferred to the city's hands, medical control was in effect divided among Cincinnati's regular medical schools. Rivalry for clinical power continued among them, however, until the trustees decreed that after 1871 no member of the hospital's staff could be connected in any way with a medical college. Clinical teaching continued, but it was conducted by the hospital staff rather than the schools.[49]

The duties of the medical staff at the CHC differed little in principle from those of their counterparts at the MGH. Before the 1860s the faculty members of the Medical College of Ohio who provided clinical instruction in medicine and surgery were also responsible for attending the hospital during the four-month school term; during the rest of the year the other professors served in the hospital two at a time. They did not ordinarily visit the wards daily. "The duties of the Faculty extend no further than visiting the patients, making prescriptions, and performing surgical operations," one attending physician defensively explained in 1851. "No one could expect them to *nurse* the patients, nor to remain with them to witness the effects of remedies. This is the duty of the resident physician; he is constantly in the house; and sees that the medicines are administered, and meets such emergencies as may arise during the absence of the Faculty."[50] After the reorganization in 1861, attending physicians were required to visit the wards every day. Residents were ordered to visit each patient at least twice daily, to keep a "regular & minute" written record of the history and management of each case, to make a register of the attending physicians' visits, to see to it that the nurse properly administered the prescriptions, and (perhaps tellingly) to make sure "that the patients are treated kindly by the attendants."[51] The patient records leave no question that at least until the 1860s many of the resident physicians at the CHC, in contrast to their counterparts at the MGH, performed their duties lackadaisically.

The CHC was a good deal larger and busier than the MGH. In 1840 it admitted 1,238 patients, compared with only 342 at the MGH; by 1846 the respective totals were 2,038 and 459. The financial and physical resources of the CHC relative to the number of patients it cared for were more modest than those at the MGH. George Cheyne Shattuck, Jr., who later became an attending physician to the MGH, toured the CHC in 1834 and observed in his diary that "the wards are not remarkably high well ventilated or clean . . . So niggardly is the administration that sufficient attendants to keep the building clean & in order are not furnished."[52] Thirty years later the superintendent of the CHC at once bragged and bemoaned in his annual report that while an average of $9.86 per week was spent on each patient at the MGH, at his institution the expense was only $6.28.[53] A visiting committee of the CHC board of trustees reported in 1861 that the hospital building was in wretched condition. "It is without proper ventilation or any modern improvement. Its contracted windows, low ceilings, crumbling walls, and dilapidated condition, render it unfit for the purposes of a Hospital. It has not a single redeeming feature to recommend it for the uses to which it is devoted."[54] The hospital's character improved greatly after 1869, when it moved into completely new facilities. By 1881 the CHC was admitting nearly twice as many patients as the MGH and had a daily average of 330.5 patients in its wards, compared with 166 at the MGH.[55]

The CHC was a rougher place than the MGH socially as well as physically. The social differences between inmates of the two hospitals contributed to this disparity but were not its sole source. Complaints against nurses recorded by the CHC's superintendent in the late 1860s typically included ignoring patients, giving the wrong medicines, staying out all night without permission and returning to the hospital drunk, physically assaulting one another, and stealing from patients. In one report in the late 1860s the superintendent described in detail a quarrel in the wards that ended when one patient stabbed another in the heart.[56] A decade later the superintendent became nearly obsessed with the "perfect recklessness" of the resident physicians. Responding to complaints from nurses and patients about their late, noisy returns from town, he began to keep a detailed log of the time each one came in, which he later turned over to the board of trustees. In his final entry before the trustees became involved, he wrote, "About 12 o'clock of noon to day the young men comprising the Res[ident] Staff—were so disorderly at their office—holloring, yellowing, and otherwise—that it was impossible to transact business—This state of affairs is not an unusual thing—While Ladies, visiting the Hospital were passing the door of the Res[ident] Staff office—they had to troad over playing cards, strewn on the Hall floor."[57]

Taken as a whole, the patients at the CHC were a harder lot than those at the MGH. As a private institution the MGH could discriminate among its applicants, giving preference to the "worthy" sick and those able to pay; but because the CHC was public, admission to it was a right of residence. The MGH could exclude the chronic drunkard and the prostitute who were common occupants of CHC beds. And the CHC's contract with the federal government brought large numbers of boatmen into its wards. A far greater proportion (three to fourteen times as many, depending on the decade) of the male medical patients admitted to the CHC had been drinking heavily just prior to entering the hospital than had those at the MGH.[58] While the proportion of patients admitted in the wake of heavy drinking bouts peaked at both hospitals in the 1880s, at the MGH these men made up just 2.7 percent of the admissions, as compared with 13.8 percent at the CHC. Recidivism was high at the CHC for heavy drinkers, who often were brought to the hospital by police or friends after spreeing. A resident physician's entry history on a patient admitted in 1842 stated, "An old inmate lately sent out from here with money from the trustees to carry him to some distant point.—Spent it in riotous living and here we have him again with face flushed—eyes turgid tongue red—nauseated—and great pentitence [sic]—with promises of future sobriety."

The profile of the level of patient occupation was significantly lower at the CHC than at the MGH. Very few white-collar patients entered the CHC prior to the 1860s, though thereafter the proportions at the two institutions were about the same. Skilled and semiskilled blue-collar workers always represented a greater proportion of the patient population at the MGH than at the CHC, where their proportion increased over time but never reached half. On the other hand, unskilled laborers made up a far greater share of the patients at the CHC than at the MGH—roughly twice as many for most decades, and thrice as many in the 1880s. Between a third and nearly half of the male medical patients at the CHC were unskilled laborers, and from the 1830s through the 1860s about a fifth of its male medical patients were boatmen, a much greater proportion than at the MGH.[59] Compared with the city's male labor force, unskilled laborers and boatmen were overrepresented in the hospital. Men from these two occupational categories together made up between one-half and two-thirds of the sampled patients at the CHC from the 1830s through the 1860s and two-fifths in the 1870s and 1880s.

Prior to the 1860s, the nativity of patients at the CHC was identified only infrequently, though it is clear from the narrative case histories that many patients in the late 1840s and the 1850s were sick or at least exhausted immigrants who had come upriver via New Orleans directly from Ireland. During the 1860s, 1870s, and 1880s the proportion of sampled patients of Irish nativity was the same at the MGH and the CHC, roughly one-third. The proportion of German-born patients at the CHC during the same decades, about one-fifth, greatly exceeded that at the MGH, where it was under 3 percent. A larger proportion of patients at the CHC than at the MGH was foreign born, but the difference was not a dramatic one. A significant proportion (4.1 percent to 12.8 percent by decade) of the sampled patients at the CHC were black, which probably was not the case at the MGH; the difference may be partly artificial, though, for often patients incidentally indicated to be black in the MGH case histories were not explicitly identified by race. While the mean ages of patients at the two institutions were similar, patients at the CHC were persistently somewhat older than their counterparts at the MGH.[60]

Diagnostic information is far less complete in the CHC records than in those of the MGH, especially for the 1850s and 1860s. Still it is clear that delirium tremens was relatively more common at the CHC and pulmonary disease somewhat less so. The overwhelming distinction between the two hospitals in disease representation was the frequent occurrence of malaria, or intermittent fever, at the CHC. The appearance of malarial signs and symptoms in patients offers a more reliable index than diagnosis to the disease's prevalence at the hospital. Save for the 1880s, when only 11.9 percent of the sampled patients at the CHC exhibited signs of malaria, between a quarter and a third of the patients fell into this category. By contrast patients displaying malarial signs were most common at the MGH in the 1880s, when they represented only 4.1 percent of the population. The large proportion of patients at the CHC with malaria reflected not only the malarial environment of the West but more especially the working environment of boatmen and laborers who spent much of their time on the docks and flatboats of the Ohio and Mississippi rivers.[61]

The patient admitted to the CHC was likely to have a much shorter stay than the inmate of the MGH. Throughout the period from the 1830s to the 1880s the mean length of stay for male medical patients at the CHC ranged from two to two and a half weeks, about one week shorter than the average stays at the MGH for the 1830s, 1840s, and 1880s and two weeks shorter for the 1850s, 1860s, and 1870s. These figures tend to overstate the brevity of stay for most patients, though, for the mean values are skewed downward by the fact that compared with those at the MGH, large numbers of CHC patients were discharged during the first week of their hospital stay, reflecting the frequency with which patients were admitted solely for drunkenness or exhaustion. The history for one patient admitted in 1844, for example, stated simply: "Drunk. He is a loafer, who has been a frequent customer of the house . . . He says he would not have troubled us this time except it is cold out." The proportion of patients discharged "cured" fluctuated widely, and a large percentage was simply listed as "discharged." The changing mortality rates at the two hospitals followed arrestingly similar patterns, increasing during the 1830s and 1840s to a peak in the 1850s (19.1 percent at the CHC and 20.0 percent at the MGH) and thereafter declining through the 1880s. At the beginning of this period, the mortality rate at the CHC was a few percentage points higher than that at the MGH (respectively 12.9 percent and 10.0 percent), but by the 1880s this was reversed (7.6 percent and 10.8 percent). The figures were never more disparate than this.[62]

The case history books from which the sample of 2,023 CHC male patients has been taken are not so complete as those of the MGH. The earliest surviving records begin in 1837, and the nineteenth-century records end in 1881. When a new house physician took up his post in the earlier year he complained in the front of the record book, "There is not a single record in the medical department, nor a single instrument in good repair." No records survive from the years 1856 to 1859, and some of the books from the 1830s and the first half of the 1860s are only partially complete. The individual case histories are also briefer than their counterparts at the MGH, rarely longer than five pages during the antebellum period and only one or two pages long in the 1870s and 1880s. The elements that went into describing a patient were roughly the same as at the MGH, but the information was not kept as systematically. Entries often were made less frequently than at the MGH, and sometimes everything except entry data and the first day's prescription was written into the record book at the time of discharge. Most of the extant CHC records from the late 1830s, the 1840s, and the 1850s are nonetheless remarkably detailed. The brief records from the mid-1860s on, when information was often entered on standardized forms and long narrative became rare, very closely resemble the contemporaneous MGH records.

What is more striking than these variations in completeness and detail between the records of the two hospitals is the difference in attitude expressed toward patients in the CHC case histories, at least before the 1860s. Unlike the house physicians at the MGH, resident physicians at the CHC at times blatantly wrote into the case histories the amusement, disgust, or scorn they felt for patients. Most often these comments were directed at drinking or at ethnicity, reflected by recording the patient narrative in dialect. The pervasive sense was that patients were on the whole stupid, lazy, and deceitful, though at times the CHC physicians' expressions of deep sympathy with the plight of exhausted Irish immigrants brought to the hospital from the boats elicit a pathos the more subdued MGH records never approach.

Describing one patient in 1837, the visiting physician typically wrote that "he is tainted with a disease more obstinate than the one of which he has been cured of—It is often discovered in many of our inmates, and may be put down under the head of 'laziness' or 'free-wohlity.' " Remarks were in the aggregate far stronger about female than male patients, and were often sexual. Of a woman admitted for delirium tremens, the case history recorded, "Patient has been in the House four weeks; Two days ago she got permission of the Trustees to go out & see about her things[,] in other words to go to Camp Washington to get *pinked* & to get drunk, where she did go & got both." The entire case history of one woman admitted in 1850 was as follows:

> Kitty had been on a 'tod' as Jack Harris says, she took too many 'nips' got 'glorious' and met with neither friends nor kin—
> Rx Dr Death & *Eau froid*
> This treatment was continued till the 8th when she was glad to find other quarters and change her medicine and her doctor.
> Farewell Kitty—in all thy ways and wanderings keep away from the 'Ospital' or Dr Death and cold water will be after you. Glad to leave on the 8th.

To the case record of a thirteen-year-old prostitute admitted in 1846 for gonorrhea the resident physician appended, "By the way, She would make a very nice go."

Therapeutic Change at the Massachusetts General Hospital and the Commercial Hospital of Cincinnati

A prefacing example will illustrate the most frequently recurring points about therapeutic change that analysis of hospital case records discloses and will underscore two caveats to generalization. Figure 4 displays the proportion of male medical patients who were bled (by venesection, wet cupping, or leeching) while in the MGH. Two characteristics of this portrait of bloodletting's demise are especially important, for they typify therapeutic change in nineteenth-century America. First, the practice diminished gradually over a period of many decades; at no point was it abruptly rejected. Second, while the frequency of letting blood unmistakably tended downward, it did not decline steadily but fluctuated from year to year. The fluctuations remain visible even when the yearly frequencies are grouped by decade.

While the general pattern depicted for the MGH is a reasonably true mirror of bloodletting's decline in American practice at large, such a conclusion must derive from a broader knowledge of practice and not merely from a study of the MGH. One of the most pronounced themes to emerge from the scrutiny of hospital records is the variability of practice. It would be perilous indeed to generalize about American therapeutic practice from one hospital's case histories, as a comparison of bleeding at the MGH with its use at the CHC, also

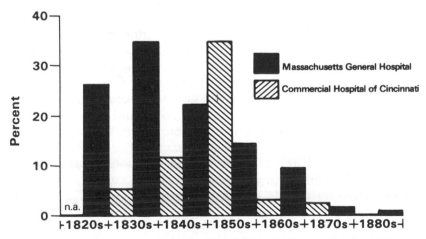

Figure 4 Percentage of cases in which bloodletting of any sort (leeching, wet cupping, or venesection) was prescribed.

shown in Figure 4, demonstrates. The surge in bloodletting at the CHC in the 1850s was a response to circumstances peculiar to the physicians practicing there, but because American physicians practiced in an enormous diversity of situations, the CHC experience was not exceptional in being singular. Substantial variability in practice among different contexts is to be expected.

The second caveat concerns an aspect of therapeutic change that statistics alone cannot reveal or even hint at. Physicians often bled with very different objectives at the MGH and the CHC, but there is no way to discover this from numbers alone. To discern changes in therapeutic orientation and to understand the meaning of the practices employed, interpretation of statistical description of change in behavior must be informed by narrative materials that give insight into physicians' thinking.

Therapeutic depletion prevailed in hospital practice in early-nineteenth-century America just as it did in private practice, but the extent to which physicians prescribed depletive therapies and the way they believed this treatment would restore a patient's system to its natural balance varied. For example, cathartics and emetics, the mainstays of depletive practice, fostered cure by serving two related but separable ends. On the one hand they were given to lower the morbidly excited system through heroic purging; on the other hand by physically expelling obstructing matter from the bowels and stomach purgatives also removed impediments from nature's way, enabling her to restore the destabilized system to its natural balance. Physicians at the MGH and the CHC sought both of these therapeutic ends through the 1850s, but the emphases at the two institutions differed. At the MGH cathartics and emetics were most commonly given to assist nature's operations, but at the CHC they were often used as powerful antiphlogistic agents to force cure by breaking up disease. The relatively more aggressive orientation at the CHC persisted until the 1860s, when practice at the two hospitals converged onto a very similar course.

Aggressive depletion at the CHC is exemplified by the use there of the mercurial cathartic calomel and the antimonial tartar emetic. (The relative frequencies of use of the therapies discussed herein are given by decade for the MGH and CHC respectively in Tables 1 and 2.)Through the 1850s calomel dominated the therapeutic experience of the majority of the male medical patients admitted to the CHC. The hospital's earliest surviving case records show that in the late 1830s nearly two-thirds (63.3 percent) of the patients ingested calomel between admission and the time of discharge or death (Figure 5). An

Table 1 Percentage of cases in which selected therapies were prescribed, Massachusetts General Hospital.

Therapy	1820s	1830s	1840s	1850s	1860s	1870s	1880s
N (no. of cases in sample)	175	250	249	251	274	341	222
Aconite	0.0	0.4	0.0	6.8	4.7	3.5	1.4
Alcohol	16.0	9.6	16.9	29.9	27.4	24.1	25.2
Bismuth	4.0	2.0	4.0	4.4	4.7	7.3	5.0
Bleeding (any method)	26.3	34.8	22.1	14.3	9.5	1.8	0.9
Blister/cantharides	46.3	25.6	9.2	19.9	14.6	10.0	6.8
Bromide (any compound)	0.0	0.0	0.0	0.0	5.8	12.9	18.0
Calomel	57.1	43.6	30.9	21.1	11.7	3.5	3.6
Chloral hydrate	0.0	0.0	0.0	0.0	0.0	11.1	7.2
Cinchona	8.6	4.8	8.8	5.6	8.8	3.8	4.1
Cod liver oil	0.6	0.4	0.4	16.7	11.0	12.6	10.4
Cupping	8.6	9.6	0.4	1.2	4.0	1.2	0.5
Diet mentioned	60.0	72.4	76.3	70.1	85.0	68.0	86.0
Diet, high prescribed	2.9	0.0	0.5	10.2	21.9	20.3	14.1
Diet, low prescribed	23.8	15.5	3.2	1.1	0.0	1.7	0.0
Dover's powder	0.0	4.0	11.7	21.9	15.7	12.3	7.2
Ipecacuanha[a]	23.4	27.2	16.9	20.3	14.6	9.1	5.9
Iron (any compound)	8.0	10.8	13.7	14.7	30.7	29.9	19.4
Laudanum	32.0	20.8	18.5	15.9	9.5	5.6	11.7
Leeching	12.6	23.6	20.1	11.6	4.7	0.6	0.5
Lobelia	0.0	0.0	0.4	0.0	0.0	0.0	0.0
Mercury (any compound)	62.9	50.8	41.4	28.7	17.2	4.4	5.9
Morphia	0.0	2.8	8.5	13.2	11.3	20.2	19.4
Opiate (any compound)	45.1	45.2	54.2	62.6	50.4	42.2	34.7
Opium (any compound)	45.1	45.2	48.2	59.0	44.5	29.3	20.7
Opium powder[b]	19.4	22.0	19.7	21.5	13.4	5.3	1.4

Table 1 (continued)

Therapy	1820s	1830s	1840s	1850s	1860s	1870s	1880s
Podophyllum	0.0	0.0	0.0	2.0	4.4	2.3	0.9
Quinine	5.7	8.4	13.7	15.1	23.4	23.2	21.2
Salicylate	0.0	0.0	0.0	0.0	0.0	7.3	18.0
Sinapisms	2.9	8.8	22.1	17.5	12.8	9.4	6.8
Tartar emetic	21.1	22.0	12.1	6.8	2.2	0.9	0.5
Venesection	8.6	10.8	6.0	2.0	1.1	0.0	0.0
Veratrum viride	0.0	0.0	0.0	1.2	3.6	0.3	0.0
Mean no. of different treatments per case	7.9	7.4	7.9	8.7	8.0	6.5	5.2
Mean no. of changes in treatment, days 1–5	3.5	3.4	3.3	2.9	3.0	2.3	2.7

a. Does not include ipecacuanha content of Dover's powder prescriptions.
b. Opium powder as an ingredient in any compound other than Dover's powder and laudanum.

Table 2 Percentage of cases in which selected therapies were prescribed, Commercial Hospital of Cincinnati.

Therapy	1830s	1840s	1850s	1860s	1870s	1880s
N (no. of cases in sample)	79	550	342	243	700	109
Aconite	0.0	1.1	1.2	0.0	0.3	1.8
Alcohol	2.5	14.6	13.7	14.8	10.6	10.1
Bismuth	2.5	0.4	0.9	6.6	12.1	11.9
Bleeding (any method)	5.1	11.5	35.1	2.9	2.3	0.0
Blister/cantharides	21.5	13.1	6.7	7.0	2.9	1.8
Bromide (any compound)	0.0	0.0	0.0	5.3	6.9	12.8
Calomel	63.3	42.2	52.5	17.3	5.7	1.8
Chloral hydrate	0.0	0.0	0.0	0.0	9.6	10.1
Cinchona	7.6	3.6	5.3	4.9	4.6	8.3
Cod liver oil	0.0	0.6	3.2	2.1	5.0	6.4
Cupping	0.0	9.1	23.1	2.1	1.9	0.0
Diet mentioned	1.3	8.2	5.9	20.6	7.3	15.6
Dover's powder	51.9	31.3	30.7	3.7	2.7	0.9
Ipecacuanha[a]	21.5	26.2	24.0	8.2	1.4	0.9
Iron (any compound)	1.3	5.1	4.4	16.1	13.3	4.6
Laudanum	13.9	14.6	14.6	5.8	8.6	7.3
Leeching	0.0	0.0	0.3	0.4	0.4	0.0
Lobelia	3.8	1.5	5.0	0.4	0.1	0.0
Mercury (any compound)	72.2	53.1	63.5	23.9	6.7	3.7
Morphia	3.8	14.7	18.1	16.5	10.3	14.7
Opiate (any compound)	78.5	59.1	53.2	41.2	24.4	24.8
Opium (any compound)	78.5	52.2	46.5	29.2	16.3	12.8
Opium powder[b]	24.1	15.6	16.4	16.9	5.0	4.6
Podophyllum	0.0	0.2	0.0	0.8	0.6	0.0
Quinine	24.1	32.4	26.0	36.2	24.3	10.1
Salicylate	0.0	0.0	0.0	0.0	3.1	9.2

Table 2 (continued)

Therapy	1830s	1840s	1850s	1860s	1870s	1880s
Sinapisms	1.3	2.6	3.5	1.2	1.6	0.9
Tartar emetic	21.5	17.3	17.8	3.7	0.9	0.0
Venesection	5.1	4.0	18.1	0.4	0.0	0.0
Veratrum viride	0.0	0.0	1.2	3.3	0.9	0.0
Mean no. of different treatments per case	5.5	5.6	5.9	4.2	2.8	2.5
Mean no. of changes in treatment, days 1–5	2.1	2.1	2.7	1.8	1.4	1.3

a. Does not include ipecacuanha content of Dover's powder prescriptions.
b. Opium powder as an ingredient in any compound other than Dover's powder and laudanum.

additional 8.9 percent of the patients who were not given calomel took some other mercurial. Calomel use dropped after 1840 but then rose abruptly toward the end of that decade. By the mid-1850s the proportion of patients prescribed calomel had fallen again to about one-third, where it remained when the records resumed at the start of the 1860s. It diminished sharply from the mid-1860s on until by the early 1880s calomel was used in only 1.8 percent of the cases.[63]

The aggressiveness of calomel use at the CHC is also apparent in the large doses clinicians there prescribed. In the 1830s, for example, when calomel was administered to half again the proportion of patients receiving it at the MGH, it was given in doses on average nearly four times as large. One index of its use is the mean dose given on the first day of a case in which it was used, figures for which are presented by decade in Figure 6. In the late 1830s the mean dose at the CHC was 21.7 grains, an amount that dropped precipitously in the 1840s, increased slightly in the early 1850s, and then progressively diminished to a mean dosage of 3.0 grains in the early 1880s.[64] Physicians at the CHC prescribed calomel in diminishing doses and with variable but generally decreasing frequency over a period of many decades; at no point did they abruptly reject the drug, but continued to use it through the 1880s.

Antimonial emetics were also used at the CHC to lower the sthenic patient. A man admitted in 1837, for example, was prescribed "Tart[ar] Emet[ic] in grain doses every hour—if that does not subdue the excitement by 2 oclock P.M. set him up in bed & bleed—Then continue

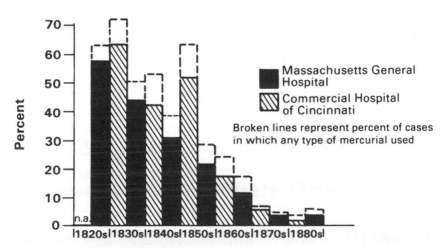

Figure 5 Percentage of cases in which calomel was prescribed, and in which any mercury-containing drug was prescribed.

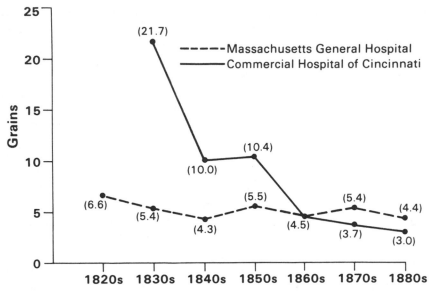

Figure 6 Mean dose of calomel prescribed on the first day it was ordered.

Tart. Emetic as before." Six days later the house physician noted, "The Tart. Emet. has kept down the excitement, so that further bloodletting was not necessary." Tartar emetic and calomel exhibit similar patterns of changed use at the CHC, being employed extensively in the 1830s and noticeably but not dramatically less frequently in the 1840s and 1850s (Figure 7). Prescriptions of both drugs had dropped very sharply by the 1860s and diminished further thereafter.

The use of depletive drugs at the CHC appears even more aggressive when contrasted with the moderate employment of cathartics and emetics at the MGH.[65] During the 1820s and 1830s daily doses of calomel-containing cathartics were common at the MGH.[66] As at the CHC, mercurials were viewed there as the most active of the common cathartics. Unlike their Cincinnati counterparts, however, MGH physicians rarely administered drastic doses of calomel to physiologically lower a patient and ordinarily gave only small amounts to impose regularity on the body's dejecta and cleanse the system.[67] Thus while the therapeutic plan prescribed for one patient admitted to the MGH in 1832 was identified as "Medicine expectante," the patient nevertheless received compound calomel pills morning and evening.

Of the drugs identified with heroic depletion, none was given more frequently during the MGH's first decade than calomel. In the 1820s

57.1 percent of the patients sampled were given calomel at some time during their hospital stay, and an additional 5.7 percent received mercury in some other form. Figure 5 shows the remarkable steady decline in the frequency of calomel use from the 1820s through the 1860s, with a leveling off in the 1870s and 1880s at about 3.5 percent. At the same time that they used mercurials less frequently, physicians also delayed longer before having recourse to them.[68]

The risk of masking important changes unavoidably results from grouping the frequencies of a drug's use by decade. While the decline in the use of calomel at the MGH was at no point punctuated by abrupt rejection, its changing employment was not quite as steady as the general schema shown in Figure 5 represents. Underlying this overall diminution were fluctuations from year to year in the frequency of calomel prescriptions, expressed in Figure 8. Two leading periods of change are evident. The first occurred between the early 1820s and the mid-1840s, after which calomel use leveled off until about 1860. The second and lasting drop occurred during the several years just after the Civil War. In no single year after 1865 was calomel given in as many as one-tenth of the admitted cases, whereas its use had fallen beneath that level in only two of the hospital's preceding forty-three years. Periodic drops in calomel use during the late 1820s and the 1830s

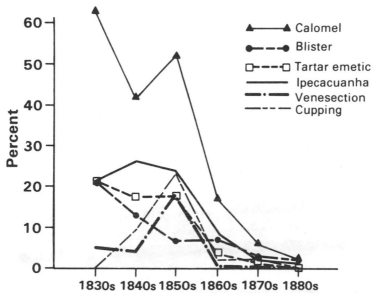

Figure 7 Commercial Hospital of Cincinnati. Percentage of cases in which selected therapies identified with heroic depletive therapeutics were used.

suggest the influence of contemporaneous Broussaisian attacks upon
mineral cathartics, an influence corroborated by the simultaneous rise
in the use of leeches at the MGH. Also suggestive is the fact that
podophyllum, an eclectic botanical drug regular physicians came to
regard as an alternative to calomel, attained its most frequent use at
the MGH in the middle and late 1850s, coinciding with the second
period of calomel's decline.

The dosages of calomel given at the MGH offer compelling evidence of moderation in prescribing cathartics even in the hospital's
early decades. The size of calomel doses (see Figure 6) declined somewhat at the MGH through the 1830s (when the mean was 5.4 grains
compared with 21.7 at the CHC) but thereafter fluctuated without
discernible direction.[69] This oscillation reflects the therapeutic mild-
ness that even in the 1820s characterized New England medicine. Once
a physician at the MGH decided to use calomel, whether in the 1830s
or the 1880s, the initial dose he prescribed was on average about the
same. Doses given during the second quarter of the century by such
physicians as Bigelow, Holmes, and Jackson were large enough to produce sure catharsis but not to drastically lower the patient. In contrast
the progressively diminishing mean doses of calomel administered at
the CHC represent the gradual weakening of a sort of heroic depletion
never common at the MGH.

Physicians at the MGH occasionally used tartar emetic as they

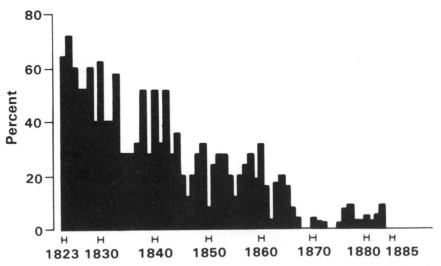

Figure 8 Massachusetts General Hospital. Percentage of cases in which calomel was prescribed.

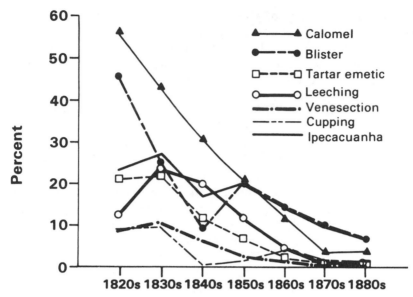

Figure 9 Massachusetts General Hospital. Percentage of cases in which selected therapies identified with heroic depletive therapeutics were prescribed.

did calomel to lower systemically overstimulated patients through depletion, but principally employed it to clean out the patient's system. Through the early 1840s tartar emetic maintained the level of popularity it had had when the hospital's wards opened in 1823, being given to about one-fifth of the patients (Figure 9). Thereafter it shared calomel's pattern of gradual decline with a permanent passage from vogue (but not from use) after the Civil War. Although physicians at both hospitals continued to prescribe purgatives, by the mid-1860s they no longer saw them as the cardinal means of righting their patients' imbalances.

The decline of heroic depletion was not marked by abrupt rejection of the mainstays of early-nineteenth-century practice, as the cases of calomel and tartar emetic illustrate, but it cannot be described by a steadily downward curve either. Indeed, any model of nineteenth-century therapeutic change that postulates a uniform, steadily diminishing reliance on depletive therapies is solidly refuted by the example of venesection's use at the CHC.

Venesection differed from the other elements in the arsenal of therapeutic depletion in several important ways. It was a surgical procedure used as a medical therapy. The heroic character of a drug such as calomel could be mollified by giving it in a small dose to produce mild catharsis instead of drastic lowering, but venesection was intrinsically a bold intervention. Almost all patients took pills, but not every patient had a vein opened. Furthermore, from the 1860s on venesection fell into a disuse more nearly complete than that of the other therapies associated with heroic depletion. At the same time, however, it was in principle the most fervently defended of all regular practices.

During the 1830s and 1840s venesection was practiced on about one-twentieth of the patients admitted to the CHC, as Figure 7 shows, but in the early 1850s its frequency spurted upward to 18.1 percent. It experienced remarkable popularity in the hospital between 1850 and 1852, dropping again to its pre-1850 level from 1853 to 1855. No records survive from the remainder of the 1850s, and when they resume in the next decade venesection has all but vanished; it appears again in the sampled cases only once, having been used to treat a patient in "extreme collapse" in 1866. A seasonably variable practice, venesection was overwhelmingly more common at the CHC in November through April than in May through October. The enthusiasm for it that reigned in the hospital from 1850 to 1852 therefore becomes even more evident when monthly frequencies are calculated, since in some of the winter months as many as half of the male medical patients were venesected during their stay.

Like most treatments, venesection served more than one therapeutic function. Much of the bloodletting performed at the CHC was designed to relieve pain, but physicians there also sought curative benefits from it. In keeping with the belief that to break up a disease by bloodletting the physician had to perform the operation early in the disease's course, nearly three-fourths (74.2 percent) of the patients venesected at the CHC were initially bled on their first or second day in the hospital. Often physicians prescribed venesection explicitly to reduce inflammation and lower fever and excitement with the objective of actively curing the disease. The antiphlogistic intent of venesecting was unmistakable when, the day after a patient was given a large dose of calomel for fever, the house physician recorded that he was "greatly improved in every respect. Medicine kept down fever so that it was not necessary to bleed."

Bleeding was an accepted way of relaxing the system; for a patient with tetanus in 1843, the resident physician recorded, "Bled him nearly to syncopy, when his muscles were released." Whatever its particular intent, venesection made a palpable impression on the system. "Pulse has become much fuller & pupils instead of being dilated are now contracted," the 1837 history of a dying patient recorded. "Carotids beat vigorously—face & body moist. Abstracted nearly 32 ounces of blood when pulse began to acknowedge its loss—then stuped—it produced some effect—as he could be slightly aroused after it by hollowing in his ears."[70]

The intriguing upsurge of venesection at the end of the 1840s and in the early 1850s was only one among several factors that made therapeutic practice at the CHC during those years extraordinary. An unmistakable renaissance of heroic depletion at the CHC began in 1849, was expressed most fully between 1850 and 1852, and was evident to a lesser extent for another two years. It was marked by an abrupt rise in the frequency with which three mainstays of heroic depletion—calomel, cupping, and venesection—were prescribed (see Figures 4 and 7). Contrast of the CHC with the MGH further highlights the heroic extent of depletion at the former hospital during the 1850s: comparative frequencies of use at the CHC and the MGH during that decade were for calomel 51.5 percent and 21.1 percent, for cupping 23.1 percent and 1.2 percent, for tartar emetic 17.8 percent and 6.8 percent, and for venesection 18.1 percent and 2.0 percent.

The elevation of faith in heroic depletion at the CHC emphasizes more forcibly than the changing pattern of use for any single treatment can the fallacy of assuming that heroic depletion followed a progressively downward path leading inexorably toward its demise. The return to depletion in Cincinnati also underscores the fact that in accounting for change, it is necessary to look not only at the animi that broadly operated on the practices of American physicians but also at the idiosyncratic social and intellectual positions of the practitioners who chose to alter their therapeutic approach. The exceptional recrudescence of heroic depletion at the CHC in the early 1850s is to some extent attributable to changes in the hospital's medical staff, but it was chiefly driven, as is elaborated elsewhere,[71] by a sociopolitical situation in Cincinnati medicine that brought threats against the orthodox profession to a desperate state of crisis.

At midcentury the sense Cincinnati regular physicians had of being under siege from sectarians reached its zenith. Perhaps in no other American city was sectarian power so prominent in municipal life and so entrenched institutionally. The outbreak in 1848 of an Asiatic cholera epidemic, especially severe in the West, highlighted the theoretical disunity and therapeutic inadequacies of orthodox practitioners and catalyzed the solidification of sectarian power in the city's medical institutions. In 1849 sectarians succeeded in ousting all regular physicians from the city board of health and in placing an eclectic practitioner at its head. Regular physicians at the CHC were especially vulnerable to sectarian assaults. In 1848 the faculty of the Eclectic Medical Institute of Cincinnati instituted a campaign to force the Ohio legislature to divide patient care in the hospital among orthodox, eclectic, and homeopathic practitioners and insisted that no student should be denied access to a hospital supported with public funds. The legislature opened the CHC to sectarian students in 1850, and even though this measure was reversed in the following year, orthodox practitioners had reason to fear that their hegemony might be subverted.

Facing very real threats to orthodox power, it was important for the attending physicians at the hospital, in their multiple roles as clinicians, medical school faculty members, and leaders of the regular profession in the West, to declare loudly that they would not capitulate to sectarian pressure. It was vital for them to display to sectarians, regulars, the public, and themselves that they were standing firm in their devotion to the orthodox faith. They saw themselves as the guardians of orthodoxy at the front lines of its battle with medical sectarianism.

The physicians at the CHC responded to the sectarian threat by sharpening the differences between themselves and sectarian practitioners rather than muting them. Preserving the hospital against sectarian taint was not merely a duty but an exercise of their identity, and the revival of heroic depletion in the CHC wards functioned as a reaffirmation of professional regularity. Certainly they must have derived some pleasure from giving clinical lectures that exhibited the beneficial effects of heroic depletion before the intruding sectarian students. More than this, their clinical behavior decisively confirmed their standing as orthodox physicians. The remedies of heroic depletion were the emblem of regular separateness, and by prescribing them CHC physicians unambiguously indicated the tradition in which they chose to root their identity. Bleeding patients and dosing them with mineral drugs served to purify the hospital that had been vitiated by a sectarian presence and proclaimed the allegiance of its staff to the regular therapeutic creed.

By returning to a more aggressive use of such therapies as venesection and calomel, practitioners at the CHC were choosing, consciously or not, to emphasize the most recognizable signs of their identity as orthodox physicians. This return to the durable core of regular therapeutic tradition must have been comforting to men who saw their professional world being pulled apart at the seams. It was a reassuring albeit limited way of preserving the self-confidence that was so essential to the regular physician's "profession" of being singularly competent to care for patients. In a period of professional instability dominated by the challenge of growing sectarian power, the Asiatic cholera epidemic may well have precipitated a crisis state that drove physicians to seek solace in a familiar touchstone of regular identity.

In this respect the celebration of heroic depletion at the CHC represented one attempt to maintain order in a time of severe professional dislocation.

The contrast between the resurgent use of depletive remedies at the CHC and their continued decline at the MGH illustrates the naiveté of generalizations about "American" therapeutic practice that fail to recognize the underlying diversity in bedside activity. Yet the imposing contrast between the relative frequencies of venesection at the two hospitals is just one sign of a profound difference in their therapeutic orientation. Physicians at the CHC were inclined to use it, like calomel and tartar emetic, to break up disease. But at the MGH, just as physicians tended to use cathartics and emetics to clear the way for nature's operations more than to force a cure, so too they seldom employed venesection primarily as an antiphlogistic agent. Instead, they used it mainly to relieve pain while nature corrected the systemic imbalance.

At the MGH venesection was never employed with as great a frequency as were other means of heroic depletion. As Figure 9 shows, during no decade were many more than one-tenth of the patients at the MGH venesected. The frequency of venesection rose somewhat in the early and middle 1830s and thereafter declined. By midcentury it had passed from common use, but it was practiced sporadically for another decade and a half. Like calomel and tartar emetic, venesection exhibited a gradual decline rather than the abrupt abandonment that would imply active rejection.

In the majority of instances in which physicians used venesection at the MGH, the primary objective was unmistakably the reduction of pain, with systemic debilitating effects expected but secondary.[72] Occasionally they venesected explicitly to lower sthenic patients, but as a principal goal this was never common. Most often it was prescribed for patients with violent headaches, but pain in the side or breast associated with internal inflammation and acute pain in the joints from rheumatism were also treated by general bleeding. The case of a fifty-year-old baker who was admitted to the MGH in 1830 with bronchitis and laryngitis (having been bled thirty-two ounces before entering the hospital) illustrates this motivation for bloodletting. Initially James Jackson treated him for pain by applying eighteen foreign leeches to his throat. The next day he consulted with the other visiting physicians and directed that "if distress become[s] urgent at any time," 6 to 13 ounces of blood should be drawn by venesection.

Physicians often resorted to venesection only after other remedies had failed to relieve pain. A young seaman from the Azores who entered the MGH wards in 1852 with acute rheumatism had already been treated with opium and morphia, but when he persisted in exhibiting a hard, fast pulse, rapid breathing, and "groaning, & frequent crying out c[um] pain," Jacob Bigelow prescribed the removal of eight ounces of blood by venesection. Some patients were bled repeatedly with relief almost always forthcoming but not lasting, leaving the physician to determine whether the reduction of suffering warranted further blood-shed.[73]

The physicians of the MGH neither used nor avoided venesection by rote. By midcentury they had largely set aside their lancets but were willing to open a vein if the patient's condition indicated it. During the 1850s and 1860s, venesection was prescribed occasionally by a coterie of physicians known for their allegiance to mild treatments and the healing power of nature: Bigelow, J. B. S. Jackson, and David Humphreys Storer. (Holmes was no longer attending physician by that time but had prescribed venesection in the MGH in the late 1840s.) Most of the patients venesected during these decades exhibited desperate symptoms such as delirium and intense pain in the head and were diagnosed as suffering from such full-blooded conditions as apoplexy, sunstroke, and cerebral congestion. What is most notable about the infrequent use of venesection during these years at the MGH is not that it had passed from common use—it had done that in the practice of most physicians by the 1860s—but rather that it illustrates how undoctrinaire medical practice was.[74]

The decline of venesection was not to any significant extent attributable to its replacement by another therapy at either hospital. There is no evidence that local bloodletting—wet cupping and leeching—compensated for the reduction in venesection, nor do the usage patterns of the cardiac sedatives, drugs that were touted as substitutes for venesection because they mimicked its pulse-slowing action, indicate that they supplanted it. Aconite was first used to any substantial extent at the MGH during the 1850s and 1860s but was applied externally as an analgesic. When it did come to be used internally as a cardiac sedative during the following two decades it was given in only a small percentage of cases. Veratrum viride, the other leading contender as a replacement for venesection, was used in a similarly scant proportion of cases in the 1850s and 1860s and all but vanished from the case histories in the 1870s. Aconite was prescribed at the CHC even less frequently than at the MGH, while veratrum's use at the two hospitals was nearly identical. Control of pain by hypodermic injections of morphia after the mid-1860s sometimes served the palliative function that venesection had in the 1820s and 1830s, but the one treatment did not replace the other.

In private practice the physician often directly witnessed the effects of his prescriptions and so could adjust dosages to produce the consequences he desired. In hospital practice, however, the visiting physician who prescribed treatment as a rule neither administered it nor observed its immediate results. Thus although hospital physicians ordinarily specified the amount of a drug to be given, they not infrequently directed that treatment be continued until some desired result was attained. The physician matched a cathartic, opiate, or bleeding prescribed in this way to the patient's condition by specifying the physiological reaction that would mark the therapy's completion, be it purging, relief from pain, or sedation, rather than a fixed dosage.

Venesection exemplified individualized therapy. At both the MGH and the CHC directions for venesection were ordinarily given in terms of physiological effect rather than of a fixed volume of blood, thereby taking into account individual peculiarities.[75] By far the majority of prescriptions for venesection at the CHC were written simply as "Bleed q[uantum] s[ufficit]," "Bleed him to produce an effect," or bleed "to such an extent as will induce some feeling of faintness." At the MGH "V.S.—p[ro] r[e] n[ata]"—that is, venesection as is needed to produce the desired effect—was one common manner of specifying the volume to be drawn. When an amount was indicated, it might be qualified by the phrase "if borne well"; or a physician could direct the letting of six ounces of blood, adding that "if P[ulse] becomes more full without faintness" twelve ounces were to be taken. Resident physicians often recorded the extent to which venesection was actually carried in functional rather than quantitative terms as well. Of one patient treated at the CHC in 1843 by John Harrison, the resident wrote, "Bled him till the strength of his pulse was some lessened," and of another, "Took blood from the arm till an impression was made upon the pulse." The fact that the mean volumes of blood drawn dropped at the MGH after the 1820s and progressively declined at the CHC from the 1830s through the 1860s suggests that over time the alterations physicians sought became less heroic.[76]

By recording the amount of blood actually extracted to produce a particular effect the resident physician preserved for the attending physician one index of the patient's systemic animation or debility. The character of the blood obtained was another indicator of condition. Although at both hospitals the condition of let blood was ordinarily mentioned, physicians at the CHC, using venesection for therapeutic manipulation of the disordered body more than for palliation, were more interested in the condition of the blood than were their MGH counterparts. The case record routinely included the physician's judgment of how firmly the blood coagulated and whether or not it appeared "buffed" or "cupped." Buffed blood and an excess of fibrine were both

indications of internal inflammation, for example, and their exhibition
in the blood of a venesected patient often directed further bleeding.
Thus a patient admitted to the CHC in 1850 whose "blood shows an
immense amount of fibrine" was venesected five times.[77]

The fact that at the MGH venesection was prescribed primarily
to palliate underscores an important characteristic of many of the treatments identified with the heroic medicine of the early nineteenth century. While the medical literature clearly presented such treatments
as cupping, leeching, and blistering as having curative value, the pre-
dominate use of all of them in both hospitals was to relieve pain. Like
venesection local bleeding by wet cups was sometimes used to reduce
local inflammation, but it was principally employed as an analgesic.
Ordinarily cups were applied to the temples or the back of the neck
and drew between 6 and 12 ounces. Leeching, rare at the CHC, was
used more extensively than cupping at the MGH. Typically between
six and fifty leeches were applied directly to the seat of pain, such as
the temples, abdomen, head, scrotum, throat, or joints. Because leeching was often repeated on different days and on various parts of the
body, some patients leeched at the MGH had many dozens of leeches
applied during their stay. Blistering with cantharides (Spanish fly), as
well as sinapisms (mustard plasters), were also used at both hospitals,
largely for relieving pain.

While these practices served similar therapeutic functions, the
changing patterns of their use illustrate the fact that the practices
linked to early-nineteenth-century heroic medicine did not rise or fall
as a single unit, as is evident in Figures 7 and 9. Blistering, for example,
did not experience the elevated use at the CHC in the 1850s exhibited
by venesection, cupping, tartar emetic, and calomel. Instead its employment diminished in a very even pattern from the 1830s onward.
At the MGH nearly half of the patients admitted in the 1820s were
blistered during their hospital stays. This treatment continued through
the mid-1830s, when blistering fell sharply in favor of leeching; it
increased again in the early 1850s and then steadily diminished through
the 1880s. The overall pattern of blistering's decline was similar at the
two hospitals, though its demise was more rapid at the CHC and its
disuse by the 1880s more complete. The use of cups, leeches, and
sinapisms also followed notably dissimilar patterns at the two hospitals, with leeching and sinapisms relatively more common at the MGH
and cupping more popular at the CHC.

The discrepancies in the use of therapies such as leeching at the
two hospitals ordinarily did not represent doctrinaire practice. The
dearth of leeching at the CHC reflects not so much a therapeutic choice
as the extreme difficulty of getting good leeches in Cincinnati. In Bos-

ton, where leeches were regularly imported from Europe, the timing of leeching's climb to fashion in the late 1820s and its gradual decline during the 1840s certainly implies a Broussaisian bent among some of the MGH physicians. Such cases as that of a patient who entered the hospital with gastritis in 1833 and was treated with six applications of about a dozen leeches each and a diet of mucilage of gum arabic displayed exemplary Broussaisian form, but most cases in which leeches were used decidedly did not.[78] Physicians at the MGH directed that leeches be applied to a variety of sites on the body, showing no particular favoritism for the epigastrum as a strict follower of Broussais might do. And far from exhibiting Broussaisian allegiances in their use of other remedies, MGH physicians even prescribed leeches and calomel simultaneously, a practice that would have been an anathema to cathartic-damning Broussaisists. Broussais's teachings certainly drew attention to the value of leeching and probably fostered its use at the MGH, but they by no means dictated the particular ways leeches were prescribed there.

The case histories kept at the MGH and the CHC bear witness to the perception of physicians that their therapies worked. Treatment by bloodletting, purgatives, and blisters induced manifest physiological changes that fulfilled their expectations. The efficacy of venesection, for example, was confirmed at the MGH when the resident physician recorded that it reduced the rate and force of the pulse, alleviated pain, lowered temperature and respiration rate, returned a livid flushed countenance to a natural condition, and relaxed the anxious patient so that he could sleep. In one case in which 10 ounces of blood were drawn, the house physician could write, "P[ulse] 90 before, 58 after venesection. Was a little faint & decidedly relieved from the headache & throbbing in temples wh had existing before"; in another, after letting sixteen ounces of blood he recorded that the "patient bore venesection . . . remarkably well and said 'his pain left him at once.' Pulse became slower, & more full. Resp[iration] reduced to 34 per minute. C[oun]t[enanc]e less anxious."

Patients occasionally dissented from prescribed therapies. An Italian mechanic with pneumonia who "speaks very little English" chose to leave the CHC rather than submit to repeated bleedings in 1850. After being venesected twice his pulse was still 108 and firm, and the attending physician prescribed venesection to twelve ounces. "But," the case history records, "he would not consent to this and got up[,] put on his clothes and left. *Discharged* by request and very much against our wishes & his welfare." A laborer who refused to acquiesce to a second application of blisters followed the same course in 1837. "Symptoms again requiring the Blister to Epigastrum it was applied," the record stated. "He feeling somewhat uneasy under it, & apprehending a repetition of them, Swore By God he would stand it no more, so he took French leave."

To a striking extent, however, patients shared the perception that therapies used in the hospitals worked. The resident physicians who kept the records filtered patients' attitudes through their own beliefs, to be sure, but some indications of patient confidence in heroic treatments are nonetheless evident. Patients helped sustain bloodletting by affirming its efficacy. After 8 ounces of blood were drawn from a twenty-year-old Boston truckman at the MGH he "became faint, but expressed himself soon after as feeling decided relief especially in head." A patient whose severe head pain had resisted other attempts at palliation reported "very little [pain] in head since being cupped"; similarly, after a patient who entered in 1825 had twenty leeches applied to his temples, he reported his "head much relieved since the leeches from heaviness." Such validation of palliative bleeding would have been impossible without patients' testimony.

Recorded instances of demand for heroic treatment far outnumbered those of resistance. A patient admitted in June 1844 reportedly "has been accustomed to be bled every year, about this time"; the attending physician directed that 12 ounces of blood be taken by venesection and an additional 6 by cupping. An Irish farmer with pain in his head was reported "very anxious to be bled" when he entered the MGH. This patient was typical, though, in that his specific therapeutic demands went unmet; the fact that he was not bled evinces a degree of physician control over therapy that was common in hospitals but difficult to exercise in private practice.

The faith patients evinced in the treatments associated with heroic depletion is further reflected in domestic medical care, in which the therapies that characterized professional practice figured prominently. Sick Americans' cardinal reliance on cathartics during the first half of the century is evident in the reports patients gave of their treatment prior to entering the MGH: those who had treated themselves reported having used cathartics more than any other therapy, and it was not unusual for a patient to be "in [the] habit" of using cathartics or to enter with a "constant dependence upon cathartic medicine." After cathartics, emetics were the remedies MGH patients most often reported having used. Purgatives, especially mercurial cathartics, were mainstays also in the self-dosing habits of CHC patients. The house physician there noted of a twenty-two-year-old man admitted in 1839, "[He] has been sick from nearly a week—effect of cold and exposure[.] Says his friends poured down the calomel without mercy."

Just as practice tended to be more aggressive at the CHC than at the MGH, so too the sick who came to the Cincinnati hospital through the 1850s by and large reported having received more heroic depletive treatment from physicians before being admitted than did their Boston counterparts. A blacksmith who entered the hospital in 1842 had been "under the care of a German Dr whose medicine says the patient purged him 19 times in 12 hours." A twenty-four-year-old laborer who had contracted bilious fever in Mobile announced to the CHC physicians that he had already "taken his *'hat fulls of medicine.'* " Some patients, especially those diagnosed with bilious fever, entered the hospital displaying severe salivation, a sign of mercury poisoning. A laborer admitted in 1850, for example, had been bled two quarts by a doctor before entry and was badly salivated; the house physician noted, "Says he had fever and ague and the Doctor done this."

As some physicians began to doubt their ability to actively cure many diseases by drugging, they also stressed palliation more and more. Especially in the 1840s and 1850s some practitioners came to regard relieving pain while nature provided a cure as the first indication of patient care. But just as physicians' judgments of the revaluation of nature and art that underlay this shift in emphasis from cure to care differed, so palliation did not attain uniform prominence in their actual practices. Reliance on palliatives appeared earlier and was more emphatic at the MGH than at the CHC, where there was no evidence of a turn to palliation until the 1860s.

The most enduringly important treatments for pain at the MGH were opiates, and their changing use best illustrates the growing preoccupation with palliation. However, several difficulties encumber generalizations about the purposes for which opiates were prescribed. Opiate use transcended broad categories of therapeutic orientation such as heroic depletion, heroic stimulation, and the expectant plan. Virtually all regular physicians recognized the power of opium to allay pain, but at various times many practitioners also claimed for it both stimulant and depressant attributes in different dosages. Opiates were further given to produce sleep (in part by alleviating the disturbance pain caused), check diarrhea, and suppress coughing. Many of the practitioners most skeptical about the power of art held opium to be regular medicine's most valuable agent. "The mere relief of suffering is in all diseases, one of the most important indications," John Ware told his classes at Harvard around 1850. "The knowledge of the proper administration of opiates, makes more difference in physicians than any other one thing."[79] Despite this diversity in their use, it is clear that from the 1820s through the 1880s in the lion's share of opiate prescriptions at the MGH the primary effects sought were analgesic.

The overall course of opiate use at the MGH, represented in Figure 10, underwent two striking periods of change that are surface indicators of deeper shifts in therapeutic orientation. The first is the increased frequency of opiate prescription during the 1840s and 1850s. This mirrors both the rising skepticism regarding the physician's ability to actively break up disease and the growing emphasis on palliation that accompanied the increased trust among elite Boston physicians in the healing power of nature. The second major change is the marked decline in frequency of opiate use that began in the mid-1860s. Opiates were given in two-thirds of all cases in the 1850s and in only one-third by the 1880s. This reflects not so much a weakening faith in opiates as the introduction of several new drugs—salicylic acid, chloral hydrate, and the bromides—that supplied the physician with potent alternatives in controlling pain and inducing sleep. These drugs to some extent supplanted opiates for certain therapeutic purposes.[80]

Underlying the smooth contours of these changes was a more complex fluctuation in the forms of opiates prescribed at the MGH. The use of *opium* compounds (*opiates* excluding the alkaloid derivative morphia) roughly paralleled that of *opiates* of all sorts (see Figure 10), but the various individual preparations of opium were more erratically prescribed, as Figure 11 illustrates. Dover's powder, a mild compound

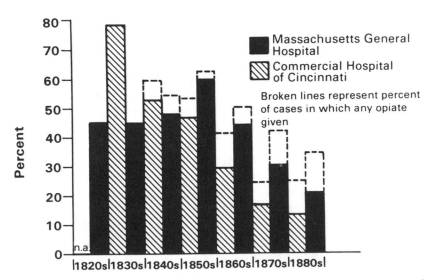

Figure 10 Percentage of cases in which any opium-containing drug was used, and percentage of cases in which any opiate (including morphia) was prescribed.

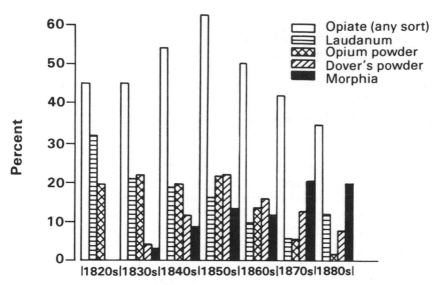

Figure 11 Massachusetts General Hospital. Percentage of cases in which selected opiates were prescribed.

of opium and ipecacuanha that first appeared in the sampled cases only in 1837, was prescribed infrequently until the mid-1840s through the 1850s, when its use grew strikingly, and thereafter diminished gradually in popularity.[81] Elevated use of Dover's powder during the 1850s was largely responsible for the rising employment of opium as a whole during this decade. Whereas physicians generally prescribed Dover's powder primarily to relieve pain and less frequently to stop diarrhea and cough and as a diaphoretic, during the late 1840s and the 1850s they also commonly gave it to promote sleep. A patient at the MGH in 1848 received the typical prescription of "Pulv Doveri 10 grs. at night, inasmuch as he says 'his nerves go all over him' "; while the prescription for another several years later read, "If no sleep by 9 PM, Rx Pulv. Doveri 8 gr."

Dover's powder may have replaced laudanum (tincture of opium) to some extent at the MGH. While the frequency with which the powder was used increased progressively from the 1820s through the 1850s, during the same period the use of laudanum declined by half. It continued to decrease through the 1860s and 1870s, reviving somewhat in the 1880s in the treatment of pain. The prescription of opium powder in other compounds remained reasonably constant from the 1820s through the 1850s, a period of greatly fluctuating laudanum and Dover's powder usages, and thereafter diminished to become very infrequent by the 1880s.

Morphia, first used in sampled MGH cases at the start of the 1830s, was prescribed for an increasingly large proportion of patients through the late 1860s, when its frequency rose sharply. About a fifth of all patients received morphia during the 1870s and 1880s. This increased use started just after morphia began to be administered by hypodermic injection rather than by mouth. In a substantial number of cases after the late 1860s, physicians actively selected morphia over the crude opium they would have used in earlier years. The frequency of opium use dropped sharply from the mid-1860s on, but that of opiates (opium or morphia) slackened only gradually. Between the 1850s and 1880s the proportion of patients who received morphia but no other opiate tripled; conversely, the proportion who received opium but no morphia diminished to a third of its earlier level.[82]

Opiates were the leading means of subduing pain at the CHC as well, but the patterns of their use there bear scant resemblance to those at the MGH. At the Cincinnati hospital there were no signs whatsoever of the heightened interest in palliation evident at the MGH in the 1840s and 1850s. Prescribed to nearly four-fifths of CHC patients in the 1830s, opium was progressively less used until by the 1880s it was given to just over a tenth of the patients (Figure 10).

Opiate use at the CHC is striking in several respects. The hospital's earliest records show that in the 1830s opium was prescribed to one-third more of the patients at the CHC than at the MGH. Opiates did not accompany the practices of heroic depletion in their signal revival in the early 1850s but continued to diminish in use during that decade. Moreover, the decline in opiate use was steadier and more rapid at the CHC than at the MGH. The failure of physicians at the CHC to increase their prescriptions of opiates in the 1840s and 1850s can in part be explained by the fact that they were already using them more frequently than were their counterparts at the MGH; nevertheless, narrative evidence and the persistently lessening reliance on opiates at the CHC make the absence of any turn to palliation comparable to that which took place at the MGH unmistakable. The gradual process of pruning opiates from practice that is evident at both hospitals was also more thorough at the CHC by the 1880s, when opiates were prescribed to a quarter of the patients there compared with a third of those at the MGH.

At the CHC as at the MGH, the popularity of various opiate compounds rose and fell on diverse schedules. There are few similarities in patterns of use between the two hospitals. Some of the differences can be attributed to dissimilar intents in prescribing a given drug at the two institutions. For example, during the 1870s and 1880s morphia decreased in use at the CHC but increased at the MGH. Prior to this period physicians at the CHC gave morphia primarily for pain but secondarily for subduing patients, a purpose not evident at the MGH. A boatman of whom the resident physician wrote "but little the matter with this fellow—worse scared than hurt" was tranquilized with morphia in 1850, and an unruly black patient was given a solution of morphia before he was finally "discharged for disorderly conduct" in 1866. By the 1870s control of rowdy CHC patients was readily effected instead by such new agents as chloral hydrate and the bromides.

The absence at the CHC of the elevated interest in palliation that occurred at the MGH in the 1840s and 1850s was consonant with the more aggressive therapeutic stance of Cincinnati physicians. Their heroic use of drugs bespoke both the desire to forcibly alter the patient's condition and the belief that doing so could break up disease. Although important, palliation was secondary to cure as a goal of therapy. Similarly, the faith in nature that encouraged physicians at the MGH to stress relief from pain was strongly denounced by many practitioners at the CHC, in part because of their peculiar social situation at mid-century.

Cincinnati practitioners' predilection to dose boldly, already illustrated by the fact that larger doses of mercurials were administered at the CHC than at the MGH, is apparent also in the doses of opium given at the two hospitals. Physicians sometimes prescribed the dosage of opiates, as they did many other remedies, in terms of effect (such as sleep or the elimination of pain) rather than amount. At the MGH Bowditch was following convention when in 1850 he directed for a patient with acute rheumatism "Pulv. Opii 1 gr ev hour until relief from pain." When dosages were specified, the mean amount of opium contained in prescriptions ordered at the CHC was consistently larger than it was in those at the MGH. Between the 1820s and 1880s the mean amount given on the first day opium was used ranged by decade between 0.9 and 1.4 grains at the MGH, whereas at the CHC it fluctuated between 2.2 and 3.2 grains from the 1830s to the 1870s, falling to 1.5 grains only in the 1880s.

As Figure 12 shows, at the MGH the mean opium dose gradually declined from the 1820s to the 1880s. The dip in the 1850s reflects the frequent use during that decade of Dover's powder, given often in modest 10 grain (containing 1 grain of opium) or smaller doses. These declining opium doses do not of course mean that patients received on the average diminishing doses of opiates, which include the powerful derivative morphia. To the extent that morphia took the place of opium-containing prescriptions, it principally replaced those containing more opium than did the dilute preparations of paregoric, laudanum, or Dover's powder. During the 1870s and 1880s these last two retained more of their popularity at the MGH than did other prescriptions containing opium. Most of the patients given opium during the 1870s and 1880s received roughly the same small dose they would have gotten in earlier decades, whereas those given morphia who in an earlier period would have gotten large doses of opium often received an ultimately more potent dose of opiate. This was especially true after the mid-1860s, when hypodermic injections of morphia came into common use.

The mean dose of opium given at the CHC did not decline progressively, as Figure 12 shows, and presents an erratic pattern compared with that for the MGH. In a general way the fact that mean amounts of opium given between the 1830s and the 1870s fluctuated within a narrow limit (2.2 to 3.2 grains of opium) does indicate that physicians tended to give opium compounds in similar doses across time. The declining mean doses of opium used from the 1860s to the 1870s and 1880s (from 3.2 grains to 1.5 grains), a diminution especially marked after the mid-1870s, reflects the increasing use of morphia for cases of severe pain in which particularly large doses of opium would have been used in earlier years.

The frequency and force with which a physician wielded highly interventionist therapies such as venesection, mercury, and opium are the most direct indices of therapeutic aggression, but not the only ones. Equally revealing is the extent to which he was prepared to tolerate

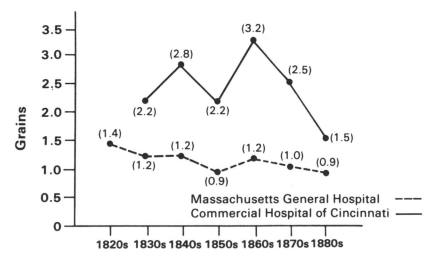

Figure 12 Mean dose of opium in any opium-containing drug(s) prescribed on the first day an opium-containing drug was ordered.

iatrogenic harm to his patients. Through the 1850s physicians at the CHC were on the whole far less sensitive than their MGH counterparts to the potential damage drugging could do. Both iatrogenic mercury poisoning and opiate addiction were reported more frequently at the MGH than at the CHC, but that does not mean that these problems were necessarily more acute in Boston than in Cincinnati. The reporting of these conditions is more telling as an index of the attention physicians paid them than of their prevalence.

Except in the treatment of syphilis, at the MGH mercury poisoning was regarded as a sometimes necessary evil rather than as a positive therapeutic good. Signs of mild mercury poisoning as a side effect of therapy included a "mercurial factor" on the breath and red, swollen, painful gums, while continued mercurial treatment could lead to ptyalism, with bleeding gums, loss of teeth, and necrosis of the mandible. The caution "if mouth gets sore stop the pills" was a common adjunct to mercurial prescriptions. Faith in the therapeutic efficacy of mercurial remedies in both hospital and domestic treatment was reflected by persistent reliance on them through the 1850s despite the danger their use entailed. Calomel made strong psychological as well as physiological impressions on patients, and many recalled its iatrogenic effects years later; thus a patient admitted to the MGH in 1878 reported to the house physician that he "took a great deal of calomel up to [the] point of salivation & loseing of teeth" when he had typhoid twenty-seven years earlier.

But while mercury was seldom given at the MGH as an alterant (to intentionally produce therapeutic mercury poisoning), its alterative use at the CHC was not rare.[83] A nonsyphilitic patient admitted in 1843, for example, was prescribed calomel "till gentle salivation." Nevertheless, a larger proportion of the patient population at the MGH was identified as displaying mercury poisoning than at the CHC. During the 1820s MGH physicians noted that nearly a quarter of the patients in the male medical wards showed signs of mercury poisoning, a proportion that declined to roughly a tenth in the next two decades and a twentieth in the 1850s. At the CHC, by contrast, mercury poisoning was reported in only about one-twentieth of the patients from the 1830s through the 1850s, with but a few instances noted in the 1860s (Figure 13).

That mercury poisoning was reported more frequently at the MGH than at the CHC is surprising, for the far greater use of calomel at the CHC would predict the opposite. In part this reflects the inclination at the CHC to give drastic single doses of mercury, since modest doses repeated over a long period of time—the usual practice at the MGH—were more likely to cause poisoning. The extensive reliance on mer-

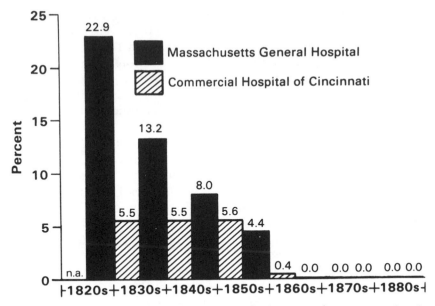

Figure 13 Percentage of case histories in which signs of mercury poisoning were recorded.

cury at the CHC suggests, however, that mercury poisoning may in fact have been more common there than at the MGH but that many instances of mild mercury poisoning were not recorded. Possibly mercury poisoning was so unremarkable at the CHC during the early years that physicians in effect did not see it. Those instances that were logged in the case record book often involved severe ptyalism and were graver than the cases of slightly sore mouth recognized as mercury poisoning by physicians at the MGH. Even if physicians at the CHC were aware that their patients' sore gums indicated mercury poisoning, such iatrogenic signs may have been expected attendants of the therapeutic experience and not strictly speaking noteworthy.

Physicians at the MGH were well aware of extensive opiate use in the population from which the hospital drew its patients. Although domestic use of opiates was not as often reported as was that of purgatives, from the hospital's earliest years many patients had been dosed with opiates by private physicians before entering the hospital. Laudanum was widely used in self-treatment, a fact attested to by the sizable number of admissions for laudanum poisoning, both accidental and intentional.

Unlike their counterparts in Cincinnati, practitioners at the MGH expressed considerable sensitivity in the case records to the problem of iatrogenic opiate addiction.[84] When a farmer was admitted with phthisis in 1840, the house physician noted that he had "been in the habit of taking opium since June, beginning with 2 or 3 grains a day & now increased to 8 or 10." Clear signs of habitual opiate use were evident beginning in the late 1830s and became more pronounced during the 1840s. Of one patient admitted in 1839 the house physician wrote, "Patient for the last 24 years has drank about 1 pt of wine daily; has also taken opium . . . Quantity of opium habitually taken, by his account, probably amounts to 5 or 9 grs daily, occasionally 10 or 12 grs." A student who had been treated previously in the MGH for neuralgia was readmitted in 1847 for the same condition, reporting that he "was obliged to resume morphine, which for a short time he had dispensed with, at first ½ gr. daily but gradually has increased to 2 gr & sometimes 4." The attending physician initially prescribed morphia and by the third day directed, "Let him have opiates at pleasure." In the CHC case records occasional instances of opiate addiction were noted, as in the case of a patient admitted in 1875 with neuralgic pains that "have been so severe lately, that he was obliged constantly to put himself under the influence of morphia & in that way has become addicted to the use of it," but addiction was mentioned only rarely.

The most sweeping movement in therapeutic practice at midcentury was the rise of support or stimulation, the mirror image of the decline of depletion. Like the ebbing of depletive therapy and increased reliance by some physicians on palliation, the turn to stimulation did not follow a uniform course in all contexts. It was clearly evident at the MGH from the outset of the 1850s, years marked at the CHC by the final celebration of heroic depletion. Because the case records of the CHC are lost for the second half of the 1850s and sparse for the early 1860s, it is not possible to locate precisely when that institution's therapeutic balance was tipped from depletion to stimulation. Signs of an inclination toward supportive therapeutics did appear at the CHC in the 1860s, but stimulating practice was never used there as extensively as it was at the MGH. Thus while the move to therapeutic stimulation became evident at both hospitals, the fact that it followed different paths and timetables in them again underscores the variability of therapeutic behavior.

The turn to stimulation in bedside practice must be discerned in the changing usage patterns of individual supportive therapies. Shattuck at the MGH employed all the leading treatments of therapeutic stimulation save quinine when in 1852 he prescribed beef tea, wine,

brandy, iron, cod liver oil, and tincture of cinchona for a patient with
typhoid fever. Just as the practices linked with depletion did not decline
as a unified block, the therapies placed in aid of stimulation were not
monolithic in their rise. Nor were treatments conventionally identified
with depletion and those connected with stimulation mutually exclusive. Bigelow demonstrated this when in 1853 he prescribed for a patient with pneumonia wine, cod liver oil, an iron compound, and opium
together with podophyllum, calomel, and tartar emetic.

Alcohol most vividly embodied the ethos of heroic stimulation
at the MGH. Figure 14 illustrates its use and that of several other
stimulants. Physicians employed alcohol as a supportive treatment
from the time the hospital opened, and few drugs maintained such
continued therapeutic popularity from the 1820s through the 1880s.
It increased markedly in use in the early 1850s, being given to two-
fifths of the patients, and then diminished somewhat in popularity,
but was still prescribed to about one-quarter of the hospital's male
medical inmates through the 1880s.

The sustained elevation of the frequency of alcohol use in the
1850s through the 1880s as compared with its prescription in the 1820s
through the 1840s is impressive. The underlying change in the ways
alcohol was employed is more striking still. Before midcentury it was
mostly given in the form of wine whey, a custardlike milk mixture
with a very low alcohol content that was a supportive nutrient but not
a stimulant.[85] In the early 1850s, however, physicians began to pre-

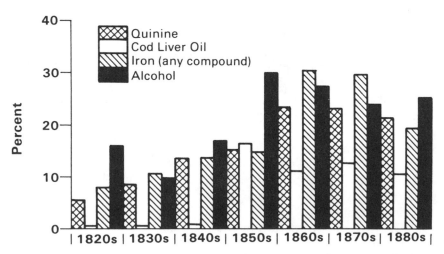

Figure 14 Massachusetts General Hospital. Percentage of cases in which selected supportive and stimulant therapies were prescribed.

scribe straight whiskey, wine, or brandy—administered in large and sometimes frequently repeated doses—explicitly as stimulants. In the 1850s and 1860s it was not unusual for a patient with pneumonia or typhoid fever to be given between 8 and 12 ounces of spirits a day and for this treatment to be continued for several days. Thus alcohol used to stimulate took up a central therapeutic role that it maintained through the 1880s.

Cod liver oil, which came into extensive use at the MGH concurrently with alcohol, had been growing in popularity as a restorative treatment since the 1840s. It was given to nearly one-fifth of the patients admitted during the 1850s and to more than a tenth of those treated from the 1860s through the 1880s. An ambitious advertising campaign for cod liver oil in the Boston medical literature accompanied its increasing use at the MGH. Patients also began to report taking it domestically before entering the hospital, as in the case of a phthisical patient admitted in 1868 who "had been using Ol[eum] Morrh[oae] [cod liver oil] freely—drinking it undiluted from the bottle without measuring the quantity." Although particularly favored in the treatment of phthisis, cod liver oil was also commonly used to strengthen the body debilitated by pneumonia and typhoid fever.

The burgeoning use of iron compounds at the MGH beginning in the early 1860s represents one facet of the same general movement toward stimulating treatment that had increased the use of alcohol and cod liver oil a decade earlier. Iron compounds were prescribed explicitly as strengthening agents for nearly a third of all patients during the 1860s and 1870s. The employment of iron to treat anemia in the narrow sense of the term reflected its broader invigorating use, but comprised only a small part of it.

Quinine use followed a somewhat similar course at the MGH, rising from the 1820s through the 1850s and becoming far more common in the early 1860s. In that decade and the next the drug was given to nearly a quarter of the patients, and the proportion dropped only slightly during the 1880s. The use of cinchona bark, the crude source of quinine that shared its dual role as a tonic and an antiperiodic, does not account for this changing pattern, but experimentation starting in 1879 with cinchonidia sulphate as a substitute for quinine more than accounts for the small drop in the eighties in the frequency of quinine prescriptions.

The shift from depletion to stimulation at the MGH is further exemplified by the changing therapeutic manipulation of diet. Attending physicians often gave dietary directions along with their other prescriptions from the hospital's opening. Like drug therapies early in the century, the diets prescribed at the hospital in the 1820s and 1830s were at times explicitly low or debilitating, with physicians directing "abstemious diet" or "antiphlogistic regimen" for roughly one-fifth of the patients and rarely prescribing high or supportive diets. But as Figure 15 shows, this situation was reversed after the 1840s: while low diet was prescribed infrequently, high diet became more common, peaking in the 1860s when it was directed in over one-fifth of the cases. A supportive diet, like the drugs alcohol, cod liver oil, quinine, and iron, was part of a restorative therapeutic regimen.

The high cost of stimulant therapies was an important restraint on their use in nineteenth-century hospitals. Beginning in the middle of the 1850s, the decade in which beverage alcohol's popularity rose so sharply at the MGH, the superintendent began to complain in his annual reports that hospital expenses were exceeding receipts. He targeted the therapeutic use of alcohol as one cause of this situation. A new system of carefully monitoring prescriptions of liquors and diet was introduced, and expenditures for wine and spirits were itemized separately in the reports. The proportion of the medical budget used to purchase alcohol decreased during the next few years but was again rising by the mid-1860s. In 1866, for example, nearly half of the budget for drugs was spent on alcohol, testifying to the physicians' high valuation of this therapy. The MGH trustees routinely urged therapeutic

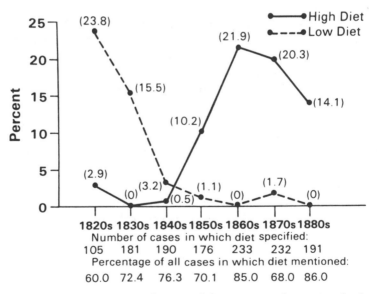

Figure 15 Massachusetts General Hospital. Percentage of cases in which either elevating or lowering diet was prescribed.

temperance in the interest of economy, but the relative affluence of the institution and the social prominence of the staff probably aided physicians in resisting such pressure.[86]

The expense of stimulant therapies may have been one reason that when the turn to stimulation evident at the MGH in the 1850s did finally occur at the CHC in the 1860s it was more reserved. Alcohol prescriptions exhibited no increase in frequency whatsoever in the CHC wards at midcentury. Alcohol use at the CHC did rise from the 1830s to the 1840s, as it did at the MGH, but its frequency (about 14 percent) was uniform from the 1840s through the 1860s. During the same period alcohol was given to roughly twice that proportion of patients at the MGH.

It is likely that when CHC physicians did begin to favor stimulating therapy, the guardians of that institution, a poorer and larger one than the MGH, more successfully dampened the inclination to prescribe alcohol than did their Boston counterparts. In 1867, at a time when by one estimate the MGH spent over half again the amount of money the CHC spent per patient per week, the medical staff of the CHC responded to the board of trustees' "expressed dissatisfaction with the expenses of the Hospital" by offering to keep a register of all dietary prescriptions, including alcohol. "In a special column all stimulants, and the quantity ordered daily for each patient will be noted, as well as the quantity and quality of special articles of diet," the staff proposed. One month later the trustees again moved "to request the Medical Staff to economize the use of brandies and wines." Feeling falsely accused but nonetheless accountable, the staff set up a committee "to make such investigations of the expenditures, and general conduct of the House, as may be necessary to exonerate the staff from the charges of extravagance." Avoidance of such censure and interference was an incentive not to prescribe alcohol when a cheaper therapy would do, and similar economic pressure surely inhibited expensive prescriptions of quinine and invigorating diet. Yet while physicians at the CHC may have been more vulnerable than those at the MGH to economic coercion, the fact that in the late 1860s as much as two-fifths of the CHC's annual budget for drugs was spent on beverage alcohol is one significant indication that physicians there too had come to rely heavily on therapeutic stimulation.[87]

The mean dose of absolute ethanol used at the two hospitals offers another index of the shift to stimulation. Figure 16 does not reflect the increased dosage from the 1840s and 1850s at the MGH that narrative evidence suggests but does indicate that the general trend over time was toward prescribing alcohol in more and more forceful doses. Two problems make mean dose a doubtfully trustworthy mirror of practice in this instance. First, the absolute ethanol content of wine whey is not readily determinable and so has been treated as a missing value; accordingly the larger doses of alcohol occasionally given to moribund patients are greatly overrepresented in the figures prior to the 1850s. Second, alcohol used to stimulate was at times prescribed by effect rather than amount. Large amounts of alcohol often were administered in executing such directions, but unless the house physician happened to record the amount given it remains unknown, thereby reducing the calculated mean from the 1850s onward.

Dosage information indicates an increasingly aggressive use of alcohol at the CHC in the 1850s and 1860s that is not discernible in frequencies of prescription. As Figure 16 shows, the mean dose increased steadily from the 1830s to the 1860s, when it peaked at 3.8 ounces of absolute ethanol, roughly equivalent to a daily dose of 7 ounces of brandy or whiskey. This spirited prescribing reflects both a shift from wine and ale to the more potent brandy and whiskey and the use of alcohol to stimulate patients rather than merely to sustain them. Even more striking is the fact that the dosage level at the CHC was consistently higher than it was at the MGH (in the 1860s almost three times as large), although by the 1880s the mean doses had converged. As in the instances of calomel use before the 1860s and opium use through the 1880s, the relatively large doses of alcohol given at the CHC suggest that when a physician at that hospital gave a drug he tended to do so more aggressively than his MGH counterparts.

Like alcohol, strengthening treatment with cod liver oil, iron, and diet was prescribed far more frequently at the MGH than at the CHC. Cod liver oil's use at the CHC increased slightly in the 1850s, but it was still given five times as often at the MGH. A portion of this discrepancy might be ascribed to the greater incidence at the MGH of phthisis. Nevertheless, nothing in the use of cod liver oil at the CHC suggests more than a gradual, never extensive rise in supportive treatment. Iron compounds give sounder evidence of a vogue for invigorating therapy in the 1860s, when the proportion of cases in which they were prescribed rose to more than thrice that of the preceding decade. Yet while iron compounds were given to nearly a third of the patients at the MGH in the 1860s, at the CHC the proportion was only half that. Physicians at the Cincinnati hospital never gave as much attention to dietary prescriptions as did their MGH counterparts. The infrequency of dietary specifications at the CHC renders them unfit for meaningful quantification, but some signs of a shift away from a lowering diet are evident. The attending physicians directed for a patient in 1837, "Put him on an Antiphlogistic regimen," for example, and in 1846 specified a "Low Diet" for another patient; by the mid-1860s,

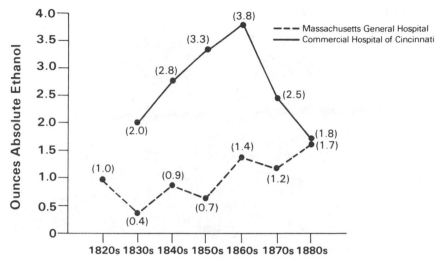

Figure 16 Mean dose of beverage alcohol prescribed on the first day beverage alcohol was ordered.

however, when diet was specified it was more likely to be a supportive one.

The epidemiological realities of the environment in which patients were treated sometimes altered the reasons a particular drug was prescribed. Differential disease prevalence at the CHC and MGH made perhaps the greatest mark on the use of quinine. In themselves the relative frequencies of quinine use at the two hospitals say little about why the drug was prescribed. Quinine was regarded not just as an antiperiodic, suited to the malarial fevers common in the vicinity of Cincinnati, but also as a stimulant and an antipyretic. In fact its rising use in the 1860s is the strongest evidence for a turn to stimulation at the CHC, but this is not self-evident from frequencies of use alone.

The pattern of quinine use at the CHC, shown in Figure 17, was quite dissimilar to that at the MGH. From the 1830s through the 1850s quinine was prescribed far more frequently at the former hospital; but while the frequency of its use there fluctuated upward and downward within a confined range, at the MGH it increased progressively from the 1820s to the 1850s (Figure 14), rising so sharply in the 1860s that by the 1870s it was given to about one-quarter of the patients at both hospitals. In the 1880s quinine's use at the CHC fell off so precipitously that it was actually more frequent in the Boston hospital.

At the MGH quinine was principally given as a stimulant, not an antiperiodic. The majority of the patients treated there with quinine

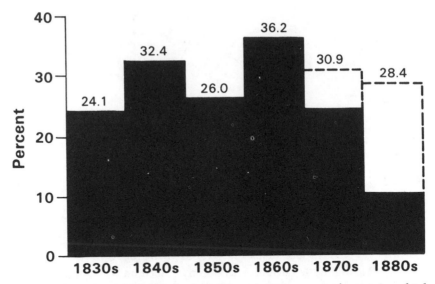

Figure 17 Commercial Hospital of Cincinnati. Percentage of cases in which quinine was prescribed (area bounded by solid line), and in which cinchonidia sulphate was prescribed (marked by broken line). The number surmounting the bar for each decade represents the percentage of cases in which quinine and/or cinchonidia sulphate was prescribed.

exhibited no evidence of intermittent fever, no malarial signs or symptoms of any sort. During the 1860s and 1870s nearly a quarter of MGH patients received quinine, though evidence of malaria was noted in only a small percentage of them.

The purpose of quinine's use was much more ambiguous at the CHC. Malaria, as Table 3 shows, was roughly ten times more frequent among CHC patients than among those at the MGH (except in the 1880s). This in itself would more than account for the greater quinine use at the CHC, but the situation was more complex. Quinine prescriptions were by no means ten times as frequent at the CHC as at the MGH, yet before the 1870s a patient at the Cincinnati hospital who exhibited no malarial signs whatsoever was more likely to receive quinine than his Boston counterpart (Table 4). And while a drop in the proportion of malarial patients at the CHC in part explains the fall in quinine use there in the 1880s, malarial incidence does not account for such other phenomena as the rise in quinine use in the 1860s. The prevalence of periodic fevers at the CHC suggests one explanation for the frequent resort to quinine there but cannot account for the changing patterns of its use.

Table 3 Percentage of cases in which malarial signs and/or symptoms were present, Massachusetts General Hospital and Commercial Hospital of Cincinnati.

Decade	Percentage of cases	
	MGH	CHC
1820s	3.4	n.a.
1830s	2.8	36.7
1840s	2.8	31.3
1850s	2.8	21.4
1860s	2.9	24.7
1870s	2.4	25.7
1880s	4.1	11.9

Table 4 Percentage of malarial and nonmalarial cases in which quinine was prescribed, Massachusetts General Hospital and Commercial Hospital of Cincinnati.

Percentage of cases in which quinine was prescribed

Decade	Malarial		Nonmalarial	
	MGH	CHC	MGH	CHC
1820s	50.0	n.a.	4.2	n.a.
1830s	85.7	42.3	6.3	16.0
1840s	71.4	66.9	12.2	16.7
1850s	100.0	68.5	12.7	14.5
1860s	87.5	80.0	21.7	21.9
1870s	100.0	55.0	21.5	13.7
1880s	100.0	15.4	17.9	9.4

The relatively small proportion of patients at the CHC given quinine in the 1880s is especially striking. A scant 15.4 percent of the malarial patients admitted to the hospital in that decade received it; as Table 4 indicates, the smallest frequency for any other decade was a much more substantial 42.3 percent. These figures are deceptive, however, for they do not reflect the use of other cinchona bark derivatives such as quinquinia, cinchonidia sulphate, and chinii sulphate. These drugs purportedly shared quinine's antiperiodic and tonic properties and especially from the 1870s onward were prescribed as cheaper substitutes for it. Cinchonidia sulphate was the most extensively used.[88] From the time it was first widely employed at the CHC in 1877 until the extant medical case records end in 1881, cinchonidia sulphate was prescribed for a fifth of the men admitted to the medical wards.[89] When Figure 17 is redrawn to display not only quinine use but also that of cinchonidia sulphate (excluding from the calculations of cinchonidia sulphate frequency those very few cases in which quinine was given along with it), it becomes clear that the use of cinchona bark derivatives at the CHC did not plummet after the 1860s as the changed prescription patterns of quinine alone would suggest.

Quinine use was less tightly linked to malaria at the MGH than at the CHC. Except in the 1830s, when there were very few malarial cases at the MGH and little quinine was used, and the 1880s, when cinchonidia sulphate had largely supplanted quinine at the CHC, the correlation between quinine use and malarial signs was a good deal stronger at the CHC than at the MGH, as Table 5 indicates. The majority of cases in which quinine was prescribed were nonmalarial at the MGH but malarial at the CHC.[90]

The exceptions to this general pattern are particularly intriguing. As Table 4 shows, a patient exhibiting malarial signs was far more likely to receive quinine at the MGH than at the CHC, reflecting perhaps the more anomalous, therapeutically distinctive character of a patient with periodic fever in Boston. And at the CHC the use of quinine as a stimulant, while not its primary application, was nonetheless important. Prior to the 1870s, when widespread cinchonidia sulphate use at the CHC reversed the pattern, in nonmalarious cases

Table 5 Correlation of quinine prescriptions with malarial signs, Massachusetts General Hospital and Commercial Hospital of Cincinnati.[a]

| Decade | Correlation | |
	MGH	CHC
1820s	0.48	n.a.
1830s	0.61	0.41
1840s	0.39	0.63
1850s	0.53	0.64
1860s	0.36	0.65
1870s	0.39	0.55
1880s	0.52	0.09

a. This table was constructed using Pearson's contingency coefficient C. The values have been divided by 0.707 so that a perfect correlation equals 1.0.

quinine was consistently given more frequently at the CHC than at the MGH. This suggests that the validation of its therapeutic efficacy that CHC physicians so often witnessed in treating malarious diseases may have encouraged them to generalize its use to other conditions. Yet the simple fact that they used quinine *less* regularly than did physicians at the MGH in treating patients who *did* exhibit malarial symptoms tends to refute the common notion that the prevalence of malaria in the West and the efficacy of quinine combined to cause its prescription there by rote.

What is most arresting is that the use of quinine in nonmalarial cases peaked at both hospitals in the 1860s, and at nearly identical levels. During that decade about one-fifth of the patients at both hospitals were given quinine solely for its tonic virtues.[91] That this period saw the zenith of such quinine use is evidence of the ascendancy of faith in stimulative treatment in Cincinnati as well as in Boston. This elevated quinine use marked a more dramatic departure from earlier practice at the MGH than at the CHC, however, reconfirming that besides occurring sooner at the MGH, the shift to stimulation there was also more pronounced.

When physicians at the CHC gave quinine, they tended to prescribe larger doses than did those at the MGH. This mirrored the pattern of more aggressive dosing at the Cincinnati hospital already displayed by the larger doses of calomel, opium, and alcohol administered there. But it also reflected the greater use at the CHC of quinine as an antiperiodic. The shift to larger doses of quinine for malaria in the 1840s is plainly evident in the rise of the mean dose to 16.9 grains, up from 11.1 grains in the preceding decade. Except in the 1830s, the mean dose of quinine remained relatively constant through the 1880s, varying between 15.8 and 17.5 grains.[92] Whenever during this period CHC physicians prescribed quinine, they tended to specify roughly the same dosage level. Although increasingly active use of quinine as a stimulant at the MGH was marked by mean doses that progressively increased from 4.6 grains in the 1840s to 12.2 grains in the 1880s, these doses remained substantially smaller than their CHC analogs.[93]

Arresting as the overall change in drug use at the two hospitals between the 1820s and 1880s is, the restructuring of clinical cognition evident in their records offers a sign of the transformation of medical therapeutics that in some ways is even more compelling. Especially after the mid-1860s a movement toward an increasingly reductionist perspective on patients is apparent. The array of parameters by which physicians logged their patients' conditions, a reliable mirror of what they thought it was important to know in order to understand disease and navigate an appropriate therapeutic course, illustrates the inclination to clinical reductionism. Case records became much shorter as physicians gave less attention to the individuating factors of social background and physiological idiosyncrasy that characterized a particular patient's natural state of health. At the same time, practitioners relied more and more on instrumental and chemical analyses to describe a patient's condition, while quantified signs and symptoms became the accepted means of gauging deviation from normality.

Changes in their approach to patient management accompanied clinicians' readjustment of their perspective. The focus at the MGH and the CHC, perceptible in case histories, was increasingly directed toward monitoring each patient's course while therapeutically manipulating only one or two specific deviant characteristics. The patient's overall physiological level was not ignored, as the persistent popularity of supportive therapies shows, but instead of using a large number of treatments to restore the natural state of the system as a whole physicians tended to prescribe a few powerful remedies narrowly targeted to effect specific physiological modifications.

Pulse and respiration rates were virtually the only patient characteristics other than age and duration of illness before entry that were frequently quantified prior to the mid-1860s. Recording a quantified pulse rate was a nearly routine part of keeping a case history at the MGH from the time the hospital opened.[94] The medical case histories of the CHC generally reflect less attention to monitoring the varying condition of patients; thus in the 1830s quantified pulse rate appeared in only a little more than a tenth of the case histories at the CHC, compared with over nine-tenths at the MGH. This disparity lessened beginning in the 1860s, when pulse rate was given for nearly three-fourths of the CHC patients. At both hospitals the frequency of recorded pulse rate declined somewhat in the 1870s, perhaps due in part to the concurrent rise in quantification of other patient signs. These new measurements in effect gave physicians other outlets for the impulse to reduce patient characteristics to numbers, and they may have encouraged them to question the worth of listing a quantified pulse rate when the notation "Pulse normal" would suffice.

Quantified respiration rate was similarly accessible but was never accorded the diagnostic or therapeutic importance attached to pulse rate. It was recorded occasionally by MGH physicians from the 1820s onward but not by their CHC counterparts until the 1840s, and always was more common at the Boston hospital.[95] Reflecting the preoccupation with quantification at both institutions by the 1880s, the frequency of logging respiration rates rose sharply in that decade, appearing in two-fifths of the case histories at the CHC and twice that proportion at the MGH.

Temperature was described almost exclusively in qualitative terms prior to the mid-1860s.[96] Thermometers were first employed in the MGH in the 1820s, but recorded the temperatures of patients' baths and surroundings rather than of patients themselves. In 1828 one of these thermometers was used to record a patient's temperature, for the house physician noted of a patient, "by thermom[eter] tempe[rature] of hands 70° room 60°," but this was an uncommon event. Only after Carl Wunderlich's work had brought medical thermometry into clinical fashion in Europe were quantified temperatures recorded for MGH patients with any regularity. From being entirely absent prior to 1865, quantified temperature came to be included in one-fifth of case histories during the second half of the 1860s, two-fifths in the 1870s, and four-fifths in the 1880s. Clinical thermometry at the CHC followed much the same pattern, though its frequencies were lower.

The graphical representation of pulse and respiration rates and of temperature depicted even more vividly physicians' desire to express patient signs in terms of measurable deviations from the normal. The first temperature graphs at the MGH were included in case records in 1867 and consisted of grids drawn by hand onto the same pages as the narrative history. Pulse rate graphs appeared by 1870, and graphical representation of respiration rates, never common, appeared only in the 1880s. By 1870 hand-drawn grids had been replaced by printed forms pasted into the record books; these forms further included anatomical diagrams that permitted visual localization of disorders detected in auscultation and percussion. A "normal temperature line" at 98.6° was printed on the forms, facilitating the physician's assessment of abnormality by glancing at the clinical chart.

At the CHC a temperature graph was drawn into a case record from the female wards as early as 1866, but that effort was curtailed after seven days when the house physician marked in the case book, "Broke thermometer." Graph keeping was not continuously practiced. In the female medical wards a number of temperature graphs appeared in 1867, then vanished, not to reappear until 1876. Pulse and respiration rate graphs never became common at the CHC, although physicians ordinarily wrote morning and evening measurements of pulse and respiration rates onto the bottoms of the temperature graphs. Graphical representation of clinical signs on the whole remained much less common than at the MGH. During the 1870s, when pulse rate and/or temperature graphs were included in 7.6 percent of the case histories at the Boston hospital, the corresponding frequency in Cincinnati was only 0.9 percent; in the 1880s, these figures were 43.7 percent and 8.3 percent respectively.

Instruments became increasingly common mediators between physician and patient. The stethoscope and the timepiece had, of course, been used since the hospitals' records began. Microscopic examinations of urine appeared for a few patients with diseases such as diabetes in the MGH case records in the mid-1840s, became common by the start of the 1850s, and were almost routine by the early 1870s. The microscope was only infrequently used to examine blood samples.[97] Clinical use of the microscope at the CHC did not begin until the early 1850s and was never as common as at the MGH. In the late 1860s physicians at both institutions began to employ the laryngoscope, ophthalmoscope, and aesthesiometer (which tested sensation) in diagnosis. Sphygmographic tracings began to appear in MGH case histories at the start of the 1870s and became ordinary by the end of the decade; by contrast, tracings were vanishingly rare at the CHC, although at least one was pasted into the record book in 1878. Very infrequently, such tracings at the MGH were placed in the service of therapeutic evaluation, as in the parallel presentation of sphygmographic tracings one hour before and one hour after nitroglycerine was given to a patient in 1881.

Physicians were keenly self-conscious when they used a new instrument in the wards, and the case records often reveal a preoccupation with the tools themselves. When the thermometer was first used to measure patients' temperatures at the MGH, for example, qualitative descriptions of bodily heat were indicated by the term "temperature" whereas their quantified analogues were referred to by the term "thermometer." Thus in 1865 and 1866 entries such as "Evg Thermometer 102 P[ulse] 112 R[espiration] 24" or "Ther[mometer] 98°" often appeared, but by the following year the quantified measurements that the no-longer-novel instrument gave were called "temperature."

Chemical analysis of patient signs during this period was confined almost exclusively to that of urine. In the mid-1840s physicians at the MGH began to request occasional urinalyses, and a separate post of hospital chemist and microscopist was established. Later in that decade urinalysis became common, and by the start of the 1850s it was nearly routine and was no longer performed only for those patients suspected of having Bright's disease, diabetes, or uremia. A urinalysis report consisted, in addition to the results of microscopical examinations, of the measurements of the urinometer, which determined specific gravity, and a quantified inventory of the urine's components or the comment that the levels of various compounds were normal (almost never "natural"). By the 1880s these reports were submitted on standardized forms pasted into the case books. At the CHC urinalysis was reported in some case histories beginning in the mid-1850s but became common only in the 1860s and 1870s. Like instrumental measurements and quantification of patient signs, chemical analyses were not used as frequently at the CHC as at the MGH, perhaps in part a consequence of the larger patient population.

One therapeutic correlate of the reduction of patient signs to measurable deviations from the norm was a more narrowly focused effort to normalize specific, often quantified processes or conditions. The growing preoccupation with antipyresis that accompanied clinical thermometry's ascendancy exemplified the association between clinical analysis and therapeutic orientation. Quinine, for example, was occasionally used as an antipyretic in nonperiodic diseases at the CHC as early as 1874. Marked on a temperature graph drawn into a case entered in that year was the label, "Temp before Administration of Quinia." In the case history of a patient admitted in the following year was recorded the comment, "On the 9th T[emperature] was 102—but under the Quinia has come down to normal." At the MGH quinine was used explicitly as an antipyretic in the early 1880s. A patient admitted with typhoid fever in 1880 was prescribed 40 grains of quinine, given in 10 grain doses every fifteen minutes to reduce his temperature. On the following morning the house physician noted, "Temperature fell after the exhibition of the quinine from 103.8° to 96°. (Vide temperature chart.)" The curve of the patient's temperature graph, falling dramatically after the quinine was administered, verified the drug's antipyretic effect.

In the late 1870s and the 1880s the inscription of antipyretic treatments onto temperature graphs became relatively common at the CHC. In addition to quinine, salicylic acid, salicylate of soda, cinchonidia sulphate, and quinquinia were also used to lower temperature. At the MGH both salicylic acid and alcohol were tried as antipyretics, but the most widely employed method of lowering temperature there was the cold sponge bath. This treatment was used especially in typhoid fever and constituted a central element of the therapeutic regimen for it. Antipyrine was not used in the wards until 1885.

The extensive use of newer therapies like chloral hydrate, the bromides, salicylate, and hypodermic injections of morphia during the 1870s and 1880s reflects physicians' search for agents that would give them specific control over certain aspects of their patients' condition. The bromides (usually potassium bromide) were first used in the cases sampled from the MGH in 1864 and from the CHC in the following year, and were prescribed to about one-tenth of the patients admitted during the remainder of the 1860s, maintaining their popularity in the next two decades. Chloral hydrate first appeared in the sampled cases from both hospitals in 1870 and was administered to about a tenth of the patients during the 1870s and 1880s. The principal therapeutic purpose of these drugs, both aggressively active agents, was to produce sleep. When bromide or chloral hydrate was given it was often the only drug prescribed, though both were at times given in conjunction with morphia.

The exercise of control sometimes extended beyond the narrow objectives of palliation and cure to creating a healing environment in the wards. When a patient with typhoid fever was admitted to the CHC in 1885, the house physician commented that he "exposes himself so indecently that nurse is obliged to keep a screen around him . . . Will not take food at night. Seems to act badly from pure cussedness. Had a talk with him & he promised to behave better." However, the following morning the case record stated that the patient "was so troublesome last night that give him c[um] desired effect" 30 grains of potassium bromide, with the added note, "Was quiet rest of night."

Salicylic acid first appeared in the sampled cases at the MGH in 1875 and at the CHC in the following year. The salicylates (salicylic acid and salicylate of soda) quickly became established and were given to nearly one-fifth of the patients at the MGH by the 1880s and half that proportion at the CHC. Physicians prescribed salicylate especially for acute rheumatism, using the compound for its analgesic and associated anti-inflammatory effects.[98] The failure of salicylate to adequately relieve pain at times led physicians to turn to other analgesics such as morphia, Dover's powder, or leeches, but their more usual persistence in using salicylate indicated that their expectations of the drug were largely fulfilled. A patient with rheumatism admitted to the MGH in 1884 was given a dose of salicylate of soda on the day he entered the wards, and the next morning the house physician could record, "Felt better from first dose, took 90 grs yesterday, 70 during the n[igh]t, and 10 grs every hour today until 9 o'clock when his ears began to ring . . . Swelling and pain all disappeared." During the late 1870s and 1880s case histories of acute rheumatism became essentially chronicles of changing salicylate dosages. Reflecting the narrowing therapeutic focus, clinicians showed scant interest in symptoms other than pain or in treatments other than salicylate, but meticulously tracked the shifting courses of these two factors.

The change in attitude that underlay these specific alterations in clinical observation and drug use was manifest in the physical appearance of the clinical records. In many case histories the majority of daily entries consisted almost exclusively of temperatures and pulse rates, and along with respiration rates and urinalysis reports these stood out as the most striking features of case records by the 1880s. Records became progressively shorter as much of the narrative description that in earlier decades had sought to characterize the patient's destabilization from a natural condition was dropped. Case records were more uniform but less discursive, contained fewer words but more numbers, were more concise but less evocative of sick individuals.

From a therapeutic perspective, the most noticeable change in the case history was the diminished prominence of prescriptions. As physicians devoted more attention from the 1860s onward to chemically analyzing, instrumentally measuring, and quantifying patient signs, the emphasis they placed on treatment in the case records diminished. Although the mean length of stay for male medical patients did not change much over time, the mean number of different treatments prescribed declined at both hospitals (Tables 1 and 2). Whereas at the MGH the mean number of treatments given per patient from the 1820s to the 1860s fluctuated by decade between 7.4 and 8.7, it dropped in the 1870s to 6.5 and in the 1880s to 5.2. The mean number of treatments given to patients at the CHC, always lower than at the MGH, was reasonably constant from the 1830s through the 1850s and thereafter steadily fell from 5.9 in the 1850s to only 2.5 by the 1880s.

The attention physicians gave to therapeutic manipulation also diminished. The mean number of times the course of treatment was changed during the first five days of a patient's stay declined at both hospitals (Tables 1 and 2). While the mean number of prescription changes at the CHC rose from 2.1 in the 1830s and 1840s to 2.7 in the 1850s, thereafter it progressively declined, reaching a nadir of 1.3 in the 1880s. The decrease in the mean number of changes at the MGH, from 3.5 in the 1820s to 2.7 by the 1880s, was more gradual but nonetheless clear. A steadier and more parsimonious therapeutic strategy characterized postbellum practice at both hospitals. To some extent clinical vigilance, embodied in the quantified monitoring of a patient's progress, was substituted for the more active emphasis on therapeutic intervention that had characterized the earlier decades of the nineteenth century.

Reflecting the diversity of regular medical activity outside hospital walls, the changing courses of therapeutic practice at the MGH and the CHC display marked differences. The broad movements in therapeutics between the 1820s and 1880s, such as the shift from depletion to stimulation and from cure and drugging to palliation and monitoring, were visible at both hospitals, but often they were expressed in different ways. The rise in the use of heroic depletive therapies at the CHC in the early 1850s contrasted with their continued diminution at the MGH is in itself sufficient to establish that the paths and timetables these movements followed were far from uniform. The growing emphasis on palliation encouraged by a reliance on nature, so evident at the MGH from the 1840s and 1850s on, appeared only later at the CHC. While a movement to supportive and stimulative treatment occurred at both hospitals, it was later and feebler at the CHC than at the MGH. Furthermore, before the 1860s depletive therapy at the CHC was far more aggressive than was that at the MGH. Relative frequencies of use and dosages of particular drugs point to this difference in aggression, while narrative case histories suggest that underlying it was a greater faith at the CHC in the physician's ability to actively break up disease by therapeutic intervention, a stronger orientation to cure than to care.

These differences establish that in the two hospitals, as in American medical practice more broadly, therapeutic activity and change in it were not uniform. Yet in some ways the shared features of therapeutics at the MGH and the CHC are even more revealing than their divergences. All of the sweeping general movements in medical therapeutics between the 1820s and the 1880s were expressed at both hospitals, notwithstanding important discrepancies in their timing and intensity. And at any given moment physicians in both institutions called upon roughly the same armamentarium. These characteristics sustain the legitimacy of making some generalizations about therapeutic change.

Certainly it can be said that by and large change took place at both institutions in very similar ways. Experiences at the two hospitals demonstrate that groups of therapies denoted by such terms as "heroic depletants" and "heroic stimulants" were not monolithic. Use of their various elements often changed independently—venesection declining substantially in use well before calomel, for example, or alcohol use rising before the stimulants iron and quinine became prominent. Therapeutic continuity is also impressive: once established, medical therapies showed remarkable tenacity. Apparent too is the gradualness of most changes. To be sure, the frequency with which physicians used specific drugs fluctuated upward and downward, and a new remedy might gain rapid acceptance, but established practices were not abruptly abandoned.

The fundamental orientation of the therapeutic enterprise also followed very similar tacks at the MGH and the CHC. Before midcentury physicians at the two hospitals sought to restore the patient's system to a natural balance. If they nudged at the MGH, at the CHC they tended to shove, but the end point they envisaged was the same. By the 1880s practitioners at both institutions instead directed much of their attention to restoring fixed, often quantified signs of well-being to normal standards.

One further important pattern transcends the specific similarities and differences in therapeutic change of these institutions. Over time, practice at the two hospitals converged. The therapeutics of the CHC and that of the MGH resembled each other far more closely in the 1880s than they had in the 1830s. At both institutions the management of patients became more standardized—in the strict sense of the word, more normalized—over time. Although there was some evidence of this trend before the mid-1860s, especially in the gradual shedding of all types of heroic therapeutic extremism, it became most pronounced in the 1870s and 1880s. This is apparent not only in the use of individual therapeutic practices but also in the way physicians looked at and described their patients. The disparity between the amount of patient information recorded at the MGH and at the CHC in the 1830s narrowed and by the 1880s had all but vanished, and this change was not just the result of changes in the conscientiousness of the two staffs. Extensive description of the individual patient's history and condition fell away as physicians at both hospitals came to place their principal emphasis on fixed criteria of normalcy, often represented by standardized measurements and frequently filled into standardized forms in the case history books. This convergence in therapeutic practice and vision reflected a broader shift from individualization in medical therapeutics to universalism, a universalism that in the 1870s and 1880s began to be associated with and in part define a new therapeutic epistemology and a new ideology of professional identity.

— 5 —

Attitudes toward Change

BECAUSE THERAPEUTICS was so central to both the professional identity and the daily tasks of nineteenth-century American physicians, the process by which it changed was inevitably complex and disturbing to them. Looking hard at the way they regarded change and at the place and meaning it held in their values and institutions helps make sense of that process. One key to understanding their attitudes toward change is to recognize how the structure of medical theory minimized the disruptiveness of permutations in therapeutic practice, a disruptiveness that the profession's institutions further mollified. Another is to see that most of the factors that molded the individual practitioner's decision on whether or not to bring change into his practice exerted dual actions. He derived incentives for both stability and innovation from sources of medical instruction such as schools, apprenticeship, textbooks, and societies and from the socioeconomic context of practice that sectarianism so strongly shaped. Such factors as medical sectary and the institutions of medical education did not unidirectionally encourage either stasis or change in therapeutics but rather exercised both conservative and progressive influences.

Medical tradition was a leading source of professional pride. The communal rituals at which physicians periodically reminded each other of the nature of their calling, such as orations presented at medical commencements and presidential addresses at society meetings, conventionally began by recounting the distinction and responsibility a noble heritage conferred. In facing the trials of medical practice, physicians could take solace in the knowledge that they were participating in a tradition of ideas and behavior handed down for many centuries. Filiopietism pervaded professional rhetoric. The frequency with which

American physicians' sons born in the late eighteenth and early nine-teenth centuries received the given name Benjamin Rush is one re-flection of a self-conscious attempt to perpetuate professional tradition.

Veneration of tradition served a more fundamental purpose than the inflation of the medical ego. Its crucial importance for professional identity is illustrated by the function of medical history in nineteenth-century America. Put simply, medical history and the values it dis-played validated the regular profession's regularity. History placed phy-sicians in a continuing lineage and affirmed the links with the past that gave them legitimacy. Orthodox physicians who wrote medical history used tradition as a professional tool to set themselves apart from the variety of alternative practitioners.

Tradition also provided confidence in practice. Compounded ex-perience since the time of Hippocrates attested to the propriety and efficacy of such treatments as bloodletting. The fact that medical ther-apeutics in the early and mid-nineteenth century had in some respects changed little from that practiced over two millennia earlier was, one point of view held, not at all a mark of inferior practice; that therapies were antiquated simply meant that they had received the validation of centuries of trial. The support of tradition for a practice indicated that successive generations of eminent practitioners vouched for its effectiveness and that it was therefore worthy of the nineteenth-cen-tury physician's faith.

At the same time, the orthodox profession was resolutely com-mitted to progress. Physicians maintained that it was the regular profession's active efforts to advance medical knowledge and practice that distinguished its therapeutics from unthinking sectarian routine. "*Conservatism* is a principle worthy of all honor," a New Orleans physician urged, "but there is a principle paramount to it, and worthy of still greater honor—and that is, a manly and enterprising *progres-siveness.*"[1] Regular physicians claimed to be singularly deserving of public confidence by merit of their assurance that the profession would readily alter its practices if such change would bring about better care.

Physicians were aware of sharing in an ideal of progress that per-vaded both the culture of science and American society. The exhibition of progress in medical institutions was one source of pride in their profession, for it was a sign that they were keeping pace with the advancement of their science and their society. "There is but little that is stationary in the present epoch, and still less in the science of medicine. 'Progress' and 'change' seem stamped on every page of med-ical literature," a Georgia physician asserted with satisfaction.[2] The expectation of progress was an integral part of right professional think-ing.

Tension between the profession's loyalty to tradition and its commitment to change in the name of progress was inevitable. On the one hand, complacent adherence to tradition could render physicians resistant to alterations in existing ideas and practices and unresponsive to innovation. An Ohio practitioner argued that medicine was singular among the various branches of knowledge in not having purged itself of "the assumptions, traditions, hypotheses, and superstitions" of the past, and as a consequence, "presents the anomalous spectacle to-day of endeavoring to harmonize the exact knowledge of several of its ministerial branches with the terms and ideals of tradition!"[3] He was wrong in seeing medicine's attachment to tradition as anomalous, but the fact that he so plainly stated his fear of tradition's oppressive influence reflected the objection of many physicians that it blocked progress. Proposals for change could always be counterbalanced rhetorically by the weight of tradition. As a Boston physician argued, "Change and progress are not always synonymous, and the wisdom of a decade does not easily outweigh that of many centuries."[4]

On the other hand, pleas for progress often carried with them assaults upon tradition. Devotion to the past could be an encumbrance to advancement that was out of keeping with the ideals of a progressive profession. If regarded as improvement, change implied a judgment of inferiority on prior ideas and practices. The ultimate tendency of faith in progress was a devaluation of the past. "The *old*," asserted one physician who took up the extreme call to "discard authority, precedent, and tradition," "is valued only as it squares with the *new*. The *past* is estimated solely by the standard of the *present*."[5] Offended by precisely this attitude, a Massachusetts practitioner charged, "Truths as old as the world itself are unheeded and trampled upon, that heresy may be paraded and flaunted in our very faces."[6] While tradition could deter progress, progress threatened to dismantle tradition.

In the realm of therapeutics, however, medical theory was remarkably successful in arbitrating the conflict between these two opposing commitments. Change in therapeutic practice did not necessarily imply any judgment whatsoever upon prior practice or the tradition that sustained it, for an expectation of change in response to fluctuating circumstances was built into the medical belief system. Physicians assumed that in the natural course of things permutations in the physical and social environments, in the nature of prevailing diseases, and in populations and their characteristics would inevitably necessitate alterations in therapeutic behavior. Just as the principle of specificity dictated the need for therapeutic discrimination over space (North versus South, America versus Europe), it also declared the inevitability of therapeutic shifts over time. Fundamental changes in therapeutic practice could thus be accommodated to an underlying allegiance to tradition.

For example, the belief that diseases were "continually alternating in type, and running into each other," or that one disease could don the "livery" of another, reflected a conceptualization that saw therapeutics, like diseases, as always in flux.[7] "Every such variation," Philadelphia clinician William Wood Gerhard observed, "requires a corresponding modification of treatment: so that the same disease in different years, may call for the most opposite remedies for its cure."[8] The general character of all prevailing diseases also irregularly shifted with the seasons. The epidemic constitution or prevailing diathesis, a collective characterization of diseases which transmutated over time, was one regulator of therapeutic change. The notion of disease as some thing malleable diminished as the idea of specific disease entities strengthened in the last third of the century, but it did not vanish even then.

Because change was built into the ordinary functioning of nineteenth-century medicine's belief system, fundamental alterations in practice could occur without disrupting the system's integrity. Therapeutic change could challenge the authority of the past without necessarily compromising an allegiance to tradition. The particular way that medical theory predicted inevitable, perpetual change in therapeutic practice made this singular rapport between change and tradition possible; it also set therapeutic change apart from change in the "basic" sciences, medical or otherwise.

To understand the dynamics of nineteenth-century American therapeutics, it is crucial to recognize that change in practice did not necessarily entail rejection, usually it did not. The passing of a therapeutic agent from use ordinarily was a gradual process, not an abrupt break in routine. It was rare—and professionally suspect—for physicians to refuse to use a practice they had formerly employed, denying that it could be or ever had been of service. Instead they simply turned away from it. Clinical criteria to support the *dis*use of an agent were, after all, even less clear than the amply ambiguous ones used to judge a therapy valuable. Rejection of a treatment on the basis of theory was equally infrequent. Theoretical objections to therapeutic practices were common but were effective weapons only against prior theories, not against prior practices. Evidence purporting to show that a therapy was less efficacious than hitherto supposed was rarely used to argue that it was bad in principle, even in the case of a practice plainly in eclipse. Such a charge would directly challenge the judgment of medical tradition and of all physicians who had ever prescribed the treatment in question.

Revolution is an inappropriate model for the process of change in nineteenth-century therapeutic practice, and not simply because physicians regarded true revolutions in practice as professionally illegitimate, though that was most certainly the case.[9] If the term *revolution* is to mean anything more specific than simply noteworthy change, then it must connote something about the process through which change is effected and the consequent discontinuity between old and new. In particular such a process must involve rejection or overturning, a radical departure characterized by some measure of violence. Taken as a whole, the changes that occurred in therapeutic practice in America between the 1820s and the 1880s ill fit these criteria. Change came rather out of an interplay between old and new in which alterations took place with the greatest possible conservation of tradition. It was characterized more by compromise with the existing order than by a frontal assault on practices deeply embedded in the professional ethos.

Some of the changes that did occur in medical therapeutics were dramatic, to be sure, and the process of change itself was sometimes punctuated with fierce debates and brutal rhetoric about theory. Yet for regular physicians this turbulent discourse and the attendant change were confined within a largely shared framework of assumptions and commitments. During the course of the century the shape of that constraining framework changed markedly, but at no point did it rupture. It was the configuration of medical theory and its relation to practice that made it possible for substantial therapeutic change to occur without the violence to tradition that revolution implied.

In the appraisal of physicians, changes in practice could be not only positive or negative but also *neutral*. Unlike most change in the basic sciences, pivotal therapeutic changes were often adjudged neither good nor bad but merely staying even in the face of mutating circumstances. Practice could be turned on its head and physicians could agree that the change was essential; yet they could at the same time maintain that practice was neither improved nor harmed by the alteration. This was a singularly useful feature of therapeutic explanation, for it soothed the anxieties generated by changes in such sociopolitically volatile practices as dosing with mercurials and bleeding.

The way physicians explained the replacement of depletion by stimulation as the predominant therapeutic strategy between the 1830s and the 1860s illustrates how the concept of neutral change functioned in therapeutic thought. Myriad explanations were brought forward to account for this dramatic twist in practice, some arguing that it represented genuine advancement over prior practice and others asserting that it was a retrogression. The most common explanation was the change-of-type theory, which postulated that the shift from depletion to stimulation came about as a necessary consequence of changing circumstances: it was not a revolution, good or bad, but just prudent adaptation.

The leading proposition of the change-of-type theory as it was formulated in the 1850s and 1860s was that since the early 1830s the general character of all diseased conditions had shifted from a sthenic or overstimulating type to an asthenic or enfeebling type. Diseases had earlier demanded depletive therapy to lower the morbidly excited system to a healthy level, but physicians observed that as the character of diseases gradually weakened, their patients could not withstand further enfeeblement by antiphlogistic therapy and required elevation by stimulants instead. Accordingly, they found less and less frequent occasion to use the lancet, tartar emetic, or calomel and employed alcohol, iron, and a supportive diet in their place. "Change in the type of fevers," an Alabama practitioner asserted, "forced this change of treatment upon practitioners, often against their will, for they repeatedly witnessed the most disastrous consequences from the use of those means, which had, in former years, proved most successful."[10]

A modified version of the change-of-type theory attributed the fundamental shift from sthenia to asthenia to human factors rather than to disease. A practitioner in a small Ohio town observed in 1852, "The grade of fever throughout the Miami valley, is decidedly lower at present, than that which prevailed here fifteen or twenty years past, and this change has been made slowly and gradually, as the face of the country, the character, habits and mode of living of the population have changed." He believed that this permutation and the concomitant decline in the use of the lancet and purgatives it dictated were due to changes civilization had wrought in the physical and social environments and their influences on the human system. The type of diseases prevailing in the 1850s, he asserted, "seems to mark an increased delicacy of living, and the introduction of those luxuries which tend to enervate the constitution, while they banish from among us those strong and robust frames, which formed as it were the pabulum of diseases of a higher grade of action."[11]

A complete list of the conditions to which the change of type was attributed would constitute virtually an inventory of mid-nineteenth-century American culture. Sedentary habits, poorly ventilated living and working conditions, urbanization, foreign immigration, travel by rail, and the social use of tobacco and alcohol were all cited as factors. Yet as striking as the multiplicity of hypothesized causes is the fact that often physicians simply commented that the change had occurred while remaining untroubled by their ignorance as to its cause. This is important, for it shows how deeply rooted was the assumption that changes such as those postulated by the change-of-type theory would occur as part of the expected operation of nature.

The paramount explanatory advantage of the change-of-type theory rested in its judgment that one of the major therapeutic transformations of the century was in its essence neutral. To conclude that the shift from depletion to stimulation was inherently negative—that it meant giving patients care inferior to that provided previously—would have constituted an intolerable assault upon the prudence of the majority of regular physicians practicing in the mid-nineteenth century. Conversely, to claim that it was positive—that it was a clear improvement over prior practice—would have been tantamount to saying that before the early 1830s most orthodox physicians were doing the opposite of what their patients' welfare required. Such a blatant affront to medical tradition was professionally irresponsible and socially perilous. The possibility of neutral change allowed for such significant changes in practice to take place without threatening tradition.

Implicit in an explanation for the rise of stimulative therapy based on the concept of change of type was the possibility that disease might at any time revert to a sthenic type, demanding a renaissance of depletive treatment. If disease had once shifted, one physician speculated, "will it last always; have we had any evidences that we are approaching the circumference of a different circle, during the revolutions of which, a more anti-phlogistic medication may be demanded? As faithful sentinels, is it not our duty to be on the alert, so that we may not be surprised by a sudden onset of the enemy?"[12] His language points to a second usage of *revolution* that was not only permissible but actually predicted by medical theory. Of the two sorts of revolution I. Bernard Cohen has distinguished in discussions about scientific change, the first, which "denotes a breach of continuity or a secular (i.e., non-cyclical) change of real magnitude, usually accompanied—at least in political events—by violence," was not acceptable in medical therapeutics; however, the second, "signifying a cyclical phenomenon, a continuous sequence of ebb and flow, a kind of circulation and return, or a repetition," was an integral component of therapeutic change.[13] The change-of-type theory underscored the physician's responsibility to be prepared to redirect his therapeutic tack in answer to altered circumstances.

Therapeutic change came about as the result of decisions made by the individual practitioner who had to act at the bedside. Even neutral change was automatic only in principle. The institutions of medicine, as well as the various elements of the socioeconomic context within which practice was conducted, all embodied both conservative and transformative forces that acted in combination to influence attitudes toward change. These forces must be analyzed in order to assess: What were physicians' motivations for bringing change into their practices (or declining to do so)? What incentives for change and stability underlay therapeutic decision making?

To a large extent a young physician's attitudes toward change were molded by his socialization while a student. The most conservative institution of medical education was apprenticeship, the core of which was the perpetuation of traditional wisdom. The principal method of learning was the student's observation and imitation of his preceptor, coupled with the repetition of tasks. Opportunities for exposure to a diversity of opinions were minimal, although a student might have intercourse with the therapeutic ideas of other practitioners by attending a medical society meeting or observing his preceptor in consultation. An apprentice occasionally treated patients of his own independently of his mentor's practice. However, when practicing as an agent of his preceptor, he was immediately accountable to him, if not actually watched, and occasions for therapeutic deviation were rare.

Besides direct observation, the other principal source of knowledge in apprenticeship was reading. Preceptors conventionally prescribed a course of textbook study for their apprentices. A detailed account of one student's reading habits is recorded in the diary of John Richardson, a North Carolinian apprenticed to his uncle.[14] Richardson began the daily log of his reading in April 1853: "I commenced reading medicine. I read forty pages in Bell's Anatomy, the subject was Ostiology. I was not much interested owing to the fact of there being so many technical terms." During subsequent months he read with scant enthusiasm Silliman on chemistry, Gunn on domestic medicine, Wood and Bache on materia medica, Furgusson on surgery, and Magendie on physiology, complaining that "the study of medicine has thus far been very dry and uninteresting." His interest was sparked in November, when he recorded, "I commenced Eberle's Therapeutics and read twenty pages. His style is superior to any medical work I have read yet. It is graphic, forcible and fascinating." Several days later he wrote, "I read fifty pages in Eberle. I learned more about medicine to day than any former day this year."

Richardson plainly took his medical reading seriously, even reading page by page the *Dispensatory*, which he found "too insipid, there is no variety." His conscientiousness was certainly driven by his uncle's practice of examining him at intervals of about every hundred pages. In general, the degree to which the student was encouraged to read and to adopt uncritically the therapeutic instructions of his text-books depended on the amount of faith the preceptor had in each book and the interest he took in the student's learning. Still, reading was the principal means through which most apprentices encountered ideas about practice other than those of their preceptors.

Whether read by the student or consulted by the practitioner, textbooks were agencies of conservatism in therapeutics. Physicians repeatedly returned to the books they had used in apprenticeship or at school for guidance. When newly graduated physicians first began to treat patients or faced unfamiliar medical conditions such as those presented by a new region of the country or by the Civil War, they frequently wrote home for their textbooks on practice. "Send me . . . my medical books, the two of them called *Woods Practice of Medicine*," wrote a young man who found himself in the Confederate army a few months after receiving his M.D. degree. "I do not want any of the others," he added, "only the two mentioned."[15] Another physician trying to set up practice in Alabama wrote to his mother, "I want one Book if you can find it—'Watsons Practice.' "[16] A few writers on prac-tice were clearly dominant at any given period: Rush and Cooke early in the century; then Watson, Eberle, and G. B. Wood; and still later, Stillé, Bartholow, and H. C. Wood. The hegemony of a few works, coupled with the fact that physicians actively used them, tended to make textbooks a source of therapeutic standardization and conserva-tism. Yet the actual influence of textbooks was a good deal more am-biguous than their ubiquity would suggest.

To the extent that each author had his own therapeutic idiosyn-crasies—Cooke's preoccupation with mercurials, Eberle's anti-Brous-saisism, Bartholow's enthusiasm for the new remedies of the 1860s and 1870s—the simultaneous use of different textbooks constituted one source of therapeutic diversity. Furthermore, numerous caveats urged students to be wary of applying at the bedside the therapeutic precepts codified in textbooks. The principle of specificity clearly drew into question the appropriateness of textbook dictums for contexts other than that in which the author had acquired his knowledge; med-ical discourse teemed with warnings against blindly using European texts in the United States or urban texts as guides to country practice.

Moreover, physicians widely regarded textbook directions on ther-apy as unreliably doctrinaire. Teaching principles rather than practices, texts were viewed as unduly conservative guides to treatment that encouraged practice by rote. Physicians in the 1860s, for example, were aware of the discrepancy between the meager use of venesection in practice and its high valuation in textbooks. "I will put away old Wat-son for awhile," a young physician wrote to a former classmate. "I think I know his treatment any way. *Bleed* & give mercury, that embraces nearly everything with him."[17] Not only did textbooks cling in principle to therapies that had declined in actual practice, but they also were generally slow in taking up innovations. A Cincinnati medical editor advised that if a new remedy was backed by the authority of a respectable physician, "we are fully authorized to adopt new modes of treatment, although the *text books* may be silent on the subject."[18] Thus although textbooks functioned as a conservative force, the fact that physicians perceived their conservatism as sufficient reason to caution against overreliance on them diluted their counterinfluence on therapeutic change.

The dual action of conservative and change-oriented factors was far more pronounced in medical school instruction. In the inaugural addresses that preceded the opening of each lecture season, faculty members conventionally told students of the antiquity and nobility of the profession into which they were being initiated and of the great practitioners whom they followed. This hagiographic exercise indicated the tradition with which students should identify and implicitly urged that emulation of these men and their practices was one worthy objective of medical study. At the same time, most addresses were also explicitly progressive. The speaker frequently recounted recent medical advances and told students that they must prepare themselves to take up those changes that constituted real progress. Therapeutic uncertainty, its causes, and its solutions were leading themes in inaugural addresses, especially from the 1840s through the 1860s. Speeches of this genre impressed upon students the need and possibilities for therapeutic progress and the expectation of therapeutic change.

The lectures on practice students listened to during subsequent months also sought to train them in ways that took into account an expectation of change. "General Bloodletting is much less frequently employed now than formerly," a student attending medical lectures in 1859 at the University of Virginia wrote in his class notebook. "Disease now seems to be Asthenic as compared with that of former times—but in those times Bleeding was good because disease was *Sthenic*. We must consider then the *Prevalent Type* of disease in the times."[19] The message of this lecture was that the student should be prepared for analogous changes in type that could call for a return of venesection to common practice. Eli Geddings, lecturing in Charleston the following year, similarly detailed how pneumonia had changed from an inflammatory to an adynamic type during the preceding two or three decades, leading to the disuse of antiphlogistic practices. "I wish you to understand," he then told his class, "that the treatment, I am now to recommend is not designed for the disease, as it now occurs. But as many of you may practice in other parts of the world, it is my duty to state to you the management of the inflammatory variety. The treatment of the later is in the main antiphlogistic."[20] Just as the Virginia professor had made it clear to his students that they should expect to change their practices in accordance with shifts in disease over time, Geddings was preparing his to alter their therapeutics as they moved from place to place.

These explicit acknowledgments of the mutability of proper therapeutic behavior notwithstanding, the implicit and probably most forceful message medical schools conveyed was conservative: medical therapeutics was a defined body of knowledge, and the student's task was to master it. The realities of medical school curriculums often led to a didacticism that belied rhetorical commitments to the tentativeness of established knowledge. At least through the start of the 1870s most medical school programs consisted of one course of lectures, generally taken twice, that covered a period of three to six months. On the whole those who taught therapeutics simply had no time to do more than sketch a set block of material, pointing out as they went along that the application of this knowledge would require modifications according to prevailing circumstances.

Therapeutic precept was included in virtually all of the classes at a medical school but was concentrated principally in lectures on the principles and practice of medicine and on materia medica. The structures of these lectures varied widely, but most were reducible to one of two general formats. In the first the professor discussed the major disease groups in turn, reviewing sequentially their etiology, symptomatology, pathology, and therapeutics. The second was organized by classes of remedies such as cathartics, sudorifics, antihelminthics, and stimulants. Within each of these categories, roughly following the arrangement and content of the *Dispensatory*, the lecturer described each remedy's chemical nature and preparation, physiological action, and therapeutic indications.[21] Thus therapeutic knowledge was rigidly codified, and the student was encouraged to take it up as a fixed whole.

Of course the imperative for students to actually absorb what they heard in lectures, much less put their faith in it, is subject to the objections that medical school education was perfunctory, that examinations were trivial exercises and degrees were guaranteed if fees were paid, and that students were therefore under little pressure to learn the information presented to them. This is certainly suggested by the widespread historiographic caricature of medical schools as institutions attended by poorly prepared and dubiously bright students and operated by mercenary professors for profit and prestige. There is much truth in this image, but it has been exaggerated. Many students worked hard at their lessons and acquired in medical school knowledge they later tried to apply in their practices.

Students' attitudes toward the examinations required for graduation provide one illustration of their motivation (beyond genuine interest) to take seriously the task of learning lecture material. Examinations were brief and oral, generally including several questions from each member of a faculty of five or six. Historians' caricatures of the examinations as worthless if not comical affairs in which ignorance posed no threat whatsoever of failure have been drawn largely from the recollections of older physicians about their student days. Such retrospective evidence is inherently suspect. Stronger evidence that at least some students regarded the examinations as real hurdles is the simple fact that they feared the tests, earnestly studied for them, and agonized over their possible outcomes.[22]

The anxiety examinations produced in many students is lucidly reflected in the experiences of Jefferson DeVotie, a student in New Orleans who described his fear of the approaching test in a series of letters to his father. "I am afraid that we are going to have a tight time when we come in the green room as these professors here have the reputation of being awfully tight on a fellow when he appears before them and modestly asks for a sheep skin," he wrote in December 1861. Becoming progressively more disturbed about the examination, he stated in early February that "I am frightened half to death about it, and to use the words of my roommate 'I feel awfully skerred.' " Two weeks later DeVotie suggested, "I would not be surprised if two thirds of those who apply were not rejected." Toward the end of the month he told his father, "I begin to feel more confident as to the result but am still 'furious' anxious and troubled." Nor did he find himself alone in his anxiety. "Most of the students are in the same predicament as myself," he asserted, "frightened out of their wits at the prospect ahead[.] I have been attentive to lectures this winter and have read as much as I could so if I get 'pitched' it will not be from waste of time on my part." After a one-hour examination, he could write to his father in early March that he had finally won his M.D. degree.[23]

DeVotie's anxieties were unusually acute, but the fact that many of his fellows shared them demonstrates that in the view of students—which is after all what mattered—the examination could establish an incentive for adopting the didactic messages of lectures. Whether professors took the examinations as seriously as students did is somewhat irrelevant to the point, although as one student noted, a brief examination did not mean that the faculty took the task of appraising a student's knowledge lightly. "I entered the Green Room, and after remaining only 25 minutes I came out a regular made Doctor—my meeting with the Professors, for I could hardly call it Examination[,] was very flattering," a medical student in Cincinnati wrote in 1835. "Each asked me 4 or 5 Questions & declared themselves perfectly satisfied with my attainments having examined me during the whole session in their respective Classes. I have had the shortest examination which has come on the Boards thus far, & we students measure the honor of our Examinations by their shortness."[24]

There was some cause for student apprehension. The vast majority of the candidates who came up for examination were, of course, passed, especially before the last decades of the century. Making examinations too difficult would have driven away students, and graduation and diploma fees were valued sources of faculty income.[25] Nevertheless, even during the antebellum period certain American medical schools regularly failed some of their degree candidates, as the minutes of faculty meetings show. "Mr A P Scott was examined for a degree in medicine but having received 3 black and 3 white balls was rejected— Thesis and graduation fee returned," an entry in the Medical College of Louisiana's faculty minutes for 1845, a typical year, recorded.[26] At the Cincinnati College of Medicine and Surgery in 1854, "The examination of Mr Hicks, not being satisfactory, his case resulted unfavorably. He subsequently sent in a request to the Faculty, to admit him to a second examination before all the members of the Faculty, which upon motion was unanimously acceded to—he was again rejected."[27] Such instances were not unusual at Cincinnati or at other schools: graduation was not the inevitable result of attending lectures and paying fees.

The fact that many students took their courses seriously implies that they at least endeavored to absorb the knowledge codified in lectures. But it does not mean that medical schools, and their proliferation from the 1830s onward, standardized medical knowledge and practice. Pupils of a particular professor were likely to be indoctrinated with many of their instructor's beliefs. Indeed, notes taken by various students on the lectures a single teacher gave often show little variation over a period of many years. What is most striking about the abundant extant sets of lecture notes on medical practice and therapeutics, however, is the enormous diversity in what was taught at any one time. It is true that a substantial degree of uniformity would be expected in the practices and ideas of students who attended, for example, Transylvania, for there they shared exposure to the teachings of Cooke, Caldwell, and Charles Short; but a comparison of the precepts held by Transylvania alumni and by students who had studied with Bigelow, Holmes, and Ware at Harvard would reveal substantial differences in therapeutic belief. In this respect the multiplication of medical schools was as much a source of diversity in medical thought and practice as it was of standardization.

Other factors further militated against therapeutic standardization being produced by the proliferation of medical schools. Physicians did not necessarily persist in holding their schoolroom knowledge. Since attending medical lectures at Transylvania in 1824, "I have visited many places, seen many medical philosophers, conversed & heard much on the subject of my profession," a young Kentucky physician recorded in his diary the following year. "When I first began to write in this Book I was full of the Theories of the Transylvania School—In fact, I knew no others—or scarcely any." He had left school fully committed to Transylvanian ideas on hepatic pathology emphasizing portal congestion, but since then "I have heard them strongly contested— And I must confess the arguments which I have last heard; have most weight on my mind. *Some* of the Theories of the philosophers appear to me still, to have a foundation in nature & in truth—Many, I have been compelled to renounce."[28]

Furthermore, preceptors, families, and medical friends routinely cautioned students to remain skeptical of what they were taught in schools on therapeutics. Many such caveats reflected the common assumption that some professors' excessive scientific zeal made their practical teachings suspect. The doctrine of specificity was often called upon, too, to warn southern students about northern schools' teachings and rural pupils about those of the city. A cultivated distrust of medical schools as a source of applicable therapeutic precepts further weakened any tendency of school instruction to engender standardized practice.[29]

Physicians' attitudes toward change and their readiness to alter their practices were shaped not only by commitments acquired during formal medical training but also by a political interaction with patients and other practitioners. The socioeconomic context within which nineteenth-century American physicians practiced was dominated by the number and variety of competing practitioners avowing differing therapeutic faiths. No factor has been singled out more often than sectarianism as responsible for the transformation of regular therapeutics. According to this view, sectarian attacks on heroic depletion in regular practice, especially the use of bloodletting and mercurials, produced a public outcry against these therapies that ultimately compelled orthodox physicians to abandon them.

The actual influence of medical sectarianism on regular therapeutics was in fact more complex and less unidirectional in its action.[30] More than any other factor, the strength of sectarianism made American regular physicians examine the meaning of their commitments to progress and to tradition in terms of their very livelihoods. While sectarianism undeniably fostered regular therapeutic change, it could also engender a dogmatic adherence to tradition that made change difficult and at times professionally suspect.

The threat sectarianism posed to regular physicians is best understood against the backdrop of the social and economic realities of medical practice. A surplus of practitioners made it difficult for many practitioners to earn a living by following their vocation. A young physician who in 1831 had just put up a sign for his new office in New Orleans wrote to his brother that "one of the old Doctors died off [and] 14 new ones arrived to divide the spoils, and those of the most ravenous kinds." He consoled himself with the prospect that "the John [a corruption of *jaune*] Fever must kill or frighten some of them."[31] Within the year he had given up on New Orleans but continued to complain from Maryland of the overabundance of physicians. "If the town should increase [in population]," he wrote, "they will be as thick here as hail. [T]he country around is swarming with them."[32]

Competition from sectarian practitioners in addition to regulars compounded the problem, and orthodox physicians routinely expected the arrival of a new species of sectarian healer in their neighborhood to diminish their own practices. "The competition now prevailing in medicine," an Ohio physician explained in 1851, "has been brought to a very [high] pitch . . . [It] is certain that even the longest established and most estimable physicians have yielded a large part and lucrative portions of their practice to homeopathy &c."[33] A recent graduate trying to establish a practice in Mississippi wrote home to his wife that "the steam doctors . . . will likely interfere with me. One has located within a mile and will get a part of the practice, as it is a new thing here and some are in favor of the system." He noted with satisfaction, however, that the recent execution by hanging of men plotting a slave uprising had weeded out the competition. "Five or six white men and about twenty negroes have been executed," he wrote. "Among these were two celebrated steam doctors, whose medicines were found to avail nothing against hemp."[34]

This intense competition greatly strained relationships among practitioners and also made them acutely sensitive to patient demand. "Popular prejudice" in the realm of treatment became a common euphemism for the threat of sectarian competition. A patient dissatisfied with the therapy his physician offered could turn to another regular physician, to one of a variety of sectarian healers, or to any number of self-help medical systems. Sectarian charges that orthodox physicians poisoned their patients with heroic doses of drugs such as mercury and the challenge this posed to public confidence in the profession were well calculated to make regular physicians malleable to their patients' therapeutic inclinations.

Public resistance to heroic drugging, encouraged by sectarian rhetoric, clearly was one source of regular therapeutic change. Orthodox practitioners, one physician commented in the mid-1850s, had begun to look at remedies like mercury "through glasses, adapted to the *focus* of popular prejudice."[35] Physicians yielded at various times to their patients' refusals to endure not only heroic bleeding and purging but also practices later in vogue such as quinine, alcohol, and hypodermic injections of morphine. After recording the case history of a patient who had just died, for example, an Ohio physician complained in his diary in 1836, "This patient was strongly opposed to the use of the lancet, & calomel," and therefore "the former was not used at all & the latter in too small quantities to do good or hurt."[36] On the other hand, orthodox practitioners frequently cited public demand for traditional treatments as a leading impediment to change. Physicians argued that their efforts to move away from massive doses of cathartics and emetics, for example, often were blocked by "the suicidal mania for being drugged" common among their patients.[37]

The most forceful sectarian impulse to regular therapeutic change came from the example of homeopathy. By drawing attention to the important role nature played in healing, homeopathic successes urged regular physicians to recognize the tendency of most cases to satisfactory resolution without heroic intervention. Homeopathy should "not be looked upon, by scientific physicians, as an *empty humbug,* but rather be used as a mirror, which, though opaque itself, may yet serve to throw light upon our errors," proposed E. D. Fenner. While perceiving "the fallacies of Homoeopathy, as a system of medicine," physicians should, he argued, recognize that "it reveals the wonderful powers of *nature* in the cure of diseases. In comparing its practice with that of Allopathy, or the ordinary practice, it shows with *how little medicine* the most dangerous diseases may get well."[38] The sectarian example nagged regulars into reevaluating their own therapeutic ways.

Internal criticism of regular therapeutics was sometimes ruthlessly direct, explicitly challenging an aspect of the traditional order, as was the case in the empiricist denunciation of rationalistic systems. In criticizing practices, however, physicians ordinarily preferred a safer approach. The sectarian example became the core of a convention for voicing the orthodox profession's therapeutic self-doubt in a way that did not threaten medical tradition. Criticisms of regular therapeutics were framed as apologies for the rise and success of medical sects and the attendant disfavor into which the medical profession had fallen.

It was within this context that regular physicians most often formulated major criticisms of their own practices and called for change.

In its general form, this convention almost invariably included three elements. The first was a statement of sectarian successes, displayed by such indicators as the large numbers of patients relying upon sectarian medical care, the often favorable outcome of cases managed by sectarians, and the relatively low standing of the orthodox profession in the public view. The second element was a disavowal of any belief in the theoretical validity or practical efficacy of sectarian medicine, coupled with a profession of faith in the principles underlying orthodox medical tradition. Regular medicine was in essence good, and sectarian medicine was bad.

The third element in this convention was an apology for the first. The success of medical sectarians, regular physicians charged, was in large measure a consequence of the orthodox profession's misuse of its therapeutic armamentarium. Typically, this self-criticism might include the proposition that bloodletting (or alcohol, or more expansive therapeutic leanings such as heroic depletion or nature trusting), although valuable in principle, had been injudiciously applied. Essays "on the use and abuse" of particular agents, which abounded, were usually of this genre. Physicians seldom implied that the therapeutic agent or strategy under criticism was not beneficial if properly used; rejection was not an issue.

Beyond spurring a reconsideration of regular practices, the success sectary achieved led some regular physicians to reflect on the adequacy of their profession's receptivity to change. Criticism from within of excessive conservatism conformed to the same general form as the apologies for sectary sketched above but attributed the rise of sectarianism not to the misuse of a specific remedy but to the regular profession's unresponsiveness to changing circumstances that should have instigated therapeutic alterations.

Samuel A. Cartwright was typical in using the example of Thomsonianism to urge the profession to be watchful and prepared for therapeutic change. Through their rigidity, Cartwright charged, regular physicians had virtually forced many of their patients to turn to sectarian treatment, the success of which stood as a reproach to a dangerous regular conservatism. "For not admitting the claims of red pepper & lobelia & the external applications of heat as valuable therapeutic agents in some complaints," Cartwright wrote in a letter to a lay friend, "physicians have driven great numbers of persons into a new system called Thomsonianism." Orthodox practitioners were likewise to blame for not recognizing the limited value of homeopathy, thereby inciting "vast multitudes" of patients to "cast away the accumulated experience of all ages & countries to get the benefit of the few rejected facts the new system of homeopathy is built upon—& they die with inflammations for the want of bloodletting, or a dose of salts, or castor oil." If "learned men" would only be open-minded and not resist new ideas, "there would be no solid ground left out side of the borders of true knowledge for Charlatans in philosophy, politics or medicine to build new systems upon."[39]

Sectarianism also constituted one source of regular innovation.[40] Implicit in Cartwright's remarks was the idea that sectarian therapies could be of value in certain circumstances and that orthodox physicians should scrutinize and exploit these treatments. A regular practitioner from Alabama who was attending medical lectures in Charleston to earn his M.D. degree wrote in his thesis that a singular characteristic of allopathic medicine was that "she receives all that is valuable of the other schools." "Having had an extensive country practice for twenty years," he wrote, "I have been thrown in the way of empyrics and therefore had ample opportunity to test the effects of different systems of practice, watching with close attention, and in a few instances condescending to consult with an empyric for the purpose of having an opportunity . . . [to] test his practice." Through this portal, he claimed, he had brought into his practice the use of lobelia, veratrum, capsicum, podophyllum pillatum, and the "compound tincture of myrrh or 'No 6,' " a Thomsonian remedy.[41] Other regular physicians agreed that these agents were beneficial when used by regular physicians, though dangerous in injudicious sectarian hands.

On the whole, regular physicians maintained that although medical sects had in some ways fostered medical progress, sectarians made contributions only in spite of themselves. Sectarian therapy was "an easy, almost mechanical thumb-rule business"[42] devoid of the exercise of judgment and reverence for specificity essential to proper medical practice. "Progress was not coming from the Homoepaths, but from men of the regular profession," one Cleveland physician told a medical society meeting in 1882. Homeopaths "as a clas were not progressive and their dogmatic principle was direct the opposite of making medicine a science."[43] A Cincinnati physician came to a similar conclusion about botanics and eclectics thirty years earlier. "Whatever may be said of the favourable treatment that is made by these irregulars in many cases," he wrote to a lay friend, "there [sic] general tendency is the destruction of all enlightened progress in medicine."[44]

In the view of orthodox physicians, one objective of such sects as homeopathy was the repudiation of regular progress and tradition. While true therapeutic revolution shattering the beliefs that gave it legitimacy was not part of proper regular change, this was precisely what homeopathy sought. For example, William Henry Holcombe, a prominent homeopathic practitioner and editor, repeatedly called for the rupturing of the old system of medicine. His dual commitment to homeopathy and Swedenborgianism forged the link between his opposition to medical and religious orthodoxies. The structures that sustained both had to be torn down before the new order could be erected: "As it is impossible for the old bottles to contain our *new wine*, I strongly recommend the immediate demolition of all Orthodox Theological Schools and all apothecary Shops."[45] Holcombe, whose diary abounds with accounts of murderous regular treatments, believed that change could not adequately proceed within the existing orthodox frameworks. "I felt how useless it is to argue with any body whose whole life has been given to the contemplation and defense of certain dogmas," he wrote after reading a regular medical journal. "The present race of Old Church theologians and of Allopathic doctors has to *die out* before the good seed can spring up on the place of those weeds in the garden of the world."[46] Here was a clear call for what no regular physician could contemplate—a true therapeutic revolution that would abolish the old order.

Such homeopathic attitudes were made especially troubling by the fact that in practice the boundaries between regulars and sectarians were often blurred. To be sure, the orthodox profession did discriminate against homeopaths by ostracizing them from regular institutions and professional interaction. They were barred from regular medical societies and thereby denied access to one source of professional distinction, knowledge, and business. The code of ethics to which society members pledged themselves also prohibited regulars from consulting with sectarians, and some members who violated this stipulation were charged with unethical conduct and expelled.[47] Similarly, regular medical schools closed their doors to unorthodox practitioners who sought M.D. degrees, revoked the diplomas of alumni who took up sectarian ways, expelled students who associated with sectarians or themselves practiced sectarian medicine between terms, and refused to allow students who had been apprenticed to sectarian practitioners to attend lectures or become degree candidates. The faculty of the Medical College of the State of South Carolina, for example, refused to consider one student as a candidate for graduation when they learned that his father, with whom he had apprenticed, had converted to homeopathy. The facts that the student had attended lectures and that the father held an M.D. degree from that same orthodox school did not alter their decision.[48]

But despite the policy of segregation, in actuality regular and sectarian practitioners were much less rigidly separated. Especially during homeopathy's early decades in America, many of its adherents were converts from orthodox medicine who possessed regular educations and degrees. Orthodox practitioners frequently charged that homeopathists often prescribed regular drugs; "the clever rogues among the homeopathists take good care to give active doses of medicine, under cover of their infinitesimal humbug."[49] Moreover, some regulars did not rigorously exclude homeopathic remedies from their practices. Still more troubling to the upholders of orthodoxy was the suspicion that, as one Ohio physician put it, "many homeopaths are sailing under false collers [sic],"[50] and that many regular physicians were complacent about this subterfuge. For example, James Otis Moore, a Maine homeopathist practicing in the Union army in 1864, represented himself as a regular physician in order to secure the post of surgeon. When a regular medical colleague learned of his homeopathic background from a mutual acquaintance from Maine, he did not report the deception but merely told Moore, "I care nothing about it of course, as long as you do your duty as well as you have done it."[51] Belying any implied rapport between the two medical orientations, however, Moore's letters to his wife chronicled his growing horror at the harm done by allopathic treatment.

Similarly, when one Dr. Gifford's eligibility for membership in a local Indiana-Ohio regular medical society was questioned on the basis of his professional loyalty, he frankly admitted that he was not "exclusively" an allopathist. "Dr. Gifford arose and said," the secretary recorded in the minutes, "that 'he was educated in the regular profession . . . ; that he used homeopathic remedies and Allopathic remedies as each case seemed to require: that he took several journals of each school, and believed there was a good deal for the regular profession to learn yet from the Homeopaths; that he had learned, as he believed, a great deal of them, and, while not claiming to be a Homeopath, nor yet strictly an Allopath, he claimed to be in its true sense an eclectic in practice." Gifford finally became a member of the society after he "repudiated Homeopathy as a *system* of medicine, declaring himself an Allopath."[52]

Many orthodox physicians were more tolerant of social and professional interaction with avowed homeopathists than the official policy of discrimination dictated. Social intercourse between regulars and irregulars was not the rule, but neither was it rare.[53] And even some unimpeachably regular physicians occasionally had professional associations with homeopathists. When James Jackson, Sr., was asked to consult with a Salem homeopathist in 1857, for example, he did not balk at the idea of consulting with an irregular practitioner but only sought to be sure that he was an honorable gentleman. In a letter boldly marked "*Private,*" Jackson asked a Salem friend for more information. "I know Dr. G[ersdoff] to be a Homoeopath, or Semi-Homoeopath. I wish to know whether there is any objection to his character," Jackson wrote. "My rule," he explained, "has always been to meet Homeopaths, as I have other M.D.'s whose practice I disapproved, provided they would adopt my plans."[54]

This ambiguity in the boundaries that distinguished among the various categories of practitioners, coupled with the serious threat sectarianism posed to the identity and socioeconomic well-being of regular physicians, constituted medical sectarianism's most forceful conservative influence on regular therapeutics. While sectarianism contributed to a convenient convention for regular therapeutic self-examination and rebuke, it also greatly constrained the ways in which such criticism could be conducted. In order to set themselves apart from sectarians, regular physicians continually had to reaffirm their regularity. Criticism of a therapy that had been in regular use was invariably accompanied by the qualification that it had done much good in the past and, appropriately applied, could be of great service in the future. Therapeutic progress was not to be made at the cost of open assaults on practices identified with orthodox tradition.

Strictures on therapeutic criticism were tightened by the regular profession's preoccupation with professional unity as protection against sectarian threats. Younger physicians coveted the practices of those who were established, while older practitioners could not help but be uneasy about the appearance of younger colleagues in their neighborhoods. Disharmony attended aggressive competition; as a Maryland physician trying to establish practice wrote to his brother, "Some of the Physicians make use of every meaness to obtain practice by undercharging and sometimes slandering each other, so that the most experienced physician is never sure of retaining his practice."[55] Since professional disagreement could tacitly validate sectarian charges of therapeutic misbehavior and drive patients from regular medicine, the appearance of unity was an essential goal that demanded carefully guarded conduct in therapeutic discourse. Criticism of existing or past practices had to be conducted in such a way that it was kept from public view.

There were, then, proper and improper forums for criticism, the chief among the former being medical journals and society meetings. Of these two loci for therapeutic discussion, medical societies were the more revealing: with their primary purpose of promoting professional unity, they were at the interface between medicine as an objectively evaluated body of knowledge and the distorting realities of daily practice. Through the stipulations of their codes of ethics, societies sought to minimize occasions for open therapeutic discord in public hearing by forbidding their members to consult with irregular physicians and by insisting that physicians never voice doubts about their colleagues' practices in the public setting of a consultation. The rules of medical etiquette adopted by the Natchez Medical Society made this point crystalline: "No physician shall, directly or by inuendo, criticise or censure the practice of any other physician before any person or persons not qualified to be a judge in the case," it ordered. "Criticism . . . should be entirely confined to the physicians, and in no case permitted to reach the public ear."[56] In practice the code of ethics was often bent, but violations could seriously damage a physician's standing among his peers.[57]

Beyond the formal conservatism written into the code of ethics, there were other incentives for therapeutic conservatism, if not complacency, within medical societies. For the young physician especially, society membership offered an avenue to gaining practice. A recent graduate who had just moved to Atlanta explained in a letter to his sister that joining the city's medical society "will introduce me [to] all the leading Physicians in the place, which of itself, will, I hope, be of benefit to me by having any cases thrown in my hands, which they haven't the disposition to treat."[58] It was, moreover, through medical society acquaintances that the young physician would be invited into consultation, a source of both financial profit and knowledge.

Therapeutic conformity, or at the least avoidance of criticism, was important to the young practitioner trying to gain approval. Certainly professional advancement could also be sought by proselytizing something new, as was the case with some physicians who lauded the healing power of nature in the 1840s or experimental physiology in the 1870s. Nevertheless, the leading tendency of medical societies was toward therapeutic conservatism, which was primarily the result of a search for professional unity through allegiance to a shared tradition.

Regular physicians' attitudes toward therapeutic change were molded by a dialectic between their commitment to progress and their loyalty to tradition. The receptivity to innovation or stubborn attachment to tried practices of the individual practitioner must be understood as a product of these interactive forces in education, decision making at the bedside, and experience in the marketplace. A tidy enumeration of the factors that caused therapeutic change in nineteenth-century America would approach being historically pointless unless it was accompanied by a counterbalancing list of those that encouraged stasis, for a force such as sectarianism properly belongs on both lists.

Yet even together they would miss the significance of these factors for the individual physician caught up in the push and pull that marked their interaction. The major domestic sources of influence on therapeutic change urged alteration and preservation simultaneously, and recognizing this fundamental ambivalence is crucial to understanding how the changing course of therapeutic practice was shaped.

— 6 —

Attitudes toward
Foreign Knowledge

However much the course of American medicine was determined
by socioeconomic forces and conceptual resources within the American environment, it was also persistently shaped by European tutelage.
American physicians abroad traveled principally to the lecture halls of
Edinburgh before the early nineteenth century and to German laboratories in its final third. In between, it was the vision of medicine
they brought back from the Paris hospitals that was the most forceful
European propellant of medicine's transformation in the United States.
In therapeutics French skeptical empiricism commanded its American
proponents to critically re-evaluate existing practices. The more detailed knowledge of the natural history of diseases generated in the
Paris clinic served as a backdrop against which Americans could assess
for themselves the efficacy of their treatments, an endeavor sometimes
ordered by the numerical method. The strongest single impulse French
medicine contributed to the reform of American therapeutic practice,
however, was directed toward moderation—greater reliance on the
healing power of nature and less on drugging. In conscious acknowledgment of the term's partially French parentage, American physicians
widely adopted the phrase *médecine expectante* to describe this posture. French medicine did not create this therapeutic stance in the
United States, but it did reinforce a tendency toward gentleness in
prescribing that had native roots. Thus even James Jackson, Sr., could
call the expectant approach therapeutics *"à la française."*[1]

Although French medicine catalyzed therapeutic change in the
United States, it did not present a model of practice Americans cared
to emulate, and profound ambivalence underlay American attitudes
toward French teachings. Physicians saw in the Parisian medical ex-

ample sources not only of medical advancement but also of ineffica-
cious therapy, moral corruption, and professional debasement. To the
American medical mind, the French school presented a dangerous model
of professional behavior and morality that threatened to vitiate the
practitioner's character. While Americans revered some categories of
Parisian medical knowledge, many facets of French patient care repelled them. Therapeutics (regarded as a body of knowledge about therapy and a program of bedside behavior, as distinguished from its
epistemological underpinnings and methods for improving knowledge)
was the weakest aspect of French medicine, in the appraisal of most
Americans. This judgment, coupled with reservations about the applicability of European knowledge to American practice that were based
on the principle of specificity, encouraged American physicians to see
therapeutic knowledge as the least valuable component of French medicine.

American physicians were highly selective about which aspects
of Parisian medicine they elected to transmit to the United States and
which ones to eschew, and nowhere was this selectivity more pronounced than in therapeutics. Many American students of French medicine energetically embraced the skeptical empiricist *epistemology* that
underlay French therapeutics and regarded it as among the most important messages of the Paris clinical school. They aggressively used
Parisian therapeutic empiricism in combatting rationalistic systems
of practice, making it pivotal to both therapeutic reform and professional upliftment. In striking contrast, American physicians who studied in Paris on the whole shunned French knowledge about therapeutic
practice as probably irrelevant and perhaps dangerous for the American
context.

The stress here on France should not imply that it was the only
important foreign source of change. Britain was the steadiest foreign
referent for therapeutic practice in America during the antebellum
period and was regarded in some respects as a more reliable source of
authority than France. But British medicine posed no substantive challenge to American therapeutics. Furthermore, Americans harbored many
of their objections against French medicine against British practice as
well, and made similar criticisms of German clinical medicine, especially practice in Vienna. The rise of laboratory medicine beginning in
the 1860s, particularly in German centers, also elicited new sorts of
criticism and enthusiasm from Americans. Despite these several currents, American ambivalence toward European therapeutic knowledge
between the 1820s and the 1860s is most clearly illustrated in the
example of the Paris clinical school.

French medical thought was brought to America by medical journals and monographs, but most powerfully by the American physicians who supplemented their training with study in the Paris hospitals.[2] It was largely they who translated and edited French medical writings for an American readership. Moreover, these physicians on their return filled an inordinately large number of professorships in American medical schools, and from these positions proselytized French medicine to students. They frequently used their own Parisian experiences to illustrate lectures and substantiate arguments at medical society meetings. It tended to be these same physicians who applied the methods of French medicine in the American context by, for example, conducting clinical and pathological researches on American patients and urging clinical instruction in medical school curriculums.

Americans considered carefully the benefits against which the sizable costs of going to Paris were to be weighed. The leading attraction of Paris for medical Americans was unquestionably its hospitals and the large number of patients, segregated by disease, their wards contained. Here American students attended the lectures of the leading French clinicians and engaged interns to give private lessons to small groups at the bedside on the natural history of diseases and on diagnostic techniques. The free access Americans were granted to French patients' bodies, living and dead, gave them opportunities unmatched in America for making pathoanatomical correlations with clinically observed symptoms and for anatomical and surgical study. The diagnostic and prognostic knowledge gained in Paris, Americans believed, gave the practitioner the self-assurance that generated patient confidence. At the same time European experience bestowed a patina of wisdom that was a source of professional distinction and in turn constituted a competitive advantage. Some Americans also sought in Paris the exhilarating sense of being at the center of activity in medical science before they settled down to practice on its periphery.

What is most striking about American physicians' expositions of what they expected to gain from study in Paris is what is missing: they did not go to France to acquire medical therapeutic knowledge, as more than negative evidence indicates. Americans writing home from Paris routinely contrasted their enthusiasm for French pathology, diagnosis, and surgical therapeutics with their apathy or disdain for Parisian medical therapeutics. In some measure these attitudes can be attributed to French lack of interest in the subject, but their roots went far deeper than that. Many American physicians deplored French therapeutic practice and perceived in French therapeutic precept a source of real danger. Why, given their high esteem for some branches of French medical science and the centrality of medical therapeutics to the professional role and identity of the American physician, did Americans regard French therapeutic knowledge as irrelevant, suspect, and even threatening?

In part their distrust was a natural corollary to the principle of specificity and the valuation of local knowledge it encouraged. Just as treatment in the northern United States might be inapplicable in the South, the epidemiological, meteorological, social, and demographic differences between Europe and America demanded that therapeutics appropriate to the one be adjusted for application in the other. A Louisville medical professor cautioned his class that "the climates of London and Paris were entirely different from our own; the diet and habits of the people altogether different; and that these with other circumstances so modified the constitutions of the people and the character of the diseases, as to make the latter totally different from the diseases of this country."[3] National differences also altered the influence of remedial agents on the body, rendering European treatments inappropriate in many American circumstances.

Most objections to the importation of French practice inspired by the principle of specificity hinged on one fact: French therapeutic knowledge, as it presented itself to American practitioners, was essentially equivalent to knowledge produced in the Paris hospitals. Although some American physicians pointed out that there might be substantial correspondence between the therapeutic needs of certain classes of Parisians and some American city dwellers, most agreed that the therapeutic requirements of patients in Paris were fundamentally different from those of rural Americans. A student attending Benjamin Dudley's lectures at Transylvania University, for example, typically recorded in his class notebook, "The treatment of Erysipelas in Paris, London and some other large cities is of the Tonic and stimulating kind, here it is directly the reverse, Depletory."[4]

Rural-urban distinctions aside, the pauperized, hospitalized French man or woman who made up the Paris school's human material was not an acceptable therapeutic analogue to the American patient seen by the physician in private practice. Charles Caldwell returned from a visit to London and Paris in the early 1840s to tell his students, "The hospitals of those great cities were very extensive and filled with persons labouring under great varieties of diseases; but they were from the very dregs of society[,] a class whose constitutions have been depraved by intemperance and want, and modified by vice, habit and climate until they possess no analogy in constitution or disease to any class in our own country." He cautioned that "from this class or this kind of cases is the student of medicine to derive his knowledge and experience in visiting the Hospitals of London & Paris; and their constitutions and diseases are so modified and so totally different from those in our own country, the knowledge of Pathology and Therapeutics to be gained by visiting these hospitals can be of but little advantage to the practice of Medicine in the United States."[5]

Underlying most comparisons of French and American therapeutic need was the belief that American constitutions and diseases were inherently more energetic than those of Europeans. The origins of this idea can be traced back at least to the late-eighteenth-century American defense against the French Buffon–de Pauw thesis, which postulated the physical degeneracy of animal life in the New World. Like Jeffersonian claims that there were live mammoths roaming somewhere on the North American continent, the supposed robustness of American physiology in health and disease served the refutation of the Buffon–de Pauw thesis by demonstrating the vigor of organic life in America on a scale unmatched in Europe.[6]

Echoing a view held by his predecessor at the University of Pennsylvania, Benjamin Rush, the Jeffersonian physician Benjamin Smith Barton noted in 1815 that whereas Americans ordinarily required depletion when sick, enfeebled Europeans usually needed therapeutic elevation. The stimulant cinchona bark, he told his classes, "has not been infrequently employed in Erysipelas particularly in Europe. But in the U. States the disease differs essentially from what it is in Europe. In Europe it is in general attended [by] prostration of strength and debility, and requires the invigorating method of cure. But in the U. States this disease is in general one of the Phlegmasia of an inflammatory character and requires the antiphlogistic method of cure." The same pattern held in other diseases; chorea, for example, assumed a debilitated form "in the enervated and enfeebled inhabitants of Europe. But in the U. States where the Blessings of Liberty are combined with the numerous other causes in developing the Physical man, this disease is usually of the tonic and sthenic character," calling for therapeutic lowering by bleeding and purging.[7] Nor was this a singularly Philadelphian position. A South Carolina student attending medical lectures at Transylvania University recorded in his class notebook that inflammation is "modified by a variety of circumstances . . . Location or situation modifies [it]. In *Paris* we would stimulate by Porter, Bark &c— In Kentucky we would bleed & Purge."[8]

Such differences in need meant that French therapeutic knowledge was not merely irrelevant in managing American patients but could be actively harmful by directing the very opposite of the treatment required. Any doctrinaire adherence to the example of French practice would be professionally irresponsible. This was easily extended to the notion that European medicine's hegemony in American institutions of medical education, such as schools, textbooks, and journals, was a source of many of the profession's problems. French therapeutic teachings, many Americans believed, could lead to inferior practice that would engender public distrust in the regular profession and foster sectarian power.

The principle of specificity also informed objections to the overarching skeptical therapeutic philosophy of the Paris clinical school. The expectant method as it was exercised in French practice implied to some American practitioners an abnegation of professional responsibility. Although a noninterventionist plan might perhaps be suited to the inmates of Paris's hospitals (and even of this Americans had their doubts), most American physicians agreed that it was not appropriate for American circumstances, which demanded active treatment. An Ohio practitioner assured his readers that he was not one of those physicians "who prate to you about not giving much medicine. Such talk betrays infidelity to the healing art."[9]

The discomfort American physicians felt with the passivity of French practice was grounded in the fear that it threatened the foundations of what it meant to be a physician. At the core of their anxiety was a distinction between knowledge and practice in defining the physician's role. The American physician's objective, members of the profession believed, was primarily practical; he might be both scientist and practitioner, but the former was to be consistently subordinated to the latter. Many Americans feared that the "scientific" emphasis in French medicine, taken to mean a primary orientation toward understanding disease rather than intervening in it, was potentially subversive of practical medicine. Even those who were most enthusiastic about the promise of French medical science tended to believe that its practice embodied an embarrassing valuation of knowledge over healing.

American practitioners widely shared the perception that the physicians of the Paris clinical school were not on the whole particularly concerned with curing patients. "The French physicians study 'Diagnocis' or the cause of deseases," a student in South Carolina wrote in his lecture notebook in the mid-1850s. "They care very little whether the patient get well or not so long they understand the cause and discrimination. They are the best discriminating physicians in the world but not the best curers, the English and American far out strip them in this part of the *science*."[10] A Cincinnati practitioner who concurred in this appraisal charged that "the temporizing course [expectant method] pursued by the French renders their therapeutics often inefficient. In anatomy, physiology, and pathology, they stand unrivalled; but beyond this they seem scarcely to look. Having made a *diagnosis*, the next most important matter is to prove its correctness; and, as this can only be verified in the *dead body*, more enthusiasm is manifested in a post mortem examination than in the administration of medicine to cure disease. *The triumph with these physicians is in the dead-room.*"[11] Parisian therapeutic apathy and the disturbing vision of medicine in which ward patients were "mostly looked upon as good subjects for the dissecting knife"[12] represented to some Americans the evil potential of French therapeutic skepticism to support the conclusion that, because little could be done to cure disease, the physician should place his energies wholly in aid of understanding it.

A variation on this perception held that French physicians actively placed science above healing. According to this view the expectant method was not merely a bedside expression of greater faith in nature than in art but could represent purposeful avoidance of intervention for the sake of pathological enthusiasm. "In the Parisian hospitals," observed a Philadelphia medical professor who had just returned from France, "there is . . . often noticed such an intense devotion to mere scientific investigations, as causes the prescriber to forget the cure of the patient, in his anxiety to study the pathology of the complaint; and there is frequently more interest apparent on the part of their students, in noticing the post-mortem appearances, than there is in observing the restoration to health."[13] Robert Peter, who traveled from Kentucky to Paris in 1839 to purchase books, apparatus, and anatomical preparations for Transylvania's medical school, wrote to his wife that "human life is not esteemed of much value in the hospitals of Paris— an experiment is worth a dozen lives."[14]

Central to what disturbed American physicians about the French emphasis on pathology was the ambiguity, to their minds, in the relationship between pathological knowledge and therapeutic activity. Most Americans were willing to concede that investigations in the Paris hospitals had properly drawn into question the *extent* to which certain therapies were efficacious but not the assumption that they could be of benefit. Some went well beyond this, however, to suggest that the pathological inquiries of the Paris clinical school offered the most promising avenue to therapeutic certainty. "The French have arrived at a greater perfection in diagnosis and pathology than any other nation, and it is entirely owing to their having paid greater attention to the post mortem appearance of diseases," one student wrote in 1839. This knowledge, he asserted, was the only sure guide to therapeutic intervention. "From a knowledge of the pathology of diseases alone are we able to direct our therapeutical remedies with correctness and efficacy." Positive contributions to treatment were distressingly elusive, though, and most arguments for the therapeutic relevance of pathological knowledge were based on future promise rather than past achievement.[15]

On the other hand many American physicians denied that the knowledge produced by the Paris clinical school had contributed positively to therapeutic practice and doubted that it would improve practice in the future. "Though we can now *talk about disease* much more fluently and satisfactorily," the editor of a Virginia journal commented in 1859, "yet we cannot *cure* it a whit the quicker."[16] The majority of the American profession assumed that superior knowledge of pathology did not necessarily make a better practitioner. This seemed to be confirmed by a point on which virtually all American physicians agreed, namely, that while the French excelled in pathology, they were inferior to Americans as healers. James Lawrence Cabell mirrored the nearly universal American appraisal of French therapeutics when he wrote to his uncle from Paris, "I am far from being disappointed in the estimate I had formed of the capacity of the French physicians in discovering the exact seat of disease under the most complicated appearances; their skill is truly wonderful; but I have little confidence in their application of remedies."[17]

Some physicians feared that this perverse inversion that ranked knowledge above healing could infect American medicine. "According to modern notions, traceable to a Gallic origin," commented a Boston physician, "it is scientific to watch the phenomena of disease, but vulgar as well as unphilosophical to make any attempts to disturb the regular laws by which they are governed. Thus it is continually said of eminent practitioners in relation to curative measures, that they do nothing at all." All "honest men," he continued, must resist this French tendency, for "those foreign opinions, which consider the most desirable issue of any disease to be one that opens an opportunity for inspecting its locality, are somewhat contagious."[18]

Such perceptions that Parisian therapeutics was inferior and inapplicable for Americans and its achievements in improving medical treatment dubious were serious indictments of France as a source of knowledge about therapeutic practice. A Cincinnati physician reviewing the investigations of Parisian clinician Gabriel Andral concluded, "We are willing to rely on Andral in Pathology, but in therapeutics we will go elsewhere for instruction."[19] There was simply no reason for Americans to travel abroad in search of a commodity that could be found better and cheaper domestically. Moreover, many American physicians saw in the characteristic French union of scientific excellence with therapeutic impotence a threatening model for themselves. Practitioners concerned about the integrity of the American physician criticized colleagues who purportedly permitted their *"pathological vision"* to blind them to their patients' real needs.[20] "Physicians should never resemble those philosophers who pursue science or literature in the abstract, either for its own sake, or to furnish materials for others to employ. All the pursuits of practising physicians should have a practical tendency," one physician argued. "They are always out of their course, when they lose sight of practical utility."[21]

The most extreme fear the Paris model aroused in Americans was that excessive scientific zeal could unfit a man for practice, replacing his responsibility to patients with an allegiance to science. "No nation has contributed more, it is true, to the progress of medical science than the French," wrote Harvard medical professor John Ware. "But their tendency is to be satisfied with the science." Such a single-minded relish for science in a physician, Ware cautioned, could "vitiate his character as a practitioner."[22] Ware's selection of the word *character* is telling, for it was as much a man's character as his knowledge that made him a proper and effective physician. It is true that in the United States during much of the nineteenth century medicine was among the best avenues to a satisfactory career for the person whose primary objective was the pursuit of science, and there can be no doubt that some of those who chose medicine for its scientific appeal found practice distasteful.[23] Nevertheless, in a profession in which therapeutic activity was at the core of professional identity and morality, the fear that devotion to science could corrupt the practitioner was a serious one, and many of the American physicians who studied in Paris were wary of acquiring its taint.

Perhaps the clearest image of the moral debasement of the practitioner through scientific devotion and therapeutic apathy was that drawn by a popular French novelist. Eugène Sue's character Dr. Griffon, a Paris hospital physician who appears in *The Mysteries of Paris* (1843),[24] embodied the worst of what Americans feared in the character of science-oriented French clinicians. Set in the ward of a large Paris hospital, the scene that Sue describes is viewed largely from the perspective of two young women patients, La Lorraine, a poor consumptive laundress who has been in the hospital long enough to know its ways and who realizes she is dying, and Jeanne Duport, a fringe-maker who has just been forced to enter the hospital after being beaten and deserted by her husband. From their beds the two women share the stories of what brought them to the hospital, consider their fate, and witness the rounds of Dr. Griffon. The "learned doctor," Sue narrates, "considered the wards as a kind of school of experiments . . . These terrible experiments were, indeed, a human sacrifice made on the altar of science; but Dr. Griffon did not think of that. In the eyes of this *prince of science*, as they say in our days, the hospital patients were only a matter of study and experiment."

What is most striking is the interaction of Dr. Griffon with his "subjects." He enters the ward accompanied by a band of students and an acquaintance, the Comte de Saint Rémy, who is distraught by the scene before him, and is reproved by Dr. Griffon, "All these fine feelings must be left at the door, my dear Alcestis. Here we begin on the living those experiments and studies which we complete on the dead body in the amphitheatre." They proceed to the bed of an actress who has died overnight, and who, as Lorraine has told Jeanne, "was wretched at the idea of thinking that she would be dissected—cut to pieces." Lorraine has already made Jeanne promise that when she dies, Jeanne will claim her body to keep her from the same end. Dr. Griffon decides to "make a man happy" by allowing one of his students to dissect the actress's body rather than doing it himself. As Lorraine and Jeanne look on, the delighted student uses his scalpel to incise his initials into the actress's arm, "to take possession," as Dr. Griffon puts it.

Jeanne watches Dr. Griffon proceed through the ward until he reaches her bedside, where he pronounces to the pupils, "a new *subject!*" She is overwhelmed by shame at answering the doctor's questions before the crowd. Aware that her two small children will be turned out into the street if she does not return to them within the week, Jeanne begs the doctor to cure her quickly. But cure is not Dr. Griffon's intent, and "completely absorbed by scientific feelings, [he] did not give the smallest heed to Jeanne's distress." Instead, he describes to the pupils the postmortem appearances they may expect to find when they cut open her corpse. Jeanne suffers further humiliation when her bedclothes are removed but submits to the eager students' eyes because Dr. Griffon threatens her: "You will be turned out of the hospital, if you do not submit to the established usages." For Jeanne, Sue reminds the reader, "the hospital is the sole and last refuge." After Dr. Griffon's thorough examination, "the most studious of the pupils declared their wish to unite practice with theory, and also examine the patient."

As the ward round continues, the Comte de Saint Rémy recognizes a young patient to be a deceased friend's daughter who has fallen on bad times. He further learns that Dr. Griffon has just proposed to perform an especially murderous therapeutic experiment on her. "If you were not a madman, you would be a monster!" the count charges in despair. " 'Confound the man! Why has he so much science?' said the count . . . 'Eh! It is simple enough,' said the doctor in a whisper. 'I have a great deal of science because I study, because I experimentalise, because I risk and practice a great deal on my *subjects.* ' "

In the appraisal of Oliver Wendell Holmes, who was not in the least pleased by Sue's novel, there was little doubt that Dr. Griffon was intended to stand for his own Parisian mentor, Pierre Louis.[25] Whether or not Louis, whom another of his American pupils called "that 'Prince of medical logicians,' "[26] was Sue's model, many American physicians believed that the novelist's image of "the prince of science" as a man devoid of the moral sentiments they esteemed mirrored, albeit in refracted form, a disturbing reality.

Maintaining a steady orientation toward practical utility was of genuine concern to American physicians who studied in Paris, but most of them were more interested in absorbing as much scientific knowledge as possible than they were disturbed by the possibility of imperiling their character as practitioners through scientific excesses. Their time in Paris was often brief and opportunities limited for scientific inquiry after they returned to the United States. The demands of practice in America often subverted scientific aspirations. James Jackson, Jr.'s, ambition to devote several years entirely to hospital observation after returning to Boston, avoiding private practice, was gently but decisively vetoed by his father. "You can not prosecute your inquires here just as you do & can easily in Paris. This is one of the difficulties in your plan of exclusive observation," the elder Jackson explained. He reiterated a week later, "There are more difficulties than you see in doing the thing *à la Louis*. Boston is not Paris nor N Eng France."[27] The perceived dangers to the American physician of overindulgence in French medical science were generally checked by financial constraints if not by familial solicitude and the restrictions of the American environment.

The fear that Parisian influences would damage a physician's character went well beyond cautions against overemphasizing science, however. Other sources of corruption were of even greater immediate concern to the Americans who went to Paris. Many reported disapprovingly of having observed in their French mentors the sort of indifference and brutality toward patients that Sue portrayed in Dr. Griffon. French surgeons were particularly notorious for their harshness and insensitivity to their patients' suffering.[28] Americans also commonly observed that because life was little valued in Paris, high mortality in the hospitals produced little distress. One American medical student whom J. Y. Bassett had known in Paris wrote to him, "The medical world appears to do nothing but experiment in amputations at the joints, & they fail as often as they attempt. They will soon diminish the population of *France*."[29] American physicians were further disturbed, as was Eugène Sue, by Parisian physicians' disregard for patients' modesty. One Georgia physician dissented from Paris clinician

Lisfranc's "entire disregard of delicacy" in his use of the speculum uteri. "Certainly M. Lisfranc never gave a thought to the additional afflictions of the female, which never fail to be added by the unnecessary wounding of her modesty," he commented, suggesting that such an insult was not quite moral.[30] Attitudes of indifference, brutality, and indecent violation toward patients represented standards of behavior Americans openly denounced as unprofessional, immoral, and fundamentally threatening. An American molded by these influences, they believed, would be debased as a practitioner.

Americans perceived a further threat to the physician's character, and thereby to his efficacy as a practitioner, in the very experience of living in Paris: he might become contaminated by local values and mores. If this corruption took a relatively innocuous form, the American student might slip in his appreciation of the moral value of work;[31] but there was real concern that the vitiated moral atmosphere of Paris would leave the physician irreparably tainted. In 1833 the young George Cheyne Shattuck carefully recorded in his diary the cautioning remarks of Dr. Mussey, one of his professors at medical school in Brunswick, Maine. "He says that Paris is a place of abominations, and but few Americans who pass any time there escape being ruined," Shattuck wrote. "The French work from five in morning to five P.M. and then go to the opera or the brothel. The laxity of the women is astonishing. One gentleman was asked by his landlady if he had ever put a woman to bed and for how many he had done that office. A female lecturer on midwifery demonstrated on the live subject. An instance was mentioned of a young Canadian who went to Paris to study medicine, boarded, with a young widow, made love to her daughter and slept between them. His constitution was completely broken down."[32]

The perceived moral laxness of Paris threatened to debase the American physician's potency not as a scientist but as a practitioner. It did not corrupt knowledge itself but the character of the man who determined how it would be applied. Parisian values and the realities of the Paris experience, in the minds of American physicians, posed a real threat to professional rectitude that could ultimately make the practitioner ineffective in his therapeutic role.

Throughout the decades when American physicians' gaze on the body of European medical knowledge focused on Paris, those who traveled to France often visited England, Scotland, and Ireland as well, and sometimes Germany and Italy. Americans' attitudes toward French medicine reflected in varying degrees their regard for European medicine in general.

English therapeutic knowledge, for example, was subject to constraints imposed by the principle of specificity comparable to those applied to French medicine. Americans in London routinely praised the diagnostic and pathological skill they observed in the hospitals, at the same time pointing out that therapeutic precepts validated there were not necessarily transferable to American bedsides.[33] A Kentucky medical professor visiting the London hospitals in 1845 was particularly struck by the very limited therapeutic use of calomel and bloodletting. "A course of practice which with us would prove successful, would necessarily be fatal here from its very activity," he noted. "That bleeding should be tolerated here to a less extent than in the United States, is not surprising; and that tonics and stimulants should find an extensive and appropriate application, is what might be anticipated from the habits of other modifying circumstances that so powerfully influence the constitutions of the inhabitants of London; and hence it is that iron, quinine, porter, wine &c, are frequently employed, when an American physician would resort to depletion."[34]

Americans generally agreed that England much more than France resembled the United States in both therapeutic philosophy and moral character. "The English, like ourselves," Harvard medical professor John Ware proposed, "are essentially a practical people. The first question with them in all matters of science is, What is the use? We owe as striking scientific results, perhaps, to the French as to the English, but who have originated the principal applications of science to the arts?" Anglophile Ware added that the social, moral, cultural, and religious similarities between the United States and England were valid reasons for preferring a medical training in England to one in France. Noting that "religious opinions and religious feelings form a highly important part of the medical character," he suggested that "the greater resemblance in the moral and religious standard of society in England to our own" would make the English-trained American a more successful practitioner than his French-educated counterpart.[35]

Compared with the French, American and British physicians shared an inclination toward therapeutic activism. "The English say, that [French] patients die from apathy in treatment," one physician noted. "On the contrary, let us not disguise the fact, that the English are charged by their French neighbors, with destroying *their* patients by the *activity* of treatment!"[36] The majority of Americans agreed that while Paris's physicians were in advance of London's in such basic medical sciences as pathology, English therapy was decidedly superior. Physician Joseph T. Webb wrote from London in 1870 to his brother-in-law Rutherford B. Hayes, "I find Medicine & Surgery more advanced here, than on the Continent, although in the Study of disease; one has greater advantages in Germany & France—but the Treatment of disease I much prefer here."[37]

The fact that despite London's therapeutic superiority American physicians more often elected to spend their time abroad in Paris reinforces the point that American physicians in Europe were primarily in search of knowledge and experience in areas other than medical therapeutics. The similarities between American and British therapeutic inclinations and many Americans' belief that Britain was the most therapeutically enlightened nation in Europe did make Americans particularly attentive to British trends in medical treatment. American literature carefully logged the changing therapeutic thought of such physicians as Bennett, Forbes, Stokes, and Todd, but from these men's writings Americans drew principally substantiation and foils for their own beliefs. They looked to Britain not so much for a source of therapeutic change as for a voice to second their own therapeutic positions. The decision to go to Paris instead was also a simple recognition of the fact that the restrictive organization of hospital teaching in London and its high expense to the student made it more difficult for Americans to gain knowledge and experience there.[38]

By the 1860s the destination of most American physicians traveling to Europe for study had begun to shift from Paris to German cities and especially to Vienna. In part this was due to changes in the structure of clinical teaching in Paris that diminished its attractiveness to foreign students.[39] The main medical attraction of Vienna was the immense number of patients gathered at the Allgemeines Krankenhaus and the exceptionally free access students had to these inmates. Joseph T. Webb, who in the late 1860s spent several years studying in Paris, London, Vienna, and Berlin, wrote to his brother from Paris, "I shall go to Vienna the first of next month[.] There is much to learn here; but I am satisfied that Vienna, is all things considered the *best*—you get more *at* the patient in Vienna, than here."[40] Seven weeks later he wrote to his brother-in-law from the Allgemeines Krankenhaus, "This is by far the grandest Hospital in the world; there is nothing to compare to it, in Paris or London,"[41] and added an important qualification in a letter to his sister: "It is by far the best Hospital *for Doctors*, in Europe—think of it *Ten thousand children born in it every year*."[42] Because of its unmatched opportunities for intensive clinical experience, teaching in physical diagnosis, instruction in the emerging medical specialties, and work in pathological anatomy, Vienna became the favored place for American students to complete their medical studies.

The therapeutic precepts of Vienna and Berlin were subjected to American criticisms based on the principle of specificity that were reminiscent of those brought against Parisian treatment. Moreover,

Americans were nearly unanimous in their belief that physicians in the German hospitals were even less interested than the French in medical therapeutics and that some Viennese clinicians such as Joseph Dietl had extended skepticism to true nihilism. "The Germans as a race," one American in Vienna wrote, "are certainly preëminent for the originality of their investigations and for their abstract ideas; but, for the practical application of their knowledge, they are far inferior to the English and Americans."[43] This lack of interest in therapeutics, many Americans held, reflected the German valuation of science over healing. Commenting on physicians of "Teutonic proclivities," one American noted that "the day of triumph for such pathologists is not in that of the cure, but while by the side of the cadaver, scalpel in hand, holding up the diseased organs with 'I told you so' beaming joyfully from all the lineaments of the face."[44] The German posture toward therapeutics plainly was not a congenial model for Americans. As Webb wrote to his mother from Berlin, "In the Hospitals the study is to know, what is the matter; then they Stop. In *'Diagnosis'*, they excel; but in *Treatment* we excel."[45]

Like Parisian medicine, German clinical medicine in some respects threatened the American practitioner. The implications of Viennese skepticism for the professional identity of American physicians, for example, were severe. Moreover, Americans found the brutality, insensitivity, and disregard for modesty that they deplored in some Parisian physicians still more exaggerated among the Viennese. A Boston physician in Vienna noted that patients were used "as if the principal purpose of their being in the hospital was to illustrate lectures."[46]

Viennese and Parisian clinicians were, in American eyes, similar in their moral and therapeutic characters. They were excellent scientists but poor healers. Some Americans were taking from German laboratories new strategies for therapeutic evaluation and advancement that fundamentally altered therapeutic epistemology in America and promised to transform practice as well. But most American physicians who went to the German hospitals did not go for therapeutic instruction and resolutely maintained their belief in the superiority of American to European therapeutic practice.

The ambivalence Americans felt toward the therapeutic relevance of French medical knowledge and methods is displayed by their attitudes toward the numerical method. The devotion of a small cadre of American students to Pierre Louis, the method's leading proponent, gave personal meaning to their proselytization of it; this in turn gives special meaning to their appreciation of its limitations. The persistent tensions between specificity and universalism, certainty and uncertainty, science and practice, and knowledge and action became still more volatile in the context of the American adjudication of the numerical method's therapeutic worth. Attitudes toward it also show that not only Parisian knowledge but also its methods were value laden in America.

There can be no doubt that from the 1820s on the numerical method had an important influence on clinical evaluation and that it provided one form of evidence to support therapeutic change. Progressive quantification has clearly been among the most obvious trends in the organization of medical knowledge since that time. But the often-proposed notion that the application of the numerical method to therapeutic evaluation provided a compelling basis for rejecting heroic therapy in America is suspect. The reservations physicians expressed about therapeutic judgments informed by the method went well beyond the common caution that some questions were not amenable to numerical assessment. James Jackson, Jr., perhaps the most devoted of Louis's American pupils, acknowledged in a letter to his father, "There are without doubt many questions that cannot be resolved by counting."[47] And Jackson, Sr., who used the numerical method in appraising therapeutic practices at the Massachusetts General Hospital, wrote to his son that "though statistics are very valuable—yet we always find that a man who placed great reliance on them in any branch of science, physical, moral, or political, is apt to make the mistake of thinking that two and two always make four—which they do not."[48] A number of factors deeply ingrained in the professional ethos constrained Americans' willingness to accept such numerical data as having any real meaning for their own practices. At the most the numerical method applied to therapeutics was very suggestive; at the least it was irrelevant.

The numerical method's most extreme advocates believed that it would revolutionize medicine. "*Disease has never, until quite recently, been investigated*," a Massachusetts physician asserted in 1836. What "has been christened medical *science*, is in fact nothing but hypothesis piled upon hypothesis; who is there amongst us that would not exult in seeing it swept away?"[49] The numerical method, he claimed, promised to bring certainty to medicine, to make it an exact science. Most enthusiasts confined such aspirations to pathology and diagnosis, but he saw the method as an avenue to therapeutic certainty as well and prophesied that the profession would witness "a *theory of therapeutics* formed which shall be as immutable as any other natural law." To do this, he urged, investigators needed only "to place the different articles in a situation where they can act upon the system, observe the results, and arrange them in *numerical order*. Thus we would carry our arithmetic along with us, not only in the *study of disease*, but in the *treatment of it*."[50]

But while a few physicians asserted that therapeutic certainty could be attained by mere force of numbers, most saw such extreme statements of revolutionary intent as dangerous assaults upon tradition. The claim that with the "French stars" disease was for the first time really being investigated, one physician charged, was tantamount to saying "that our revered Hippocrates, Boerhaave, Cullen, and other eminent physicians, knew nothing about induction or generalization, were ignoramuses in pathology and therapeutics, unable to reason correctly, and that their works are less than useless to the medical student!"[51] Practicing physicians could not hold their decisions about treating patients in abeyance until their therapies received numerical approbation. More than this, they were not prepared to accept even in principle the proposition that they should discard existing therapeutic beliefs and practices, validated by both tradition and their own experience, on account of somebody else's numbers.

Many of their objections turned upon the principle of specificity. However applicable knowledge produced by the numerical method might be in the context within which it was generated, counting ceased to count when removed to a different locus. "Time and place," one physician observed, "may render the statistics of different epochs, or localities, wholly valueless for comparison with others."[52] The variability that characterized disease, the human constitution, and the physical and social environments meant that statistically determined therapeutic precepts had only very limited applicability even to the time, place, and category of patients from which they had come. Because the numerical method was by necessity most often applied to the urban poor in large hospitals, the therapeutic knowledge it produced was in some ways irrelevant for the daily tasks of physicians in private practice.

The principle of specificity undermined pretensions of the numerical method's advocates that it could bring about therapeutic certainty. "Some modern French writers," a physician reviewing Louis's work on typhoid fever stated, "are constantly trying to make us believe that medicine is capable of being rendered an *exact* science, and that we must not admit any positions in our reasonings on disease but what can be proved by actual observation." Reflecting the professional importance of observing specificity, he noted that "this is a most foolish and dangerous doctrine. As in moral and political philosophy, so in medicine, there are no permanently fixed and unalterable rules which are inevitably true at all times and under all circumstances."[53] Bennet Dowler, a New Orleans advocate of the hygienic relevance of vital statistics, pointed out that the extreme changeability of therapeutic indicators meant that physicians could never agree on treatment sufficiently to establish certainty. "Mathematicians, physicists, and astronomers agree, because the fundamental laws of terrestrial and celestial mechanics are fixed, known, demonstrable," he argued. "But the changeful conditions of morbidity, and the apparently variable actions of medicinal agents, certain enough in themselves, exist in relation to the human understanding as probabilities of varying intensities which cannot be defined and reduced to axioms."[54]

A persistent argument against the usefulness of the numerical method was the objection that practitioners treated individual patients, not populations. In part this was simply a variation on the theme of specificity. "We do not treat numerous sufferers in a mass, without separate, individual examination, but fully consider all the peculiar circumstances of each, which should modify treatment," asserted the young Austin Flint, who became a leading American proselytizer of Parisian methods of physical diagnosis. "In formation of rules of treatment, the numeric system disregards these peculiar circumstances."[55] The responsible physician attended to "the individuality of each case"; anything less was unprofessional routinism. "No depth of observation, no accuracy of numbers, no vastness of tables, and no grasp of memory, will ever enable the practical physician to reduce the case before him to real rule and measure," one physician asserted in 1860, "or to dispense with the necessity of considering each patient by and for himself."[56]

More than just a commitment to specificity drove the objection that the numerical method's products were of little help to the practitioner, however. Underlying prejudices against the method were the broader propositions that French medicine had contributed nothing to treatment and that excessive attention to the intricacies of science could enfeeble the physician's efforts to heal. Many American practitioners assailed Louis's work on the distinction between typhus and typhoid fevers for its failure to contribute anything to treatment.[57] One physician quipped, "As to therapeutics, Louis ordains the remedy nearest at hand—quinine, opium, warm or cold water, *ad libitum*—or nothing at all. Then make up the mortuary statistics and decide on treatment."[58] Enthusiasm for numerical tabulations could, some physicians argued, distract attention from the peculiarities of a case and lead to inferior care. Jackson, Sr., even claimed that he did not preserve copious records of his cases because note taking prevented him from giving adequate attention to his patient's needs.[59]

The numerical method was also discredited as a revealer of therapeutic truth by its tacit link to sectarian therapeutics. In the eyes of many regular physicians, numerical assessments of homeopathic practice yielding cure rates that compared favorably with those of regular practice plainly indicted either the numerical method or the way it was used. Their suspicion was aggravated by the fact that a few orthodox physicians used these homeopathic statistics to argue that homeopathic therapy (regarded as equivalent to letting nature act unhindered) was in no way inferior to regular treatment. Such claims were easily discounted by the argument that any physician who would intentionally allow a patient to be treated homeopathically was professionally irresponsible and therefore an unreliable reporter. Nevertheless, physicians came early to the conclusion that statistics could be manipulated and perverted to support whatever conclusion their user wished to establish. "Statistical argument," Dowler noted, "is virtually neutralized by the significant fact that every mode of treatment from the heroic to the infinitesimal claims its protection and takes shelter under its autocratic sanction."[60] That many American physicians virtually rejected the validity of the numerical method as a way to gain therapeutic knowledge in part because of its homeopathic associations is a clear instance of the social context of medical practice influencing physicians' epistemological allegiances.

Louis's own numerical assessment of venesection in pneumonitis, while it undoubtedly raised questions about the extent to which bloodletting was beneficial under various circumstances, did not challenge venesection as a practice of great therapeutic value. Few Americans, even the most enthusiastic followers of French medicine, were willing to draw very extensive practical conclusions from Louis's work. Jackson, Sr., who confirmed Louis's researches by applying the numerical method at the Massachusetts General Hospital, noted in his preface to a translation of the Frenchman's work, "If any thing may be regarded as settled in the treatment of diseases, it is that bloodletting is useful in the class of diseases called inflammatory; and especially in inflammations of the thoracic viscera. To the general opinion, or belief on this subject M. Louis gives support by his observations; but the result of these observations is that the benefits derived from bleeding in the diseases, which he has here examined, are not so great and striking as they have been represented by many teachers."[61] The conclusions Louis drew about the efficacy of bloodletting were cautious; a practitioner who followed the implications of his work to their fullest extension might bleed in pneumonitis to mitigate the severity of the disease or to relieve pain rather than to cut the disease short but might bleed nonetheless. On the whole, although the numerical method could produce provocative conclusions that encouraged re-evaluation of prior practices, objections to it were too thoroughgoing for the method to be able to dictate changes in practice.[62]

Furthermore, American physicians repeatedly emphasized that the value of the numerical method was far greater in all other areas of medicine than in therapeutics. When Joseph LeConte forcefully asserted that statistics represented the most promising means of advancing medical science, for example, he defined medical science in a way that excluded therapeutics.[63] On the whole, Louis attained higher regard in the eyes of the American profession for his pathological studies distinguishing between typhoid and typhus fever than for his therapeutic researches on bloodletting. As one practitioner reviewing his writings noted, "It is well known that this gentleman, however high he may be regarded as a morbid anatomist, cannot be appealed to as an authority on practical subjects."[64] Alfred Stillé wrote bluntly to G. C. Shattuck (both of them were devoted pupils of Louis) in 1842, "I confess that I do not think the numerical system very applicable to therapeutics."[65] Most Americans who applied the numerical method to therapeutic evaluation drew conclusions from their work only with great reserve. The majority of American physicians clearly agreed, though, that applications of the numerical method in the United States, whether to pathological or to therapeutic inquiry, would be of much greater value to American physicians than was European research.

American physicians were far readier to embrace French therapeutic epistemology and the methods of advancing therapeutic knowledge founded upon it than they were to accept actual therapeutic knowledge produced in France. Such selectivity was entirely in keeping with the localistic, in this case nationalistic, criteria for therapeutic relevance that the principle of specificity decreed. The Paris school's emphasis on empirical clinical observation made a critically important contribution to the transformation of American therapeutics; the impact made by the example of French practice was by comparison modest.

The openness of American students to the therapeutic epistemology of the Paris school made them less rather than more receptive to French teachings about therapeutic practice. According to the French point of view, therapeutic change would come about through empirical observation of diseases and the actions of remedies on them. This belief, reinforced by the underlying faith in the principle of specificity, encouraged the notion that therapeutic knowledge suited to the American context was best generated and validated by observing the operation of therapies on American patients in American environments.

The Parisian emphasis on empirical clinical observation was therefore inherently inimical to American acceptance of French therapeutic knowledge.

This antagonistic relationship is apparent, for example, in reactions elicited by New York physician Martyn Paine's *Medical and Physiological Commentaries* (1840), which, in the appraisal of Louis's Boston pupil Henry Ingersoll Bowditch, was "a violent attack" on the numerical method and on Louis in particular.[66] Paine's explicit objective, according to another observer, was to "un-numericalize" the American students of Louis.[67] A prolonged dispute between Paine and Bowditch ensued. One central thrust of Paine's assault accused the numerical method of ignoring the differences in disease and therapeutic need imposed by differing circumstances, especially by variations in environment and type of patient. Louis's method, he charged, "rejects all observation that is not founded upon it, brings pathology and therapeutics under the dominion of mathematics, regards not the various considerations which relate to climate, constitution, habits, age, sex, &c., and practically knows little else than a *balance sheet*."[68]

Bowditch's rebuttal was in effect an affirmation that Louis believed in the principle of specificity. "It must be always kept in mind that Louis collected his facts in Paris, and from them deduced his results," Bowditch noted. Louis had derived his statistics from observation in the Paris hospitals, and Bowditch contended that no one, least of all Louis, would wish to suggest that conclusions drawn from them were applicable to a situation defined by a different location, warmer climate, or distinct patient population. As to the differences between the Paris hospitals and other contexts, Bowditch stated, Louis "left that for others and future observers to decide."[69] The ultimate implication of these remarks for American physicians was that while Louis's method was useful and its underlying empiricist epistemology sound, conclusions derived from his application of the numerical method to therapeutic evaluation in Paris were at best only suggestive for American practice. If American physicians wanted therapeutic knowledge meaningful for their practices and patients, they would have to find it themselves.

The Parisian emphasis on empirical observation fostered the notion that in such realms of medicine as therapeutics, knowledge could best be gathered and transmitted from the patient to whom and the place to which it would ultimately be applied. This in turn encouraged American physicians to place their trust only in facts that had been seen in America and interpreted through American eyes. "The school of Louis," Philadelphia physician Robley Dunglison charged in 1839, was apt to make the physician rely on his own observation to the exclusion of all other practitioners' experience. It could, in other words, "convey the too exclusive idea, that self-observation is alone necessary to make the accomplished pathologist and physician."[70] Dunglison's remark was singularly perceptive. French clinical empiricism as it was used in the United States redoubled the commitment to the principle of specificity and its localistic implications.

American physicians, drawn to Paris by the opportunities offered in its hospitals but suspicious of its therapeutic practices, took up and used French medicine very selectively. Parisian clinical empiricism contributed substantially to a remolding of therapeutic epistemology in the United States, urging American practitioners to observe for themselves the effects of their therapeutic efforts. At the same time, it strengthened the American profession's therapeutic nationalism by reinforcing the principle of specificity and the notion that foreign therapeutic knowledge was of dubious value for local practice. The ultimate irony of American physicians' relationship to French medicine was that they could use the epistemology of the Paris clinical school to invalidate the usefulness of much of its knowledge, especially its therapeutic knowledge, for their own use.

— 7 —

The Arbitration
of Change

TENSIONS BETWEEN the commitment to progress and loyalty to tradition became particularly acute in the discussions about therapeutic change that flourished in medical circles from the 1850s through the 1870s. The function of these discussions was at once explanatory and normative, for through them physicians sought to account for the dramatic transformation that had taken place in practice since the early decades of the century and to establish a consensus for current and future practice. Evaluation of past therapeutic change and disputation of present therapeutic truth were parts of a single endeavor. This endeavor is illustrated here by an analysis of the profession's discussions about the decline of the two treatments most securely linked with early-nineteenth-century therapeutics, general bloodletting and calomel, and about a drug brought forward to replace venesection, veratrum viride. Such discussions clearly exhibit physicians' reasoning about change and the range of factors they regarded as meaningful in explaining, judging, and advocating it.

The potential of therapeutic criticism to indict both professional tradition and current efficacy was high, and regular physicians observed certain tacit rules commensurate with the risk. Internal therapeutic criticism rarely drew into question the value in principle of established remedies. (In contrast, sectarians generally charged that orthodox therapies were in themselves damaging.) Discussion among regulars ordinarily dwelled instead on theory, the rationale for therapeutic beliefs, and the extent to which particular practices were or were not useful in certain defined conditions. Even if the actual use of a practice was modified or the theory sustaining it changed, its value could nonetheless be fully upheld in principle. Criticism of theory and practice could thus bring about what was regarded as progress with only minimal threat to tradition.

A further stricture upon internal criticism was that it be kept as far as possible out of public view. External criticism was by nature and calculation conducted in a manner that drew public attention; a primary objective of sectarians was, after all, to discredit orthodox practice in the public view. Regulars realized that internal discord could inadvertently serve the same end, and therefore they established rules for conducting therapeutic discussion that were designed to blunt its potential harm. The committee on ethics of a local Ohio medical society was typical in the advice it gave its members on maintaining the appearance of a unified therapeutic front. Disagreements that arose in consultation, for example, were to be discussed and resolved without allowing the public to become aware of professional disharmony. "Neither the subject-matter of such differences nor the adjudications of the arbitrators," the committee concluded in 1853, "should be made public as publicity in a case of this nature may be personally injurious to the individuals concerned and can hardly fail to bring discredit on the faculty."[1]

No therapy occupied a more prominent position in the ideology of early-nineteenth-century medicine than did venesection. Yet even in the 1820s the attitude of most regular American physicians toward general bloodletting was ambivalent. Professionally respectable physicians did not challenge its value in principle and accepted as a solidly established truth the proposition that it could be of substantial therapeutic worth. Many did, however, question the measure of venesection's therapeutic benefits as well as the vigor with which it was practiced.[2]

During the 1830s and 1840s a heretical challenge to the principle of bloodletting was also voiced, but only by those outside the regular profession. Sectarians assailed the notion that it could ever be of therapeutic value. This assault encouraged both regular physicians and the public to reassess its use but also elicited from regulars a defensive reaffirmation of bloodletting in principle. Orthodox physicians, reflecting in their thinking the simplistic dichotomy between good and evil typical of sectarian conflicts in general, attributed the sectarian attack on venesection chiefly to irregular ignorance and duplicity, yet accorded a portion of the blame to regular excesses.[3]

By the 1830s most regular physicians agreed that bloodletting had been abused. It was perhaps the profession's most valuable treatment, according to this view, and did inestimable good when judiciously employed. But, as one Cincinnati student explained in 1831, "many Physicians bleed indiscriminately for, finding they have a certain remedy in many dangerous diseases [they] conclude from its power, not fully apprehending its qualities[,] that it may be useful every where."[4] In the appraisal of physicians, the rote use of venesection fueled the sectarian assault on orthodox treatment and debased the profession before the public. It also encouraged the public to place blame for harm done by venesection on the practice itself rather than on its users, where it belonged. "The truth is," one physician asserted, "that it is the improper application of remedies and not their inapplicable character, that renders them useless or injurious."[5]

Yet bloodletting retained a cardinal symbolic importance for the regular medical profession. Since the time of Hippocrates, physicians ceaselessly reminded each other, it "has had the endorsement of each age and generation through which it has passed."[6] Venesection was an insignia of the regular physician, a function evinced by the names of medical journals such as the *Western Lancet*. External attacks on the principle redoubled its symbolic significance, for faith in bloodletting was a clearly recognizable badge of professional regularity. It was therefore important to regular physicians that bloodletting not be rejected in principle, whatever might be its status in actual practice. When a petition to the legislature of New York in 1852 called for a legal enactment against it, one physician responded that while it was not his purpose "to advocate the once general practice of blood-letting; such practice has, with much propriety, . . . long since fallen into disuse," nevertheless "to abandon it under all conceivable circumstances would, we apprehend, be running into fatal error."[7]

The meaning of the strident affirmation of bloodletting's worth in principle is best understood against the backdrop of the sharp decline in its actual practice. Though there was no definitive break in the use of venesection, by and large the mid-1850s through the early 1860s saw its eclipse in American therapy. These years rather than the preceding decades (during which the rate of venesection's decline was quickest) marked precisely the period when the discussion on bloodletting among regular physicians became most intense. The timing of the discussion—which was energetically pursued only after bloodletting's decline in practice was an accomplished fact that nearly all regular physicians acknowledged—is important. It suggests that the objective was less to establish normative rules for practice than to rationalize the evident disparity between principle and practice and understand its implications for professional tradition. Physicians felt constrained to account for the change in practice, to judge its merits, and to reconcile it with the standing of venesection in principle.

What was new in the mid-1850s was that for the first time the possibility seemed very real that bloodletting might vanish from medical practice. Up to this point there had been virtually no internal questioning of the principle, though physicians had vigorously debated how useful or harmful bloodletting carried to various extents might be for diverse disease conditions, stages, and environments. The discussion that thrived from the 1850s through the mid-1870s was of a new type from that which preceded it. With its virtual abandonment in practice an acknowledged possibility, it became necessary to ask whether general bloodletting itself was a good therapy. And if its value was affirmed in principle, it was then necessary to explain its decline in practice.

Physicians conducted the bloodletting discussion principally in medical society meetings and through journals. Occasionally discussions on bloodletting were scheduled in advance on medical society programs, but more often they arose spontaneously in response to a paper delivered on the treatment of a particular disease. The journal literature not generated by society proceedings commonly was prompted by a fear of overreaction against venesection and its complete abandonment. The other principal context in which the discussion emerged was in response to foreign debates and claims about venesection.

What provoked many physicians to take part was a desire to defend their medical forefathers. Most who contrasted their own disuse of bloodletting with its active employment by their preceptors were unwilling to indict either present or past practice. "Are there no cases in which bleeding is absolutely required?" one physician asked. "Were our forefathers entirely mistaken?"[8] Defending the efficacy of bloodletting in prior practice also had awkward implications, however. Reflecting the other side of the physician's dilemma, a Massachusetts physician asked in 1865, "Are we willing to admit that physicians of to-day can accomplish less than our medical fathers of fifty years agone?"[9]

To a large extent physicians avoided making a choice between principle and practice by agreeing that bloodletting was a valuable therapy in principle and restricting their debate to its use in practice. Thus at the close of an energetic debate in 1859 on the use and abuse of bloodletting among members of the St. Louis Medical Society in which all participants concurred that the lancet was only infrequently used, one physician concluded that "few, if any, of our members are opposed to blood-letting in toto, and . . . those who do object to it, only oppose general bleeding and depletion in specific fevers; . . . we find none opposing blood-letting, and judging from that, we must conclude, that the lancet holds the same place as a remedial measure, among well educated medical men, that it ever did."[10]

The pivotal questions in most discussions were: Why had the change in practice occurred? And was the change a good thing? In answering, physicians unavoidably passed judgment upon both present and past practice. Their criticisms and explanations made very little difference for actual therapeutic behavior, but the symbolic importance of bloodletting was such that their assessments had serious implications for the supportive relationship that existed between therapeutic tradition and professional identity. Physicians' answers to these questions were deeply imprinted by their dual commitment to progress and to tradition and by their assumptions about the nature of proper therapeutic change.

Some physicians, to be sure, held the decline of venesection in practice to be a mistake. They recognized that bloodletting had been abused and acknowledged that to the extent that earlier excesses had been moderated, the change was for the better. They maintained, however, that the therapeutic deficit resulting from an overreaction against bloodletting outweighed this benefit. "The tendency to abandon the practice of general bloodletting, in the treatment of disease: Is it evidence of an advance or retrograde movement in Therapeutics?" a speaker to the Medical Association of the State of Georgia began his address in 1860. The orator, like most physicians, held that the decline had righted prior abuses, but also feared that the reaction against it was "apt to bury, in one common tomb, the evil and false—the beautiful, the good, and the true."[11] Those physicians who went further charged that the move away from bloodletting was "a concession to the various shades of empiricism,"[12] an unprofessional therapeutic surrender to popular prejudice and sectarian pressure. Nevertheless, only a small minority was prepared to conclude that the practice of medicine was the worse for the alteration.[13]

Diverse explanations for the change in practice shared the conclusion that while venesection was in principle sound, the decline in its employment nonetheless represented progress. Overzealous devotion to rationalistic systems had seduced many physicians to abuse a fundamentally good therapy, and the change in practice redressing this imbalance was judicious. The sources of reappraisal (and thereby change) that physicians identified included a new allegiance to empiricism and clinical observation, the application of medical statistics to therapeutic evaluation, a better appreciation of the healing power of nature, the example of homeopathic successes, and improved knowledge of the natural history of diseases against which the curative influence of remedies could be measured.

All the constituent elements of this accounting for change were subject to criticism, and in the context of the bloodletting discussions physicians rehearsed their assaults on unthinking empiricism, the doubtful relevance of statistical findings to treating the individual patient, the threat of inactivity perceived in overreliance on nature, the illegitimacy of the homeopathic example as a source of knowledge, and the inapplicability of clinical knowledge derived from one setting to practice in others. Still, this type of explanation for change had substantial appeal and was widely endorsed. It sustained the idea that bloodletting was good in principle. It also accounted for the overuse of bloodletting in the past and acknowledged that harm had been done without directly charging that regular physicians had given their primary allegiance to an injurious therapy. Change in medical therapeutics was expected, and it was not necessarily an indictment of tradition for members of an avowedly progressive profession to say that practice had progressed.

A further variant on explanations that sustained the principle of bloodletting proposed that new or newly popular therapeutic agents had come into use which physicians had found to equal or surpass venesection in meeting many indications. Chief among these were the cardiac sedatives aconite and veratrum viride. Similarly, in the South and West many physicians argued that the rise to fashion in the 1840s of large doses of quinine had fostered disuse of the lancet. Although physicians disputed the propriety of calling such practices substitutes or replacements for bloodletting—and even in the 1870s most would have felt discomfort at a New Orleans physician's claim that such drugs were rendering venesection "obsolete"[14]—they acknowledged that therapeutic alternatives to bloodletting had diminished its use. This claim neither implied that prior use of bloodletting had been bad (it may have represented the best of available therapy) nor questioned its value in principle, yet it did affirm that the change in practice represented progress.

A very different explanation proposed that an advanced knowledge of physiology, pathology, and chemistry had disclosed the error of bloodletting, properly leading to its disuse. Pathophysiological investigation had illuminated the processes involved in inflammation and its resolution, this view held, showing that bloodletting could not effect the therapeutic benefits physicians had hitherto ascribed to it. This stance was premised on the notion that reasoning from knowledge about basic science was a proper guide to therapeutic action—an epistemological step most physicians, committed to clinical empiricism, were hesitant to take.[15] Although this explanation for venesection's decline recruited relatively few proponents, its seeming heterodoxy gave it singular visibility. Most of the physicians who used knowledge of basic science to deny bloodletting's therapeutic value were young and enthusiastic about the promise of laboratory science to transform medical therapeutics, and they looked to a particular kind of scientific knowledge rather than to the authority of tradition for support.

This explanation had devastating implications. At its core was the assumption that scientific knowledge had proven bloodletting to be bad in principle; the practice itself was therapeutically useless or harmful. Such an explanation carried an open indictment of the practices of all physicians who had used and were using venesection, a call for the rejection of bloodletting from practice, and a vindication of sectarian attacks. In the appraisal of one physician, this position was "a candid confession of previous ignorance, incompetency, and maltreatment."[16] This explanation did unambiguously affirm that the decline of bloodletting was progressive, but it was progress not harmonized with medical tradition but rather accomplished through its desecration.

Opposed to this account for the change in practice was the change-of-type theory, which held the transformation in practice to be a prudent adaptation of treatment to changing conditions. Whereas the systemic overexcitement characteristically witnessed in patients before the 1830s had demanded depletive therapies such as bloodletting, the debilitated conditions observed in subsequent years required supportive or stimulative treatments. As they did most explanations, physicians ordinarily argued the change-of-type theory in conjunction with other rationales for change. Still, of all the explanations for the decline of bloodletting offered from the 1850s to the 1870s, the idea of a change of type was by far the most common.

The change-of-type theory was undoubtedly the most reassuring rationale for venesection's decline. The principle of specificity created an expectation of change in treatment over time as well as place and condition. Accordingly the disuse of a therapy did not necessarily draw into question its inherent value but only its suitability for the therapeutic needs that prevailing circumstances dictated. Despite the transformation in practice, therefore, the principle of bloodletting was preserved inviolate; former practice had been appropriate to the needs of its time, and the current disuse of bloodletting was equally correct since venesection was no longer often called for. If a physician elected to include in his brief supporting the change of type the idea that prior use of bloodletting had been regrettably extreme (a step not logically necessary though usually taken), then he could affirm that its decline was progress. But that affirmation did not indict the practice itself. Even a judgment that former practice had not been excessive implied that the change was neutral, not retrograde, and was fully consistent with a confident belief that the current disuse of bloodletting was as it should be.

The change-of-type theory provided an explanation for the decline of bloodletting so exquisitely comforting to the medical profession that the temptation is strong to dismiss it as a post hoc construction put together to explain away a potentially compromising disparity between principle and practice. Unquestionably it was to an extent a device designed to save professional face: only in the 1850s, after bloodletting's employment had substantially diminished, did physicians widely proselytize the change-of-type theory as a formal doctrine. As the secretary of the Cincinnati Academy of Medicine noted in the 1860s following a discussion on bloodletting that had dwelled upon the change of type, the subject was "discussed to death."[17] The experience and testimony of physicians whose careers spanned the period of supposed change made up the theory's entire evidential foundation; the phenomenon of a change in type could not be refuted by younger physicians. But while older physicians did tend to embrace the change-of-type theory, many younger ones supported it as well.

In part the singular vogue for the change-of-type theory in the 1850s and 1860s can be accounted for by the heightened attention accorded during these decades to all explanations for the decline of bloodletting; the idea of change of type was merely chief among them. The change-of-type theory did not spring forth only after the transformation in practice had substantially run its course, however. During the early 1830s some physicians had claimed that the type of prevailing diseases was changing, necessitating a turn from depletive to stimulative therapy of precisely the sort that was later ascribed to those very years. Articulations of the change of type in the early 1830s were far less stylized than the formal expressions that abounded after midcentury, but the idea they contained was nonetheless whole.

Although the supposed change of type closely followed the first cholera epidemic in the United States in 1832, on the whole physicians simply noted that cholera coincided with or at most initiated the change; all fevers, not cholera alone, purportedly partook in the shift to asthenia. " 'The Cholera,' I believe, has left us," a North Carolina practitioner wrote to his son in 1832. "Nothing of it appears now in the diseases that are prevalent; and the character of the season seems to be changing—Our fevers at this time are less inflammatory, & most of them call for tonic & stimulating remedies."[18] Claims about the subsiding inflammatory diathesis and increasing tendency to debility persisted through the 1840s. There was little novelty in a Cincinnati physician's confident assertion at the start of the 1850s that "the med-

ical constitution of this whole continent, if not of the world, is asthenic."[19]

Whatever existential epidemiological changes might have fostered
the notion that disease was changing in type, there can be no doubt
that its popularity was linked to physicians' perception of the increasing frequency of typhoid fever. In part the link was semantic, reflecting
the equivalance of sthenia with an inflammatory type of disease and
asthenia with a typhoid type. Most physicians, however, were careful
to distinguish the typhoid type of fever and the disease typhoid fever
when discussing the rising frequency of the latter. The medical literature traced the appearance of what was termed typhoid fever in the
South and West in the 1830s and its ascension in the 1840s to become
what many held to be the prevailing nonperiodic fever.[20] Many physicians regarded the typhoidization of the West and South as the most
significant epidemiological change of the 1840s and viewed it as one
source of bloodletting's decline in these regions.

Typhoid provided a model of disease for which mild treatment
was indicated. It was par excellence the disease associated with expectant practice. While many physicians vehemently disputed the propriety of such a therapeutic course, at least by the 1840s there was a
stronger consensus favoring therapeutic moderation and support for
typhoid than for any other fever.[21] A shift in the prevailing fever to
typhoid, physicians held, would be expected to mollify heroic use of
antiphlogistic therapies. An Alabama student writing his medical thesis at Transylvania explained the change in practice that had been
necessitated in his region when typhoid fever first prevailed there in
1838. After "many fell victims to the active and bold remedies, which
had been used," practitioners became convinced that calomel, ipecac,
and the lancet had to be replaced with more supportive treatment.[22]

In discussing the decline of bloodletting in American practice,
physicians gave scant credit to French therapeutic thought and only
infrequently borrowed arguments from French medical writers. They
often mentioned Louis's statistical studies on bloodletting in itemizing
the factors that had taken part in its changing use, but by the 1850s
Louis was cited as a supporter of bloodletting as often as he was identified as an early doubter.[23] This eschewal of French medical opinion
reflected the prevailing American suspicion of Gallic therapeutic values. In contrast, Americans drew heavily on the British discussion of
bloodletting's decline. In fact, the single debate over bloodletting and
its waning that American physicians most discussed was Scottish, the
debate of the mid-1850s in which the leading antagonists were the
Edinburgh physicians William P. Alison and John Hughes Bennett.

Although statements by the participants of the polar positions that characterized the debate were in print earlier, the Edinburgh controversy was most vigorous between 1856 and 1858, when the combatants exchanged attacks at meetings of the Edinburgh Medical-Chirurgical Society and continued them in the *Edinburgh Medical and Surgical Journal*. Both men agreed that the use of bloodletting for pneumonia, the discussion's principal focus, had declined markedly since the early 1830s, but their explanations and judgments of this phenomenon differed. Alison, the elder statesman of the profession in Edinburgh and a professor at its medical school since 1820, held that the earlier use of bloodletting had been beneficial, that its employment had declined because of a change in disease or in people to an asthenic type, and that bloodletting remained in principle a valuable therapy. Bennett, a Continent-trained holder of the prominent chair of the institutes and practice of medicine at the Edinburgh Medical School who was in his early forties when the debate commenced, rejected the change-of-type theory. He asserted instead that recent pathophysiological studies of inflammation had shown that bloodletting was not an efficacious remedy (a claim he supported by clinical statistics and his own microscopical studies of inflammation) and had always been inert or injurious. This particular debate, by no means unique in either content or form, drew inordinate attention because of the prominence of its participants and because they took up the two assessments of the principle of bloodletting that implied the most violently conflicting judgments of tradition.[24]

American physicians followed the Edinburgh debate closely, and many were quick to choose sides. Like Edinburgh physicians, most Americans favored Alison's stance. The few, characteristically young physicians who defended Bennett did not generally take up his arguments whole but rather saw in him a rallying point for contesting the change-of-type theory. In 1860, for example, James F. Hibberd, a young and patently ambitious Indiana physician, published a thirty-page defense of Bennett in reply to a pro-Alison piece written by a prominent Cincinnati practitioner. Hibberd denied that a change of type accounted for the "almost abandonment" of venesection. "In sober truth," he asserted, "the advocates of the doctrine of a change of type in inflammation have furnished not one iota of pertinent evidence to sustain themselves, except their individual opinions, purporting to be based upon clinical experience."[25] Yet so important was bloodletting in principle "that in many instances learned physicians, past the meridian of life, who have long been authors or teachers, or both, find it impossible to bring their minds to the conviction that the labors of their earlier years must be acknowledged not only vain, but worse than useless. Consequently, as a rule, neither our textbooks nor our systematic lectures reflect the actual state of enlightened practice in the treatment of acute inflammation." Drawing on Bennett's arguments, Hibberd decried this disjuncture of principle and practice and denounced the change-of-type theory as an artificial construction "flattering to the innate vanity of man."[26]

Unlike Bennett, Hibberd did not maintain that advances in pathology and physiology had led to bloodletting's decline. He cogently suggested instead that the repudiation of bloodletting by homeopathists and Thomsonians had fueled a popular clamor against the practice that in turn had induced a change in the practice of those regular physicians "found upon the borders of scientific practice" who "treat disease in great measure according to the desires of their patients."[27] The better regular physicians, he continued, "were not slow to observe that inflammations treated without blood-letting certainly did as well as those which were treated according to the most orthodox venesection." These physicians "had an influence that soon made itself felt throughout the profession, and the result was, not only the gradual abatement in the extent of blood-letting in the treatment of inflammation, but a general softening down of all heroic practice in the management of disease."[28] Hibberd also asserted that although the pathophysiological advances acclaimed by Bennett had not caused bloodletting's decline, they had revealed that the practice was and had always been useless.[29]

Americans who took Alison's side held that clinical experience over the course of years by men of "sound judgment, discrimination, and accuracy"[30] had established the change of type as a fact. "The degeneracy into a comparatively adynamic condition, which Dr. Bennett denies," the editors of a Charleston medical journal claimed in 1859, "is acknowledged as a fact by every physician of our own age and standing in these United States."[31] This was the position taken by Leonidas Moreau Lawson in the attack on Bennett that had first prompted Hibberd's rebuttal. Lawson, who founded the *Western Lancet* in 1844, had entered practice around 1832, visited the hospitals of London and Paris in the mid-1840s, and returned to hold teaching positions in Lexington and later Cincinnati. When in 1860 he published his denunciation of Bennett—what he termed "the Edinburgh defection"—he was professor of the principles and practice of medicine at the Medical College of Ohio and among the recognized elders of western American medicine.

Lawson asserted with Alison that past approbation of bloodletting could not all be wrong. "No amount of speculative pathology or ingenious hypotheses can subvert the clinical experience of the great body of our profession," he claimed. Reflecting his dismissal of Bennett's pathophysiological findings as valid criteria for judging the change-of-type theory, Lawson noted that "the evidence that the type of disease fluctuates in intensity, must be derived from personal observation and experience, in relation to the conditions of the general system, rather than the revelations of the scalpel or the microscope, concerning the minute changes in inflammation." He quipped that "closet-practitioners, and men striving for notoriety, may weave a thousand intangible but spacious [sic] theories, but it requires the crucible of clinical experience to separate the dross from the gold."[32] Lawson's allegiance to accumulated experience as the touchstone of therapeutic authority that permeated his arguments was put most plainly by a physician participating in the Philadelphia County Medical Society's discussion on bloodletting in the same year: "We cannot afford to do without the past."[33]

A major thrust of the American attack on Bennett and his fellow travelers caricatured him as a speculative pathologist who had allowed theoretical commitments to distort his clinical judgment. Like the rationalistic systems of the early nineteenth century, critics held, his rationalism and especially his reasoning from microscopical investigations of pathophysiology would lead to routine practice and extremism. Without naming Bennett, a Boston medical editor who several months earlier had reviewed the Alison-Bennett debate and labeled Bennett's views as "extreme" charged that there was "a strong tendency to routine practice . . . in the abandonment of certain modes of treatment," and denounced those "practitioners who *systematically* abstain from depletion."[34] The damning implications were clear when physicians such as Bennet Dowler in 1858 and Lawson two years later charged Bennett with setting up a new "system" of practice.[35] "All cases are to be treated in the same manner; discrimination is at an end," Lawson wrote. "This I call unmitigated empiricism." Charging Bennett and Hibberd with endorsing doctrinaire practice that disregarded the principle of specificity, he asserted that treatment "must be regulated by the condition of the patient, and not by any theoretical rules."[36]

The American critique of Bennett also displayed antagonism toward the rationalism implicit in laboratory science's therapeutic pretensions, an antagonism that would be expressed more frequently and forcefully in subsequent decades. Dowler, for example, denounced Bennett's rejection of bloodletting in principle on the basis of pathophysiological theory as "subversive," arguing that "in speculative science there can be little harm in such a fancy, but it is far different in practical medicine, when the question stands out at the bedside in the most salient form, help! help! or I perish?"[37] Dowler was himself an active experimenter in physiology but made little attempt to draw therapeutic conclusions from his researches. Indeed, basing therapeutic principles on an inappropriate foundation was precisely the crime of which he accused Bennett, whom he termed "some closeted microscopist whose facts and theories concerning the cells, their anatomy, physiology, combinations, growth, life, and decline are truly interesting, yet do not afford a basis for medication."[38]

Lawson went beyond Dowler to discredit Bennett's statistical evidence against bloodletting. In clinical statistics, Lawson claimed, "each partisan will find his theory fully sustained . . . But the judicious practitioner will perceive that some unseen agency has modified the results, and that the mere figures are but so many fallacies." Lawson further objected that the application of statistical knowledge was but another form of indiscriminate routinism: "In this blundering, if not criminal procedure, individuality is ignored, and the practitioner prescribes for a mere *name*, leaving the patient to the mercies of chance or fate."[39] He closed by pointing out with untempered glee that by one report, Bennett had recently been afflicted by an inflammatory affection for which he was venesected. "Thus, the hand of Providence becomes a more potent teacher than statistical tables or microscopical revelations."[40] Hibberd was equally unrestrained in ridiculing Lawson's model of divine retribution for scientific presumption. "The inference is," he gibed, "that God afflicted Prof. Bennett with inflammation as the most efficient means of convincing him of the error of his therapeutic opinions."[41]

It is paradoxical on the face of it that despite the notoriety Bennett gained from his challenge to bloodletting, American physicians widely favored his restorative plan of treatment for internal inflammations. Moreover, while some physicians held with Lawson that Bennett's therapeutic extremism made his statistics suspect, many Americans openly admired his statistical work. But after all, his statistical indictment of bloodletting in current practice could be judged sound and still be reconciled with the change-of-type theory. Physicians could affirm the prudence of Bennett's restorative plan and at the same time reject or ignore his reductionist rationale for using it, and most chose this course. Although some physicians condemned Bennett's treatment either as heroic stimulation or do-nothing, most recognized it as supportive, moderate therapy that meshed very well with the central currents of American practice in the 1850s and 1860s, and many cited Bennett as confirmatory authority for their own practices.[42]

Even in the 1850s some physicians worried that although the declining use of bloodletting was proper, it was going too far. This concern about overreaction grew through the 1870s and 1880s into the fear that although few regulars had rejected bloodletting in principle, it had been virtually discarded from practice. "When a remedy, once so popular, and regarded for nearly 2000 years by the most eminent and enlightened men as so essential to success in the treatment of disease, has fallen into utter desuetude," Samuel D. Gross observed in 1875, "it behooves us, especially the older members of the profession, to pause, and to inquire seriously whether there is not something wrong in all this depreciation; whether we have not fallen into the opposite error, and condemned a remedy which, if judiciously employed, is capable of doing vast good."[43] His question, Have we gone too far? was echoed repeatedly in the 1870s and 1880s. The articles with titles such as "A Plea for the Lancet" that proliferated rarely urged the extensive use of bloodletting, but they called on physicians to consider whether venesection might not on occasion be the best remedy in their armamentarium. Older practitioners who had been known in their youth as therapeutic moderates vocally affirmed the lancet's worth.[44] Just as physicians had criticized the extremism of routine bloodletting early in the century, they came to lament the opposite extreme, its routine abandonment.

Although the use of mercurials declined concurrently with that of bloodletting, the changing usage patterns of the two practices were far from parallel. Still, the discussions on decreasing mercurial prescriptions that thrived from the 1850s through the 1870s resembled those on bloodletting's decline in some of their leading concerns. In both instances the delicate problem of avoiding violence to medical tradition dominated discussion. Because mercury, especially calomel, was after bloodletting the remedy most emblematic of regular therapeutics and as such the drug most reviled by sectarians, the marked diminution in its use during the first two-thirds of the century was an important sociopolitical as well as therapeutic event, and one that demanded from physicians a judgment and accounting.[45]

   In assessing calomel's decline, regular physicians used all the kinds of explanation they brought to bear on the wane of bloodletting. Yet the discussion generated from the 1850s through the 1870s by the question, Why has the use of calomel declined? differed in character from that produced by the analogous question posed about bloodletting. Certainly the use and disuse of calomel was discussed even more than was that of bloodletting, but on the whole this discussion lacked the urgency, the sobering import that attended the bloodletting debate. In part the difference can be ascribed to the fact that there was less to explain in the case of calomel: despite its symbolic importance, it was a less distinctive practice at the bedside. The physician either venesected or he did not, and if he did the intervention was a dramatic one unmistakable to the patient and onlookers. Letting a smaller volume of blood when the vein was cut open diminished the physiological impression of venesection without fundamentally altering its psychological impact. The decline in calomel's use, on the other hand, made a less visible impression on the therapeutic tableau. Mercury could be given with reduced frequency or in diminished doses, and as a drug rather than a surgical procedure it could be blended psychologically as well as pharmacologically with other drugs that might be prescribed.

Furthermore, despite mercury's declining use, it was not threatened by total abandonment between the 1850s and 1870s in quite the way bloodletting was. While phrases such as "large doses of" and "continued use of" preceded the term *calomel* in rhetoric questioning its suitability for certain conditions, no such qualifiers ordinarily softened the criticism of venesection. Nor was calomel subjected to a direct, all-encompassing challenge to its value in principle of the sort Bennett posed against general bloodletting.

Two of the most severe attacks on the use of calomel in the mid-nineteenth century and the response they elicited from American physicians illustrate both the criteria physicians regarded as appropriate in judging a therapeutic agent and those they held to be illegitimate. The first of these assaults was Surgeon General William H. Hammond's proscription of calomel (and with it tartar emetic) from the Union army's supply table. In his Circular No. 6, issued on 4 May 1863, Hammond claimed that reports of field inspectors had shown "that the administration of calomel has so frequently been pushed to excess by military surgeons as to call for prompt steps by this office to correct this abuse." To curtail its use, he directed that it be stricken from the standard list of medical supplies. Hammond, who was only in his mid-thirties and had studied in Germany, added that "this is done with the more confidence as modern pathology has proved the impropriety of the use of mercury in very many of those diseases in which it was formerly unfailingly administered." He concluded, "No doubt can exist that more harm has resulted from the misuse of both these agents, in the treatment of disease, than benefit from their proper administration."[46]

In substance, Hammond's order was merely a singularly publicized and institutionally powerful criticism of the kind American physicians since the 1820s had been bringing against therapeutic excesses engendered by mechanical adherence to theory and habit. Some physicians read the circular this way and applauded it,[47] but most regular practitioners condemned Hammond's order, which was denounced in all regions of the United States within weeks of publication. A Chicago medical editor charged that Hammond "has perpetrated a slander on his profession," while one in Philadelphia called the order "foolish, unjustifiable, and wholly untruthful."[48] The most violent attack came from physicians in the West and especially in Cincinnati, where calomel was extensively used and where the regular profession felt itself seriously under siege by powerful sectarians. At the Medical College of Ohio in late May, L. M. Lawson chaired a meeting of the regular physicians of Cincinnati that called for Hammond's resignation. Two days later members of the Cincinnati Academy of Medicine seconded this demand, insisting as well on revocation of the "calomel order." Both demands were reaffirmed at the state medical society's meeting in the following month, and delegates further called on the American Medical Association to expel Hammond. Lawson returned from the American Medical Association's annual meeting to report that only his earlier adversary J. F. Hibberd had defended the order and the proposition that calomel should be thrown out of medical practice.[49]

Orthodox physicians particularly resented the support that Hammond, speaking in authoritative medical post, had implicitly given to sectarian disparagements of calomel. Reports of Thomsonians, eclectics, and homeopathists rejoicing that the surgeon general had vindicated their denunciation of mineral poisons became common.[50] The order, according to one regular resolution, was "a virtual endorsement of the false charges which have been made against the scientific profession by the representatives of the various empyrical systems."[51] The inescapable conclusion of such reasoning was that Hammond's action was professionally unethical and his character and standing as a regular physician nullified. "The difference now between the Surgeon-General and the Eclectics and Botanics is so slight that the profession of the United States can not discover it," one physician charged. "He should go over to the Eclectics, *et id omne genus*, where he belongs."[52]

Underlying most attacks on Hammond was the consensus that his order was a model of irresponsible, unprofessional criticism of regular therapeutic practice displayed in full public view. It indicted in a public forum the skill of physicians and broadcast the harm done by prescribing calomel. Hammond's order would diminish public faith in regular practitioners and remedies, many physicians maintained, and lower the reputation of the American medical profession abroad.[53] As one editor reviewing the affair a year later commented, Hammond "had dishonestly violated his faith to his profession."[54]

Change could not be mandated in this fashion, physicians asserted: Hammond's order directed the disuse of calomel by rote and was therefore incompatible with the ideals of regular therapeutic discrimination. To a profession so aware of the damage done by doctrinaire practice and extremism, this sweeping rejection of calomel represented a plainly illegitimate type of therapeutic change. "The characteristics of all so-called systems of medicines as homoeopathic, hydropathic, eclectic, botanic, &c., is their restrictiveness, while the regular medical profession is characterized by its broad spirit of liberality, permitting its practitioners to select their remedial agents from every department of nature."[55] The surgeon general was autocratically revoking the practitioner's prerogative to exercise therapeutic judgment. "The regular medical profession claims the right to use all agents, regarding them as potential and relative," a Cincinnati editor asserted. "Empirics regard medicinal agents as specifics and poisons. Dr. Hammond's order has attempted to degrade his profession to the level of this latter class."[56]

Practitioners also resented what they saw as Hammond's valuation of laboratory science and pathology over clinical experience and practice, a flaw in his professional values that stemmed from his allegiance to German science. "The country wants a practical man (as Surgeon General), and not a mere theorist," a Philadelphia physician wrote.[57] "He has neither the age nor the clinical experience entitling him to any such claim," a Cincinnati colleague echoed. "We care not for his acknowledged scientific acquirements, [and] we maintain that he has done his profession a great wrong."[58]

Some physicians did defend Hammond, or at least sought to squelch an embarrassing overreaction against his order. An assistant surgeon in the field, for example, wrote to a Philadelphia journal that "in the abstract, I think, the Surgeon-General is right," commenting that all diseases he had observed among the troops were of an asthenic type for which calomel was contraindicated.[59] A Chicago editor pointed out the same fact and proposed that Hammond was acting as a responsible physician by issuing the order in keeping with his own therapeutic judgment. He feared, moreover, that by creating "an excitement" over the order, the profession would further draw public notice and make matters worse than they were.[60] J. F. Hibberd seconded all of these arguments in an article sent to the *Cincinnati Lancet and Observer* in response to the local regular profession's unanimous condemnation of Hammond, charging that the tenor of discussion in Cincinnati resembled that "emanating from a ward meeting of pot-house politicians." Consistent with his earlier defense of Bennett's claims that pathophysiological investigations had invalidated bloodletting, Hibberd agreed with Hammond that "modern pathology" had established the inappropriateness of mercury's use in many conditions and favored its banishment from a "civilized country."[61]

Unlike Bennett, Hammond did not reject an established practice in principle; he asserted only that the damage done by calomel's abuse far outweighed the good derived from its use. Still, by insisting on the indiscriminate disuse of a drug so extensively employed and politically resonant as calomel, he had launched a frontal attack on therapeutic tradition, indicting both past and current practice. The deepest objection to Hammond's order was lucidly expressed in the title of a later review article: "Shall We Reject the Fathers?"[62]

A very different kind of challenge to calomel emanated from British investigations into mercury's physiological action. In 1867, at the urging of Bennett, the British Medical Association set up a committee of five prominent Edinburgh physicians, including Bennett and early experimental pharmacologists Robert Christison and Thomas Richard Fraser, to study the cholagogue action of mercury. Up until this time it had been to mercury's cholagogue action—its ability to stimulate the flow of bile—that much of its therapeutic power was attributed. For the next two years the Edinburgh Committee experimented on dogs at facilities provided by the Edinburgh Medical School to assess the action of mercury on the liver. In 1869 Bennett reported the committee's conclusion that mercury in small doses did not increase biliary secretion and in large or continued doses actually diminished it.[63] This was not the first suggestion that perhaps mercury did not increase biliary secretion, but both its experimental support and the publicity conferred by the British Medical Association's sponsorship forcefully brought the report to the attention of the American medical profession.[64]

Bennett's wording of the report strongly implied that by demonstrating "the fallacy of the opinion everywhere present as to the cholagogue action of mercury," the committee's findings called for a change in the therapeutic use of calomel. This conclusion was in keeping with Bennett's negative appraisal of mercury before the study had commenced.[65] During his travels abroad a decade earlier, E. D. Fenner had observed that even then Bennett was "preparing to beard the Sampson *calomel*, and will soon attempt to prove that this fearfully popular drug is utterly worthless as a remedial agent—that *it does not act on the liver*, nor any other organ in a beneficial way."[66] Also, in 1859 British physician George Scott published the results of his experiments purporting to show that calomel did not increase biliary secretion in dogs, a conclusion that was a foundation for both Bennett's views and the Edinburgh Committee's work. "Among the effects of medicine which are usually considered to be well established, the action of mercurial preparations in increasing the flow of bile has been admitted without question," a Boston medical editor commenting on this work noted. "If these experiments should be confirmed by future ones, a revolution may be expected in the treatment of diseases."[67] This was precisely the change Bennett hoped to effect by the committee's report, but on the whole American physicians did not share his convictions.

Many simply rejected the experimental evidence as inconclusive, leaving the question of calomel's cholagogue action unresolved. "Certainly these experiments [on dogs] cannot be said to prove that mercury does not increase biliary secretion in men," one physician asserted in a paper given before the Buffalo Medical Association.[68] In the discussion that followed, members affirmed that they had been educated to believe in calomel's action on the liver and remained convinced of this doctrine's truth.[69] L. P. Yandell, Jr., professor at the Louisville Medical College, told his students in 1874 that Bennett and his coworkers "who by their Experiments proved that Calomel does not act upon the liver . . . [are] unreliable, the Experiments being in those cases made upon the lower Animals." Yandell added that while mercury "has up to the present day done more harm than good," it was nonetheless "one of the most useful and efficacious medicines we have."[70] In a discussion at the Cuyahoga Medical Society in 1876 on mercury's therapeutic use, one practitioner, the secretary recorded, said that "he had seen references to a report of the Edinburgh Committee on the action of mercury wh militated against the view that mercury has a chologue action but he had not been able to find the report and was not inclined to change his views."[71]

The challenge the Edinburgh Committee posed to calomel elicited from American physicians almost none of the vehemence that had met Bennett's attack on bloodletting a decade earlier. Most held that however physiologically valid the committee's report might be, it simply made no difference for practice. "Whatever good effects may be obtained by using mercury, are still facts which no change of theory can alter," a Philadelphia editor commented on the report. "Modern researches only alter our interpretation of the facts, and not the facts themselves; and if mercury does not increase the amount of bile secreted by the liver, as has been hitherto supposed, but, in reality, diminishes the supply, it follows that we must look upon our results from a different point of view, and admit that our knowledge of the action of this drug, as of most others, is simply empirical."[72] As a Massachusetts physician commented two years later, "much as we may deprecate the indiscriminate use of mercurials, and much as we may theoretically condemn their exhibition altogether, cases will continually occur in which [they are demanded]."[73]

Only a small portion of the difference between the reactions against Bennett's challenge to bloodletting and his challenge to calomel can be ascribed to softening commitments to these remedies during the decade that separated the attacks. The disparity principally represents differing responses to a challenge to *principle* in the case of bloodletting and to *theory* in the case of mercury. Challenges to principle threatened the profession in a way that assaults upon theory did not. The vehemence of the reaction to the Edinburgh Committee's report was also mitigated by its lack of novelty, for regular American physicians had suggested earlier that mercury might have little cholagogue effect.[74] In addition, the report was not backed by the statistical evidence that gave special force to Bennett's attack on bloodletting. And in contrast to Bennett's sweeping repudiation of bloodletting, the committee questioned only the theory of calomel's action in one of its several purported functions; that it was in principle a useful remedy remained well assured, diminished use notwithstanding. In a discussion on mercury at the Clark County [Ohio] Medical Society in 1871, for example, one physician could declare "that although calomel is much less used now than formerly—used in a less number of diseases, and also in less quantities in any particular disease—yet in the certain limited number of cases in which it is a proper remedy, it is more firmly established, and more strongly entrenched in the confidence of the medical profession now than ever."[75]

While practitioners were striving to explain the diminished use of depletive therapies, they were prescribing supportive treatments with growing frequency. These simultaneous movements did not generate the same explanatory problems, and the former disturbed physicians far more than the latter. The eclipse of a once-prominent remedy drew therapeutic principle into question but the increased use of established treatments did not. Accordingly physicians devoted much more energy to explaining the decline of venesection and calomel than they did the rise of alcohol. Even though a construct like the change-of-type theory explained both therapeutic movements equally well, ordinarily the primary objective of its use was to account for the decline of antiphlogistics in practice in a way that did not question their value in principle, not to justify the ascendance of stimulants. Some physicians decried the extent to which alcohol was prescribed, and a few urged that its moral and physical iatrogenic effects argued against its use; but practitioners generally accepted that it was in principle a beneficial agent. Discourse on the rise of stimulative therapy in the 1850s and 1860s therefore lacked the implicit threat to tradition that gave the concurrent discussion on bloodletting and mercury such urgency.

The introduction of a new therapy marked a more discrete alteration in practice than did the increased use of one already in the armamentarium but still did not necessarily challenge tradition. Physicians

expected the discovery of new remedies to be one channel for therapeutic improvement. The prospect of a new therapy's rise was ordinarily less threatening than was that of an established treatment's
abandonment, but bringing a new remedy into a physician's practice
did disrupt habit. Generational factors clearly influenced willingness
to accept or reject a new therapy, for the longer habits had been entrenched in a physician's routine, the less inclined he would be to bring
change into his practice. Nevertheless, a practitioner's age alone seldom determined his rejection or acceptance of a new treatment.

Only when some physicians claimed that a new remedy should
replace an existing one was tradition, not just habit, seriously brought
into question. During the mid-nineteenth century physicians advocated a number of "substitutes" for the leading antiphlogistic treatments, chief among them podophyllum, veratrum viride, and aconite.
To the extent that these new remedies were recommended as substitutes for traditional therapies like bloodletting, they implied that such
practices were in principle inferior.

The case of veratrum viride, which became an important drug but
never a mainstay of regular practice, is particularly revealing. Veratrum, or the American Hellebore, had occupied a very minor place in
the regular materia medica since the early nineteenth century, when
it was recommended principally for its emetic power rather than for
the pulse-slowing property that was to be the basis of its new popularity
after midcentury.[76] In 1850 Wesley C. Norwood, a practitioner in Abbeyville, South Carolina, first drew the regular profession's attention
to veratrum's therapeutic properties as an arterial sedative (it reduced
the action of the heart and lowered the pulse rate and thereby seemed
to calm the system) when he published instructions for its preparation
and use. During the subsequent few years he advocated this use in a
variety of febrile diseases and offered to send a sample of the plant to
any physician who would try the new remedy.[77] By the mid-1850s it
had secured a substantial following.

The American reception of veratrum illustrates not only the difficulties that any new drug encountered but also the particular animosity engendered by the common suggestion that veratrum was an
effective substitute for venesection. As with all new remedies, veratrum's advocates and detractors freely exchanged accusations of extremism—routinism on the one hand and overenthusiasm for novelty on
the other. "There are," one advocate of veratrum asserted, "old fogies
in every community, occupying a high position in public confidence,
who, without trial, condemn everything that breaks in upon their routine of practice, and whose influence operates vastly to the prejudice
of this remedy."[78] Another practitioner replied that he had been called

both a "country doctor" and an "old fogy," and was "willing to accept the latter designation so far as it may be applied, because I show a firm adherence to the things that are old until the things that are new shall have been proved better."[79] The pivotal questions were, How could the value of a new remedy be established? What did physicians regard as relevant criteria in judging a new therapy, and what did they accept as valid authority?

The paramount indicator for most physicians in assessing veratrum viride's therapeutic promise was the source of its advocacy. The testimony of Norwood, a physician in a small South Carolina town, carried little therapeutic authority. Veratrum's early proponents lamented that the profession would have been much more attentive to its introduction had it been first announced in Europe rather than America or the Northeast rather than the South. Indeed, early discussion of veratrum was far more active in southern journals, though during the second half of the 1850s this regional difference all but vanished.[80] The therapeutic reputation of an individual physician also colored his testimony in the eyes of the profession. In a St. Louis discussion of veratrum, for example, one physician could dismiss John Hughes Bennett's distrust of veratrum by saying that "he thought, though Bennett was a very learned man, he was a better pathologist than practitioner, and relied more on nature than remedies in every case."[81] Some physicians also suspected veratrum of having a sectarian past and were wary of embracing a "quack" substitute for bloodletting.[82]

A few physicians, characteristically young, turned to animal experimentation as one way of evaluating veratrum's action. H. Gatch Carey, a thirty-two-year-old practitioner, presented his findings on the "Toxical Action of Veratrum Viride on Dogs" before a Dayton, Ohio, medical society in 1858. In the animated discussion that ensued, two young physicians noted with satisfaction that the sedative effect on the heart's action Carey had observed in dogs coincided with clinical observation. Nevertheless most practitioners regarded this evidence as physiologically curious but therapeutically irrelevant. One older physician who proudly affirmed that he had never used veratrum denounced the enthusiasm of "his young friend" Carey and asserted that "the experiments made upon the innocent dogs had no practical value, and shed no ray of light on the therapeutical properties of veratrum."[83] He was not, the society's secretary recorded, "prepared to admit that a medicine forced down the throat or up the rectum of a *well* dog would produce the same symptoms that it would do in one of us if we were sick and took it . . . He had no faith in this cruel and fatal drugging of dogs." Animal exprimentation "would add nothing to our stock of scientific knowledge," he claimed, and could not be meaningful as a source of therapeutic authority.[84]

The source of authority cited most often by physicians engaged in the discussion of veratrum was empirical observation at the bedside. Occasional attempts were made to use medical journals and society meetings to organize the profession's evaluation of veratrum. A Massachusetts physician, for example, distributed samples of Norwood's tincture to all the members of the Middlesex East District Medical Society in 1856, asking them to test the drug in their practices and report their findings.[85]

Most physicians credited personal rather than collective experience as the most reliable authority for judging veratrum. An Alabama practitioner reported in 1853 that during the year he had used veratrum with success in treating over a dozen different diseases, while other physicians denied its therapeutic value after trying it only once and finding it wanting.[86] There was no common referent for judging veratrum's worth beyond what each individual practitioner believed experience had revealed to him, a circumstance that guaranteed dissension. The secretary of one medical society summed up its discussion on veratrum's therapeutic value by saying, "Some regarded veratrum as an agent of immense value in the treatment of sthenic forms of disease, others regarded it as highly valuable in asthenic cases and some were of the opinion that it was of no value in any case."[87] The legitimacy of personal observation and opinion was at stake, and accordingly rhetoric both supporting and condemning veratrum was strong. One physician in the Dayton debate hailed veratrum as "the greatest remedy of the age," but another denounced it and proclaimed the conflicting testimony of its supporters "amusing," commenting dyspeptically "that veratrum was a humbug, that those who believed in its wonderful efficacy are humbugged, that Norton [Norwood?], who revived the use of it, is a humbugger, and that the poor patients who have to swallow it are egregiously humbugged."[88]

More common than strident arguments for either extreme position was concern about the dangers of extremism. Excessive enthusiasm and execration commonly characterized the reception of a new remedy, many physicians held, and the response to veratrum was no exception. While some practitioners defended trials with veratrum by pointing out that only through openness to change could therapeutics be advanced, others decried the overenthusiasm of veratrum's more zealous advocates. "If veratrum viride had a voice," one practitioner proposed, "it would exclaim, 'Save me from my friends.' " Its advocates "seemed to have laid aside all reason and moderation in their admiration of the wonderful virtues of this drug."[89] Eli Geddings, though he acknowledged veratrum's therapeutic value, told his students in 1861 that its unmistakable power to control the pulse had led some enthusiasts to regard it as a "specific." "The adulations of this remedy," he urged, "induce me to believe that our professional brethren have lost the light of pathology and have become empirics."[90]

It was not veratrum itself but the proposition that it was a substitute for venesection that elicited the most energetic protest. The medical profession's weighing of veratrum in the 1850s and 1860s coincided with the substantial disappearance of bloodletting from therapeutic practice. Although some practitioners undoubtedly began to give veratrum at about the time they ceased using the lancet, the drug's introduction played only a small role in the decline of bloodletting. Nevertheless, the fact that its sedative influence overlapped with the therapeutic actions attributed to venesection suggested that it might be a substitute for general bloodletting.[91]

The idea that veratrum was a substitute for venesection could, of course, be interpreted as an improvement in practice that in no way questioned the propriety of bloodletting's earlier application: venesection was an efficacious practice, and veratrum viride—hitherto unknown as an arterial sedative—was simply better. But this notion could also be interpreted as implicitly condemning venesection by suggesting that a good practice was replacing a bad one. One physician who adopted this interpretation in 1858 saw the search for "substitutes" for bloodletting as a response to criticisms from what he called the quack "systems," an illegitimate source of regular therapeutic change. Using the example of its effects in pneumonia, he acknowledged veratrum's therapeutic worth but denied that it was a substitute for venesection. "I shall pronounce any man who professes to have found a 'substitute' for venesection in inflammatory affections, a libeler on the character of medical science,—an imprudent pretender, alike ignorant of what medical science is, and of what it should be," he stated unambiguously. Instead, he insisted that pneumonia had changed to a type in which veratrum was useful but venesection was not. "Blood-letting never was admissible in cases of this kind," he claimed, "and to talk of a 'substitute' for it is ridiculous."[92]

While many physicians shared his reasoning about the change of type of disease and consequent decline of bloodletting, the fact remained that though their therapeutic effects differed, both veratrum viride and venesection sedated. Veratrum's use was most often accommodated to the change-of-type theory by the suggestion that despite the fact it was indeed a cardiac sedative, it did not induce substantial systemic debilitation. Therefore in sthenic conditions depletion by bleeding was indicated to control the heart's vigor, whereas in asthenic cases veratrum was more appropriate.[93] A more subtle theoretical position postulated that the ongoing change in type was only partially complete by the late 1850s. Disease had lost much of its inflammatory action and could not tolerate the depletive treatment it had once demanded, but it still retained its high vascular excitement. It "seems to assume a type intermediate between a sthenic and an asthenic character," an Alabama physician argued in 1858.[94] Regarded in this way, veratrum was not a substitute for venesection, for it lacked the latter's great depressing effect, but it was neatly fitted to the peculiar therapeutic needs of the time.

By the late 1850s veratrum viride was becoming firmly established in American medical practice, although—in part because of the high risk of lethal overdose—it never became the therapeutic mainstay its more sanguine advocates predicted.[95] The coincidence of veratrum's ascendant popularity and the eclipse of bloodletting, coupled with the idea that it was a substitute for venesection, drew inordinate attention to veratrum in discussions about bloodletting's demise. The theme of regret so common in the retrospective appraisals of bloodletting that proliferated in the 1870s extended to veratrum as well, and a number of older practitioners lamented that the profession had gone too far in taking up veratrum just as they had erred in laying aside the lancet.[96] Even after the new drug was accepted, it retained the stigma of a challenger to venesection. Most of the charges of extremism brought against veratrum in therapeutic discussion after the 1860s did not, however, hold that the drug was overused. Instead, they simply targeted veratrum as one factor to blame for the bloodletting's virtual abandonment.

The discourse on the decline of antiphlogistic agents, the rise of stimulants, and the introduction of new remedies such as veratrum was varied enough to show that the therapeutic discussion that flourished in America from the 1850s through the 1870s was not all cast in a single mold. The problems physicians sought to work out in their discussions of various practices and the vigor that informed their endeavor depended on the particular place an individual treatment occupied in the broader therapeutic schema. Yet common elements recurred again and again in these discussions about therapeutic change. Physicians consistently strove to exercise their dual commitment to progress and to tradition. These allegiances were not always in conflict, but when they were the tension generated dominated therapeutic discussion. Most often the defense of tradition pivoted on preserving therapeutic principle: physicians could explain change in both theory and practice in ways that did not draw the correctness of prior therapeutic judgment into question, but change in principle constituted a serious threat to the profession.

Several tacit rules further ordered the proper conduct of therapeutic discussion. Physicians were sensitive to the outward appearance of their deliberations, and therefore medical etiquette dictated that so far as possible adjudications of change be kept from public view. The acknowledged arbiter of good practice was experience, but because it varied among practitioners, it was an unstable referent and a difficult one to refute. This meant that therapeutic criticism often consisted of questioning the veracity or reliability of an opponent's experience, of his ability to judge. The centrality of personal reputations in therapeutic debate gave physicians special reason for shielding it from public sight. Experience worth heeding had come to be closely identified with empirical observation, and the therapeutic discussions of the 1850s through the 1870s clearly illustrated physicians' predominant allegiance to methodological empiricism and reviling of rationalism, whether it be rooted in speculative systems or in laboratory science. An overarching odium of extremism also characterized therapeutic deliberations, for excessive use or disuse of a particular therapy represented practice by rote that physicians uniformly saw as dangerous. Not dogmatic conservatism or enthusiasm for change but the middle path represented the therapeutic ideal.

PART III

Therapeutic Reconstruction

— 8 —

Physiological Therapeutics and the Dissipation of Therapeutic Gloom

THE PROPOSITION that experimental laboratory science should inform therapeutic practice and advancement became securely established in the twentieth century. During the two decades following the Civil War its acceptance was far from certain, however, for it represented but one of a number of programs envisaged for therapeutics. Physicians' expectations about the future of medical therapeutics were as diverse as were their perspectives on its past and present so evident in their discussions about change. Most practitioners agreed that the empiricist pruning of rationalistic systems had greatly improved practice, but by the 1860s they also concurred that progress along this axis had slowed to a near standstill. Therapeutics had begun to stagnate, many physicians believed, and the profession had fallen prey to therapeutic gloom. Concern over this state of things made these decades a time of exceedingly active reflection about what was to become of therapeutics, marked also by bickering about the most promising plan for escaping pessimism.

Between the mid-1860s and the mid-1880s programs for therapeutic change abounded. Some advocated the selective revival of remedies earlier in vogue, while others urged physicians to emphasize hygienic more than drug therapy, to improve practice through intensified empirical observation of drug effects, or even to turn their attention from healing individuals to the greater promise of state-sponsored preventive medicine. Of all the designs for therapeutics put on the market, the one that was most forcefully to remold medical enterprise held that knowledge produced by laboratory experimentation should become the new foundation for medical therapeutics.

In many ways this plan was also the most radical departure from

235

the past. It postulated a new source of therapeutic knowledge and authority, defined a new epistemological category for therapeutics, and carried with it an aggressive optimism its advocates contended should signal the dissipation of therapeutic gloom. It had fundamental implications for therapeutic practice and professional identity and morality, and these are analyzed in Chapter 9. To understand the therapeutic claims of experimental science, it is necessary to know why the New Rationalism that characterized "experimental" or "physiological" therapeutics so appealed to some physicians and so repelled others. Recognizing how much the epistemological implications of this new program mattered to American physicians is crucial to understanding its reception.

Beginning in the late 1850s physicians increasingly complained that even though basic medical science was swiftly progressing, medical therapeutics was by comparison static. "It seems that every other branch of medicin has gon on to great perfection but the treatment of disease . . . would seem almost dormant," a medical student in Charleston began his thesis in 1859.[1] Dissatisfaction with this state of affairs grew during the two decades following the Civil War. Although not new in form, this complaint far exceeded in strength anything witnessed earlier in the century. Frustrated by the contrast between stagnancy in therapeutics and brisk advancement in experimental physiology, biological chemistry, and microscopic pathology, practitioners saw the gap between medical knowledge and therapeutic activity widening.

Postbellum physicians generally agreed that therapeutic practice had improved since the early decades of the century, but this judgment revealed a disparaging appraisal of prior practice more than contentment with its present state. They nearly universally deemed the demise of rationalistic systems and their concomitant extremism to be signs of progress. They had learned from a fuller knowledge of the natural history of disease and the healing power of nature what they could and could not accomplish by drugging. In the 1830s only an elite minority had defended the notion that most diseases were self-limited, but half a century later this had become commonly accepted wisdom.[2] Such a stance did urge attention to patients' hygienic management, but its main practical message, as most practitioners understood it, was to do less.

Although physicians recognized the heightened appreciation of the limitations of their art and the tendency toward therapeutic moderation as progress, they saw it as *negative* progress. The impulse of skeptical French empiricism that had changed American medicine for the better was in its essence destructive. "In the use of medicine, the knowledge attained has been negative," one physician wrote. "Physicians have ascertained what medicine cannot do, rather than what it can do."[3] Henry Ingersoll Bowditch, reviewing the history of medicine in the United States at the nation's centennial, proposed that the period from the early 1830s through the end of the 1860s was best typified by the skeptical empiricism of men like Louis, Bigelow, and Bartlett. They had greatly improved therapeutics by demolishing the speculative systems that had once dominated practice, he believed; "all will admit that Louis's school was needed, in order to sweep away all theoretical systems." Yet they had contributed little positive to therapeutics. "Their mission was chiefly destructive," Bowditch asserted. "Their scepticism, like all scepticism, was iconoclastic."[4]

Therapeutic progress made by pruning past errors without nurturing the growth of anything vital in their place was not fully satisfying. Lecturing to medical students at Harvard in the early 1860s, Bowditch warned, "You are entering the profession at a time perhaps the least satisfactory to a young mind."[5] A program of demolishing the unsound edifice of traditional practice was limited in the good it could accomplish. Without some blueprint for building new, sound structures in the place of those that had been razed, the profession would be left with only a wasteland. As physicians came to believe that such a negative plan of improvement had reached its limits, a tinge of despair colored therapeutic rhetoric.

Therapeutic empiricism did in fact suggest a plan for gaining new knowledge, not just one for testing the old. In keeping with the allegiance to the principle of specificity, therapeutic knowledge was to be augmented and refined by careful clinical observation (perhaps ordered by the numerical method) of therapeutic trials on groups of patients whose distinguishing characteristics and environments were discriminated with increasing precision. In principle observant physicians could eventually discover the treatment best suited to each possible specific circumstance. Some physicians during the 1830s and 1840s had envisioned the empiricist program as a platform for elevating therapeutics to the status of an exact science. James Jackson, Sr., who was far more cautious than the most enthusiastic proselytizers of Parisian methods, commented in 1833 on the work of Louis, "If he and his successors will continue in the same course the French will, in 50 years, be as much more exact in their knowledge of therapeutics, as they now are in pathology. They have laid and are laying an excellent foundation."[6]

Well before Jackson's fifty years had elapsed, many American physicians realized that any quest for therapeutic certainty mounted on clinical empiricism was certain only to fail. The allegiance to specificity to which the empirical program was welded gave medical therapeutics a distinctive epistemological status that emphatically set it apart from the universalized basic sciences. "In surgery, in anatomy, in physiology and in chemistry, there is a large degree of certainty," an Ohio physician affirmed in 1877. "But in the application of remedies to diseases, uncertainties, exceptions, disputes and defeats are interminable; and there is no authorized tribunal to which these imperfections can be referred for adjustment."[7]

The principle of specificity forestalled the possibility of therapeutic certainty, a simple fact that physicians acknowledged frequently and openly by the early postbellum period. Furthermore, it had grown steadily clearer that severe clinical empiricism made a better sword than plowshare: it was more powerful in disclosing errors in therapeutic practice that should be cast out than in discovering new methods of treatment. Positive progress in therapeutics would come only slowly. So long as physicians subscribed to the principle of specificity, the troubling disparity between the basic sciences and therapeutics would be an unavoidable consequence of the nature of things, and the rift between knowledge and action would continue to widen. Far from being the extreme reaction of the skeptic, therapeutic pessimism seemed to many physicians a prudent outgrowth of the realities of their art.

By the 1860s, then, the dominant path to therapeutic progress warranted little optimism, and most physicians foresaw only dismal prospects if they continued to pursue it. Yet by seeking a new model for positive change, they could avoid despair; American physicians began very deliberately to redefine their program for therapeutic progress. They were overwhelmingly agreed that medical therapeutics had been improved during the middle third of the century by the dismantling of the old; they now redirected their energies toward building up the new. This was a major shift in emphasis. While medical thinkers were of one mind in regarding the progress of the past as predominately negative, however, they were much less agreed on how to cultivate positive progress. Some doggedly held that empirical clinical observation remained the only valid method of therapeutic discovery, while others proposed radical alternatives.

A large number of reflective physicians observed between the early 1860s and the 1880s that medical therapeutics was in a period of transition. One exemplification of their awareness of critical change was a marked propensity, stronger than ever before in the century, to divide the history of therapeutics into stages, situating their own time at a major transition. Sometimes these stages were explicitly Comtian and traced the stepwise progress of therapeutics toward becoming a positive science; more often, though, American physicians used the language of positivism without consciously adopting a Comtian framework. Ordered in this way, the history of therapeutics functioned as a normative statement about future advancement and justified each author's particular program for reconstructing therapeutics by presenting it as part of a heroic historical progression.

Young Boston physician David W. Cheever produced an early illustration of the growing inclination to categorize various branches of medicine into their appropriate stages in order to underscore the relative stagnancy of therapeutics. Cheever graduated from Harvard Medical School in 1858 and entered the profession at a time when empiricist iconoclasm in therapeutics was well advanced and concern about the lack of positive progress was mounting. In 1859 he published a sobering assessment of the limitations of the numerical method as a way of improving therapeutics. "Medical science has conducted its inquiries through two distinct stages, and is only partially within the borders of the third. These stages, according to M. Compte [sic] (*Philosophie Positive*) are, First, fiction and faith; Second, speculation; and Third, positive science." He proposed that "anatomy, physiology, surgery, and morbid anatomy are either firmly established in, or have already entered upon the third stage . . . while therapeutics, worst of all, remains, but for a more or less fallacious empiricism, as firmly rooted in fiction, faith and speculation as ever."[8] It was inevitable that therapeutics would remain behind the other branches of medical knowledge, he stated grimly, and the clinical application of statistics could not alter this situation. The value of statistics "descends in accuracy by a progressive ratio, and in the following order: Mortality and Births; Hygiene; Etiology; Pathology; Therapeutics," he asserted. "The last is infinitely less certain than the first."[9] Like others after him, Cheever concluded that the study of public and private hygiene held out more promising prospects than medical therapy for professional progress.

In subsequent decades, while physicians shared a remarkably unified view of therapeutics' course over the first two-thirds of the century and of the stage it was on the verge of departing, they depicted their differing visions of the future with increasing force. Their expectations for therapeutics followed five general models of progress. These included the notions that physicians would selectively recover their faith in the heroic therapy of the past; that slow but sound advancement would be effected through empirical clinical observation; that hygienic therapy fostering the healing power of nature would gain precedence over drugging; that state preventive medicine would increasingly occupy energies frittered away on efforts to cure; and that experimental laboratory science would provide the foundation for a rational therapeutics elevated to a universalized science with real promise of certainty.

Postbellum calls for therapeutic progress through the resurrection of older practices mirrored some of the attachment to tradition that had led physicians in the 1850s and early 1860s to charge that the empiricist critique of therapeutics had gone too far. The physicians who argued in the 1870s and 1880s for renewed attention to such therapies as venesection and calomel cannot, however, be dismissed as merely reactionary older practitioners. Robert Edes, for example, was thirty-two when in 1870 he told a Massachusetts medical society that although the demolition of prior fallacies had benefited the profession, the time had come to assess traditional remedies anew. Like most he lamented the disparity between progress in the basic sciences and progress in therapeutics, but he predicted a "counter-reaction" in which disused therapies would be reevaluated in light of improved knowledge and optimistically prophesied that "instead of a routine use, or almost equally routine neglect," their power would be prudently harnessed.[10] "The present age is . . . one of skepticism, but skepticism does not mean disbelief," he asserted. "We have rejected the systems and theories of our ancestors and are to reconstruct our science, as we hope, on a new and firmer basis. We may use their material, but the plan must be a new one."[11]

A second position reaffirmed the view that empirical clinical observation on the French model could indeed generate positive contributions to therapeutics and that this was the only legitimate avenue to progress. Older Paris-trained physicians often favored this posture, but it had the support of others as well. Speaking before a Maine medical society in 1869, for example, a thirty-year-old physician who had never studied in Paris noted that "the theory and practice of medicine are now in a transition state." He divided the history of medical treatment into stages and proposed that therapeutics had just entered the stage of "rational empiricism." Skeptical criticism had been salutary in clearing the way for "a well-grounded faith, which can arise only after a complete destruction and reconstruction of the tottering fabric." Now this therapeutic reconstruction would be completed by "rational empiricism," especially empirical observation of disease and the effects of remedies.[12]

The French impulse in American medicine helped shape another program for positive therapeutic advancement as well. By the 1860s many practitioners saw progress in hygienic management as the best means of furthering clinical practice. Studies of the natural history of disease that revealed the limited efficacy of drugs also underscored the benefits to be derived from fostering nature's healing efforts by carefully managing hygienic factors such as diet, fresh air, rest, exercise, and cleanliness. Hygienic therapeutics would fill the void that the disarmament of the regular drug arsenal had left.

Although it deemphasized drugging, hygienic therapeutics was fully consistent with prevailing therapeutic ideals. Progress, according to this model, would come through empirical clinical observation, often numerically ordered. After all, physicians widely agreed that of all branches of medicine hygiene was the most amenable to the statistical revelation of new truths. Moreover, hygienic treatment was entirely compatible with faith in the principle of specificity. "Hygiene more than any other department of medicine leads the observer to place something like a proper value upon individuality in the management of disease," one physician claimed in 1878.[13] Surgeon Paul Eve, lecturing to medical students in Nashville two years earlier, noted that "just as every one is recognized by some peculiarity in his personal expression, so has he peculiarities in his constitution which may require careful study before prescribing for him." Hygienic treatment, he argued, was singularly adaptable to the individual patient's needs. "We are not in search of supposed specifics, or even remedies; but rather engaged in studying hygiene, the laws of health, so as to oviate [*sic*] the necessity to resort to the use of medicines at all . . . Our great aim is to assist nature in relieving the case."[14] Furthermore, hygienic therapeutics maintained an active role for the physician, for assisting nature involved sometimes aggressive manipulation of the patient's environment.

The stress on hygiene over drugging also led to a fourth, more radical vision of the future of therapeutics, the notion that individual treatment should give way to public or state preventive medicine as the profession's primary focus. Willard Parker, a New York supporter of public hygiene, expressed a not uncommon position in 1875 when he wrote to Eve, "I have learned that *prevention* of *disease* is a higher position in science than the treatment of disease."[15] No one expected the bulk of practitioners to cease treating patients and turn to preventive efforts on behalf of the state instead, but some physicians did argue that energy directed toward promoting health would be better rewarded than attempts to solve the more intractable problems of cure. Some public health enthusiasts followed the implications of this creed to the conclusion that the chief avenue to medical progress lay not in private treatment but in public prevention.

Bowditch advocated this stance in his "Centennial Discourse on Public Hygiene" before the International Medical Congress that met in Philadelphia in 1876. In 1869 Bowditch had become the first chairman of the Massachusetts State Board of Health, the first of its kind in the nation. In his speech he dramatized the new order of endeavor he envisioned by dividing medicine in the nation's first hundred years into three epochs. The earliest, which extended from 1776 to 1832, he called "the epoch of systems of medicine." Typified by the systems of Cullen, Brown, Rush, and Broussais, this era was dominated by confidence in art and distrust of nature. The second epoch, which had ended in 1869, was that of observation, epitomized in the thought of Louis, Bigelow, and Bartlett and especially in their emphasis on nature's healing power. During this period the empiricist allegiance to facts "led not only to a thorough overthrow of all the imaginative theories that preceded it, but it has gone still farther . . . [toward a] most unhappy degree of scepticism as to the precise value of the very medical art so highly vaunted in the preceding epoch, and especially as to the use of drugs." This period was unmistakably one of destruction, good in that it razed speculative systems but bad in that it swung too far toward skepticism. The third and final epoch was that of "State Preventive Medicine," which Bowditch immodestly maintained had begun when the Massachusetts State Board of Health was established and extended "into the far-off future."[16] The way out of the middle epoch's excessive skepticism and gloom was hygienic improvement under state auspices.

Bowditch did not call for an end to efforts to improve medical therapeutics; he believed that eventually clinical experience coupled with physiological experimentation would generate more precise knowledge of drug action, but such progress would be very slow. "It may take centuries to develop, even to a small extent, the future materia medica," Bowditch commented in his essay *Preventive Medicine and the Physician of the Future* (1874). In the meantime, "the profession will learn that a system of therapeutics dependent on materia medica simply, is much less valuable than that which seeks to defend its patients from the insidious approaches of the causes of disease."[17] Anticipating the same kind of objection that had been brought against nature trusting—that it would render the physician superfluous—Bowditch noted, "It may be asked, What is to become of the physician and his practice, when the public takes care of its own health more than it does at present? Will the profession be useless?" No, it would be elevated rather than debased by the transformation. "It will be the prophet of the future, and will direct men how to govern their own bodies in order to get the full amount of work and of joy that is possible out of each body that appears in life."[18] The chief therapy the physician of the future would provide was education, instructing the public and the state on the preservation and improvement of health. Bowditch's thinking clearly reflects the contribution therapeutic frustration made to the efflorescence of public health activity in the 1870s.

The treatment of individual patients provided both livelihood and identity for most physicians, and what Bowditch proposed to erect on the purified but vacant plot left by the middle period's destruction was unsatisfying to them. His position was threatening in its de-emphasis of the practitioner's therapeutic role and inadequate in its failure to offer a strong program for positive clinical progress. Yet several of the major currents in therapeutic thinking supported it. Bettering health by creating a hygienic environment was justified by faith in the healing power of nature. Like hygienic therapeutic management of an individual patient, it was premised on the notion that nature would preserve and restore health if given suitable encouragement. The plan also pushed recognition of the limitations of medical art to its extreme, even though by this time Bowditch himself believed that the skeptical trimming of drug therapy had already gone too far. Moreover, the third epoch as Bowditch portrayed it was to be squarely grounded in the statistical analysis of empirical observations, an approach physicians agreed was singularly suited to hygienic questions. (Fittingly Bowditch dedicated his address to the memory of the numerical method's founder and his mentor, Pierre Louis.) Nevertheless, the desire to effect progress in state preventive medicine more than in clinical therapeutics remained a decidedly minority sentiment.

A fifth plan for escaping pessimism identified experimental laboratory science as the wellspring of a new therapeutic epoch. Physiological experimentation would produce the critical knowledge needed to rebuild therapeutics and would ultimately direct physicians' prescriptions at the bedside. Americans who favored this view commonly believed the program for therapeutic reform that had dominated the century's middle third had exhausted its capacity to improve practice. But "the passage of physiology, from a speculative to a positive science," New York physician William Draper asserted in a distinctly Comtian tone, was "the signal for a revolution in the practice of medicine."[19] Unlike the revolution the French school's teachings had instigated, this one was to be constructive. By offering a new platform for therapeutic reconstruction and the promise of boundless progress, its proponents held, this vision more than any other warranted optimism and the dissipation of therapeutic gloom.

In one respect the plan to base therapeutics on experimental physiology was not as radical as the idea that public hygiene should take precedence over curative efforts, for it preserved the primacy of the practitioner's therapeutic role. Epistemologically, however, the expectation that experimental science would transform therapeutics was nothing short of revolutionary. Basing therapeutics on the results of reasoning from physiological experimentation in the laboratory, not exclusively on empirical observation in the clinic, meant that rationalism was to regain its sovereignty over therapeutics. And with the New Rationalism's ascendancy would come the restoration of all that the American empiricists had toiled so hard since the 1820s to banish. The reconstruction of therapeutics on the foundation of experimental science would uplift therapeutics to the level of the universalized basic sciences, physicians committed to this program believed. It would supplant the limitations of therapeutic specificity with the prospect of universalism, fixed laws, systems, and even an approach to certainty. By offering a pathway out of sterile clinical empiricism the New Rationalism would bring about a therapeutic renaissance.[20]

The program for therapeutics rooted in experimental science was expressed in its canonical form in Parisian physiologist Claude Bernard's *Introduction to the Study of Experimental Medicine* (1865). Like so many American physicians, Bernard emphasized the novelty of his approach by implicitly dividing the history of medicine into three stages. The first, prescientific medicine, appeared in his treatise only as an implied contrast to the scientific medicine that succeeded it. In the second stage medicine became a science, but only one of empirical observation. "Medicine so conceived can lead only to prognosis and to hygienic prescriptions of doubtful utility," Bernard asserted. "It is the negation of active medicine, i.e., of real and scientific therapeutics."[21]

Unlike those few Americans content to develop the potential of hygienic therapeutics and preventive hygiene, Bernard insisted that the treatment of disease must also become more certain and more active. He argued that medicine based on experimental physiology would be elevated to a third stage—experimental medicine—in which the rigid laws of scientific determinism rather than the uncertainties of clinical observation would direct bedside behavior. Medicine must adopt laboratory science as its foundation, Bernard claimed; "only by basing itself on experimental determinism can it become a true science, i.e., a sure science. I think of this idea as the pivot of experimental medicine, and in this respect experimental physicians take a wholly different point of view from so-called observing physicians."[22]

Bernard did not reject clinical observation as an ingredient in therapeutic advancement but made it an adjunct to experimentation rather than the principal method of discovery. In experimental therapeutics clinical inquiry remained essential in determining the natural course of the diseases on which remedies were tried and in confirming the actions of therapies on human patients. Practitioners would also have to rely on observational knowledge to direct treatment until more exact experimental knowledge was produced. Bernard acknowledged that in practice the observational and experimental ways of knowing should be "fused," but his denunciation of observational therapeutics as inferior was nonetheless vehement. In particular he disparaged therapeutic truths determined by statistics as no better than their underlying observational foundation. "I acknowledge my inability to understand why results taken from statistics are called *laws;* for in my opinion scientific law can be based only, on absolute determinism, not on probability," Bernard asserted. "If based on statistics, medicine can never be anything more than a conjectural science."[23] The stridency of Bernard's attack on clinical statistics is understandable given that it was against the reigning emphasis on such clinical empiricism that he set his program for experimental medicine. At the same time, his vehemence underscores the extent to which his prescription for therapeutics challenged, and did not simply supplement, the Paris clinical school's entrenched ideals.

Enthusiasm for the medical value of experimental physiology was by no means novel to Americans in the 1860s. The crucial new element in that decade was the idea that knowledge produced in the physiology laboratory could direct therapeutic behavior, not just explain it. Physicians at midcentury commonly used physiological knowledge to account for the actions of remedies, legitimize their theories, and lend authority to their clinical practices, but they did not as a rule believe that laboratory science could test the clinical worth of therapies or guide therapeutic change.[24] Bennet Dowler, who in the 1840s and 1850s actively pursued physiological experimentation, was typical in his general failure to claim that the knowledge he produced would alter the course of therapeutic practice.[25] Americans who began to advocate experimental therapeutics were distinctive not so much in their attention to the laboratory as in their efforts to define it as a leading source of change in practice.

Bernard was the most forceful spokesman for therapeutic reform based on physiological experimentation. While the American proponents of experimental therapeutics acknowledged their very real debt to his ideas, they differed from him in a way that made their program fundamentally distinct from his: they virtually all practiced medicine.[26] American practitioners, ever driven by the imperative to act, could not remain so aloof. For most of those who shared his vision of the relationship between experimental physiology and therapeutics, there was an urgency about actualizing physiology's potential missing in Bernard's thought. The American case for experimental therapeutics was characterized by a conviction that the enactment of therapeutic reformation by scientific enlightenment was imminent.

What Bernard termed "experimental therapeutics" American physicians most often called "physiological therapeutics." According to the "physiological method," experimentation in the laboratory would elucidate physiological processes in health and disease as well as the actions of remedies. On the basis of this information, the practitioner would know how processes in the patient's body deviated from normal and what adjustments would be required to correct them. By understanding the specific alterations various therapies induced, he could then select a treatment that would precisely alter the deviant process to restore physiological normalcy. The term "physiological method" as Americans used it encompassed experimental physiology, physiological chemistry, and much of the work on in vivo drug action later subsumed under experimental pharmacology.

The methodological pivot on which progress in physiological therapeutics turned was vivisection (a term referring to all experimentation on living animals and not strictly to procedures that involved cutting). Measurement of the alterations drugs induced in laboratory animals was the operational core of the physiological method. Vivisection "is the only path to a knowledge of functional life," and the only sure source of knowledge about drug action, one physician asserted in 1868. "All other employment of remedies is purely empirical, and must remain so. Therapeutics without such investigations never can advance one step."[27] Vivisection, an epistemologically and emotionally volatile subject, became a central issue in debates over the legitimacy, morality, and practical relevance of physiological therapeutics. Clinical observation of disease's natural history and of drug action on human patients was to supplement knowledge gained in the laboratory, but it was already an accepted source of knowledge and its role in physiological therapeutics was much less a source of contention than was vivisection.

Physiological therapeutics sought to elevate therapeutic knowledge to a fundamentally new epistemological category. The chemical and physiological principles derived from experimentation in the laboratory and their use to guide practice reintroduced rationalism as a foundation for therapeutic knowledge. Therapeutics was to be advanced by reasoning from the laboratory to the bedside. In 1884 Horatio C. Wood, professor of materia medica and pharmacy at the University of Pennsylvania and a leading American spokesman for what he called "the modern physiological school of therapeutics," sketched out the role of reasoning from the laboratory to the bedside in this approach to prescribing. "The general principles which underlie rational therapeutics," he explained, were (1) "to know what can be done and what it is desirable shall be done," which meant assessing how the patient's physiological processes deviated from normal and what would be required to correct them; (2) "then to know the means at command," that is, to know from laboratory experiments which drugs induced particular physiological changes in laboratory animals; (3) "and, finally, to adapt the means to the end," reasoning from therapeutic possibilities to treatment.[28]

The New Rationalism was the hallmark of physiological therapeutics. It was both the rallying point for those who saw in experimental science a way out of therapeutic stagnancy and the principal target of those who perceived it as an invidious revival of the rationalism they had labored so long to dispel. The proponents of the physiological method countered that experimental physiology's rise made a rational therapeutics legitimate and desirable.[29] Between the 1860s and the 1880s therapeutic rationalism was a prickly issue that consistently underlay debates on such varied topics as the place of vivisection in medical research, the proper methods of training students for practice, the therapeutic legitimacy of laboratory knowledge, the possibility of therapeutic certainty, the value of clinical experience to the practitioner, and even the physician's professional identity.

In advocating physiological therapeutics, physicians often accentuated the potential of the New Rationalism by contrasting it with the limitations of empiricism. Like most American practitioners, the proponents of the physiological method acknowledged that the expulsion of some prior errors by empirical clinical observation had improved therapeutics; but empiricism had led to a dead end, for it was incapable of creating a science of therapeutics. Only rationalism could do that. " 'Empirical' experiences do not constitute a science of life and therapeutics," one physician stated flatly.[30] Methodological empiricism's critics linked it to superstition and fettering tradition in much the same way as the pupils of the Paris clinical school had earlier associated rationalistic systems with those evils. Empiricism was not rejected from therapeutic investigation, but it was derided as inferior. Thus Roberts Bartholow, an early proselytizer of physiological therapeutics, noted in 1865 that the use of bromide of potassium could be studied from both "the rational and empirical points of view, since some of the uses of this agent are derived directly from its chemical and physiological actions, and others have been discovered by its empirical employment." But, he added decisively, "I prefer the former method, because of its scientific accuracy, and for the further reason that a rational therapeutics whenever attainable, is preferable to a blind empiricism."[31]

Underlying this preference was a new conception of what constituted science in medicine that became more common during the next
two decades. The scientific basis of therapeutic practice increasingly
came to mean laboratory experimentation. In 1884 Wood told his materia medica class that because knowledge of disease and the action of
remedies was incomplete, the practitioner was forced to supplement
rational principles derived from the laboratory with "pure empiricism."
Medical practice was in part still an art, Wood acknowledged. "The
best therapeutic practice of to-day is therefore a mixture of science and
empiricism."[32] The message of his implied contrast was clear: empiricism was not science, nor were the ways of gaining knowledge that
therapeutic empiricists esteemed, such as clinical observation and
medical statistics, truly scientific. The "modern scientific therapeutist" had found more promising avenues to therapeutic truth. "The
great therapeutic departure of the last decade," Wood claimed, "is the
general abandonment of the statistical method of therapeutic research,
and the substitution therefor of the so-called physiological method."[33]
In the judgment of Wood and like-minded disciples of the physiological
method, making therapeutics more rational by basing it on laboratory
experimentation meant making it more scientific.

In so doing these physicians hoped to accelerate the progress of
therapeutics by linking it to that of physiology. "Physiology is rising
to the dignity of a positive science. If we grant its postulates, we may
accept its prophecies as true," one physician observed in 1874. "The
practice of medicine, resting as it does, and as it must to be completely
successful, upon physiology, is making progress, *parsi passu*, with the
advance of physiological science, becoming more and more rational
and scientific."[34] Bartholow made the same point several years later
when he claimed that "scientific therapeutics must always follow the
course of discovery in physiology."[35]

The aspirations of physicians like Bartholow and Wood for therapeutics went still further. In grounding medical therapeutics in experimental physiology, they hoped ultimately to elevate it to the level
of the basic sciences. "It was not until the birth of modern physiology
that scientific therapeutics became possible," Bartholow explained.[36]
Such a scientific, experimental therapeutics, as they envisioned it,
would be lifted out of the separate epistemological category that had
excluded therapeutics from the rapid progress of the basic sciences.

One liberating effect anticipated from placing therapeutics on the
same epistemological plane as the basic sciences was a shift from therapeutic specificity toward universalism. This change was enabled by
the idea that the physiological and therapeutic actions of drugs were
comparable. Experimental therapeutics redirected the physician's at-

tention away from the myriad peculiarities of patient and environment toward specific physiological processes. If normal physiological processes were known and the patient's departure from normalcy determined, and if the physiological actions of drugs were defined, then in principle the patient's physiological deviance could be engineered back to normal by selecting the drug that would precisely effect the needed adjustment. The physiological method posited that both normal physiological processes and the physiological effects of drugs were knowable and constant, and that therefore in a fully developed experimental therapeutics the principle of specificity would lose its sway.

Accordingly in physiological therapeutics the individuating factors governed by the principle of specificity forfeited their earlier significance. "In seeking a remedy," one physician asserted in 1874, "it is logically legitimate only to consider the physiological requirement."[37] The experimental therapeutist's attention was closely centered on a physiological process rather than an individual patient, and in some respects it made relatively little difference whether that process was going on in an Irish immigrant or a laboratory dog; therefore whether the physician was prescribing for an immigrant or a native-born patient mattered very little indeed. In the epistemological category medical therapeutics had previously occupied, specificity had imposed what some practitioners had come to see as "humiliating" limits on therapeutic knowledge.[38] In experimental therapeutics these restraints were lifted, for the therapeutic value of rationalism had again been asserted, and oppression by the powerful coalition of the principle of specificity and empiricism overthrown.

At the same time the turn to the laboratory for instruction suggested that therapeutic universalism of a sort was both desirable and attainable. Treatment was matched to a particular physiological process more than to the individual's constitution and background. If that process and drug action were both linked to a universalized basic science, then treatment too became in principle universalized. Physicians had never doubted that the basic sciences such as chemistry, physiology, and anatomy were universalized in their generation and validation, and the advocates of experimental therapeutics were simply arguing that the principles of basic science should to an extent supplant empirical observation as the guide for therapeutic practice.[39]

Even in the ideology of the most extreme proselytizers of physiological therapeutics, the receding importance of specificity and the rise of universalism were qualified. Medical therapeutics could not be derived exclusively from laboratory science. Clinical knowledge of the natural history of disease remained an essential component, and it was through this portal that the modifying variables of patient and environmental peculiarity crept back into the therapeutic scheme. For those practitioners who saw in experimental science the surest source of new, practical therapeutic precept, however, these distorting influences were minor modifying considerations, not ruling forces in therapeutic activity. Medical lecturers and writers continued to teach the principle of specificity through the 1880s,[40] but from the 1860s onward claims for its influence on prescribing became infrequent and enfeebled.

The movement in therapeutics from empiricism and specificity toward rationalism and universalism was accompanied by a growing belief that the quest for invariant therapeutic laws had again become a legitimate enterprise. "Let the discovery of a single fact," a practitioner proposed in 1876, "lead on to the establishment of some certain and specific method in therapeutics. In this way, by long and continued labor and perseverance, I firmly believe that we will at last attain absolute certainty in the treatment of most diseases." The profession, he continued, needed "great men who possess philosophical minds and strong reasoning powers . . . to establish unerring and inflexible laws in practical medicine, which will lead to uniformity of practice, and harmony among all intelligent and regularly educated physicians."[41] Once the actions of remedies and disease processes were known, another physician predicted the following year, "then we will be in possession of a rational therapeutics. The science will be fixed. It will no longer be subjected to the assaults of the ignorant, or the superstitious."[42]

By the early 1870s advocacy for a rational *system* of therapeutics had re-emerged in regular medical discourse. In the laboratory, some physicians believed, principles would be established capable of bringing a measure of certainty to prescribing, which had heretofore been governed by the vagaries of empirical observation. Unlike the early-nineteenth-century rationalistic systems, these therapeutic systems were not to be premised on a unitary theory of disease. Instead, the new system builders looked to knowledge about physiological processes for unifying principles.[43]

The kind of fixed therapeutic rule that proponents of physiological therapeutics wanted as a basis for a system of practice is best exemplified by the development of the idea that specific treatment was possible and proper. Physiological therapeutics suggested that treatment might be specifically matched not to disease entities but to objectively measurable signs of physiological or chemical abnormality within the patient's body. "I use the term specific in an adjective not substantive sense," a physician calling for "specific treatment" qualified his remarks. "I mean something far above and beyond the vaunted nostrums and advertised specifics of the present day."[44] Specific treatment regarded in this way depended on laboratory-derived knowledge of physiological normalcy and drug action that was the nucleus of physiological therapeutics.

At least through the 1880s most talk about creating a rational system of specific therapeutics based on experimental science was programmatic. The principle of physiological antagonism, however, was one concrete product of the laboratory search for therapeutic laws that was elaborated during this period. Certain drugs exerted directly opposed actions on particular organs or tissues, the proposition at the core of this principle held, as an antidote acts in poisoning. If poison and antidote were administered simultaneously, the opposing physiological actions they produced in the body could in effect cancel each other out. Examples of antagonistic drug pairs commonly cited included opium and belladonna, atropine and physostigmine, and chloral hydrate and strychnine. In the principle of physiological antagonism, the limited use of this knowledge in treating cases of drug poisoning was extended to its broader therapeutic potential. Knowledge of such antagonistic actions could directly target a particular drug to the specific abnormal physiological action to which it was opposed. Discrete pathological conditions such as elevated temperature, lowered arterial tension, or increased heart action could thereby be specifically normalized. Some of the experimental work used to establish this principle can be traced back to François Magendie's animal experiments early in the century. It was only in the 1860s, though, and especially after a committee the British Medical Association set up under John Hughes Bennett's direction to experimentally investigate the antagonism of medicines drew attention to the subject in the mid-1870s, that discussion of it became widespread among American physicians.[45]

The principle of physiological antagonism was deeply satisfying to the advocates of physiological therapeutics, for even more than constituting a model of specific treatment, it seemed to prove the therapeutic worth of studying drug action in the laboratory. Roberts Bartholow, who had been an enthusiastic proponent of physiological antagonism since the 1860s, was among those who saw in this principle a rational foundation for a system of specific therapeutics that would bring therapeutic certainty. As one admiring reviewer of Bartholow's textbook on practice observed bluntly, "Prof. Bartholow's system of treatment is founded upon *rationalism*."[46]

In 1880 Bartholow summarized in a series of lectures both the evidence demonstrating physiological antagonism and the causes for optimism that physicians committed to physiological therapeutics saw in it. "There is still present the notion that observation and experience should be the sole foundations for the construction of a therapeutical science," Bartholow noted. "The advocates of this empirical method are fond of asserting that the observations on animals can not be applied with any certainty to man."[47] But the bedside application of physiological antagonism scotched such thinking, to Bartholow's mind. Knowledge about the physiological actions and antagonisms of drugs could have its inception only in vivisectional experimentation. Reasoning from laboratory findings to the human patient, Bartholow claimed, had established the principle of physiological antagonism's practical usefulness and validated its epistemological presuppositions. "While the notions of the actions and uses of drugs engendered by experience and observation are constantly changing, the deductions of experiment have the same value as the same methods in other experimental sciences," Bartholow asserted. "To this end we should direct our best efforts, and rest satisfied with no less certainty than that which belongs to the exact sciences, until we have attained to such a degree of perfection that, the disease being given, the remedy follows."[48]

Proponents of specific treatment often contrasted their plan of therapeutics, informed by reasoning from experimental science, with the expectant method that clinical empiricism encouraged. Treatment guided by empirical clinical observation, they argued, often merely allayed symptoms as they arose while relying on nature for cure. In contrast the practitioner employing the specific method began by determining the physiological abnormality at the root of the patient's illness, frequently relying on chemical tests and instrumental measurements to do so. Then, drawing on laboratory knowledge of the physiological effects of various drugs, the practitioner found the best fit between the physiological alteration needed and the drug that would accomplish it. One physician explained in 1885 that the plan of treatment he was advocating "is known in distinction from the expectant or symptomatic treatment as 'specific.' It is more direct and immediate in its aim. When it shall have become entirely established, ... the practice of medicine will take its place among the sciences which are called exact."[49]

The contrast between specific and expectant treatment was but one sign of the energetic therapeutic optimism that characterized the writings of those committed to physiological therapeutics. Often this attitude was explicitly set against the pessimism still widespread among American physicians. Advocates of the New Rationalism blamed skepticism and therapeutic minimalism on empiricism in much the same way that Paris-trained empiricists had held overly exuberant rationalism responsible for heroic drugging earlier in the century.

By informing universalized therapeutic laws based on experimental physiology, the New Rationalism dispelled the causes of gloom about the future. "We should not sit down in the ashes and mourn over uncertainties and doubts," Bartholow asserted in 1873, arguing that the physiological method justified therapeutic optimism.[50] Physiology would lead to boundless therapeutic progress, unhampered by the principle of specificity. Skepticism may have been justified as long as the value of drugs could be assessed only on the basis of clinical experience, a Boston physician proposed in 1871, but now, "as we are beginning to [understand], the real unquestioned effects of certain medicinal agents on the parts affected, a ray of light falls upon the healing art, and the practice of medicine begins to be something more than the observation of cases." He concluded that "the expectant treatment, and the treatment of symptoms must yield, and be followed by the scientific appliance of remedies whose effect can be predicated to the removal of diseases."[51]

The American physicians who spoke for physiological therapeutics typically shared several characteristics. They tended to be younger than many of those who denounced their views and especially than the ardent exponents of therapeutic empiricism in the tradition of the Paris school against whom they saw themselves arrayed. They also tended to be actively seeking professional distinction and advancement at the time their vocal advocacy of the physiological method began. Furthermore, they tended to look to Germany more than to France for medical instruction, and many had studied in German laboratories and clinics. They clearly regarded German laboratory medicine as the harbinger of medicine's future, and they emphasized the sterility of the Paris clinical school despite the fact that they were themselves clinicians who sought to relate laboratory work to their own activity at the bedside. Finally, they tended to be among the most intellectually elite and ambitious of their generation. Support for physiological therapeutics was certainly encouraged by educational and generational factors; it may also have served the young, ambitious physician as a way to distinguish himself through association with novelty.

Above all these factors in determining advocacy of physiological therapeutics stood a permissive one: the younger physicians who embraced the New Rationalism had not fought the empiricist battle against rationalistic systems of practice that had so preoccupied intellectually engaged American physicians from the 1820s through the 1850s. They did not see therapeutic rationalism as an evil to be overcome for the good of the profession. One major division between supporters and opponents of physiological therapeutics was certainly generational, but to regard this as a simple opposition of old conservatives to young progressives would be to miss the point. The central intellectual experience in the professional careers of many older physician-intellectuals had been the overturning of rationalism, an experience their younger colleagues lacked. During the second quarter of the century some of the Paris-trained American physicians had prided themselves on being epistemological iconoclasts, but by the 1850s much of their crusading zeal against rationalistic systems had waned; empiricism was no longer a banner of radicalism but a standard of the dominant standpoint.

Older physicians were not freely able to take up physiological therapeutics and its underlying rationalism because they were committed to a hard-won therapeutic empiricism that they saw as being at odds with it. Their younger colleagues, who lacked the zealot's allegiance to empiricism, were more inclined to take empiricism for granted and condemn its shortcomings. Although virtually all American physician-intellectuals shared a growing sense by the 1860s of therapeutic stagnancy and the limitations of clinical empiricism, not all were emotionally or epistemologically prepared to turn to experimental science and therapeutic rationalism as an alternative.

Because physiological therapeutics threatened dominant assumptions about the proper sources and nature of medical knowledge, criticism of it was both widespread and severe. By far the most usual objection was that knowledge generated in the laboratory simply made no difference in actual practice, a charge examined in the next chapter. Beneath this utilitarian dissent was the belief that it was epistemologically illegitimate to base therapeutics on experimental physiology. Sometimes this objection was explicit. Philadelphia medical teacher and clinician Alfred Stillé was typical in his denunciation of the idea that the basic sciences could do anything more than explain therapeutics. Stillé, who had studied in Paris with Louis, held that empirical clinical observation alone was the legitimate foundation for therapeutic activity. "The domain of therapeutics is, at the present day, continually trespassed upon by pathology, physiology, and chemistry," he asserted in the preface to his *Therapeutics and Materia Medica* in 1874. "Not content with their legitimate province of revealing the changes produced by disease and by medicinal substances in the organism," he charged, these sciences "presume to dictate what remedies shall be applied, and in what doses and combinations. Their theories are brilliant, attractive and specious, and they seem to satisfy a craving experienced by every reasoning man for an explanation of the phenomena which he witnesses; but, when submitted to the touchstone of experience, they prove to be only counterfeits. They will neither secure the safety of the patient nor afford satisfaction to the physician."[52] Medical therapeutics was properly governed by clinical experience, not laboratory experimentation; by the principle of specificity, not universalism; by empiricism, not rationalism.

Critics of physiological therapeutics in the 1870s often cited Stillé's treatise as a model textbook on therapeutics, usually contrasting his prudent trust in empirical clinical observation with the reliance such authors as Bartholow and H. C. Wood placed on the products of physiological experimentation. Cincinnati physician Thomas Minor, for example, adopted this approach in reviewing Bartholow's *Materia Medica and Therapeutics* (1876). "We are aware that it has become the fashion, among latter day American and German writers, to sneer at what is called rational empiricism," Minor observed. He placed Wood and Bartholow in this category, noting that "both authors exhibit a marked preference for physiological experimentation, in order to determine the therapeutic value of remedies."[53] But, he asserted, "the practitioner at the bedside of his patient . . . does not care to indulge in medical metaphysics." The physician who gave quinine for malarial fever, for example, did so "simply because experience has taught him that it will 'break the chill.' His conclusions are deduced from rational empiricism; he cares not what the action of quinine may be on the capillary circulation of a dog's caudle appendage, and that that useful article may cease to wag under the influence of the drug; he cares not that quinine lessens reflex action in the frog and curbs the hopping propensity of the innocent bacterian. No! He leaves that all to the speculative medical experimentalist." By contrast, Stillé's book remained the most useful to the practitioner, in Minor's opinion, for it was solidly based on "rational empiricism," discriminating observation at the bedside. The task of "the modern speculator," by which Minor meant the physiological therapeutist, was "as hopeless a one as that of the infant trying to grasp the crescent moon to see what makes it shine."[54]

Minor's reference to the advocate of therapeutics based on laboratory physiology as "the speculative medical experimentalist" made his tacit comparison of this "modern speculator" with the Enlightenment system builder unmistakable. From the perspective of critics there was much to sustain the fear that physiological therapeutics meant the return in new guise of many of the characteristics of the rationalistic systems of practice the profession had struggled since the 1820s to divest. In the new therapeutics they saw not only a revival of rationalism but also claims to therapeutic universalism; the notion that a system of practice was a desirable, legitimate goal; and the extreme enthusiasm and confidence that had characterized therapeutics at the start of the century. Elisha Bartlett in the *Philosophy of Medical Science* (1844) had unreservedly denied that therapeutics could

be derived from the more basic sciences; "The former cannot be deduced from the latter. It rests wholly upon experience. It is, absolutely
and exclusively, an empirical art."[55] Bartlett's work "should be considered a sufficient answer to hypothesis-mongers of all sorts," Stillé
approvingly wrote to a Paris-trained Boston physician when the book
first appeared. "It shows . . . a certain dignified inflexibility becoming
one who has undertaken to call to account the worshippers of idols."[56]
With the rise of the New Rationalism, Stillé and like-minded physicians feared that the laboratory was a workshop wherein new idols
were being fashioned by those among their professional brethren who
had defiled the empiricist faith.

To an extent the critics of physiological therapeutics were right.
In no respect did the physiological therapeutists more closely approx-
imate the rationalistic medical systematists of the previous century
than in their faith that certainty was possible. Bartholow made the
renewed quest for certainty clear in 1876 when he delivered the annual
oration before a Maryland medical society on "The Degree of Certainty
in Therapeutics." At the time he was a medical teacher, clinician,
experimenter in physiology and chemistry, and ardent proselytizer of
physiological therapeutics, and in the same year he had published a
textbook on therapeutics founded on the physiological method. He was
known for his therapeutic optimism and notorious for his clinical experimentation. Studying in Europe, Bartholow had become deeply committed to the German vision of laboratory medicine, and although he
openly admired such men as Bernard and Bennett, he took every opportunity to snipe at French clinicians. It was scarcely by accident that
Bartholow, ever contentious, implicitly set his new vision against those
of the Parisian empiricist philosophers by using a title for his address
similar to those of well-known treatises by Pierre-Jean-Georges Cabanis (1797) and Elisha Bartlett (1848).[57]

Since the start of the nineteenth century, Bartholow began his
address, increasing scientific knowledge about disease had drawn into
question the value of remedies, while faith in drugs had been bolstered
by nothing more substantial than empirical experience. As a consequence practitioners had become skeptical of the power of drugs. "In
the ruin of their own faith and the refutation of their own experience
they see an end to certainty in therapeutical knowledge," he noted.
"Beginning with a blind confidence, these simple souls end with an
unreasoning skepticism."[58]

Experimental therapeutics based on laboratory physiology constituted the legitimate foundation for recovering certainty, Bartholow
believed. "Therapeutical writers," he acknowledged, "are by no means
agreed to the relative merits of the empirical and physiological meth-

ods." He cited the textbooks of Stillé and G. B. Wood as representative of these respective positions.[59] To illustrate the empiricist stance, Bartholow quoted from Stillé's preface to the fourth edition (1874) of his treatise, in which he stated that he had "contended against the mischievous error of seeking to deduce the therapeutical uses of medicines from their physiological action" in the first (1860) edition of his text. "Continued study, observation and reflection have tended to strengthen his convictions upon this subject, and to confirm him in the faith that clinical experience is the only true and safe test of the virtues of medicines," Stillé wrote.[60] This had been precisely Bartlett's position, and Bartholow belligerently denounced it as "reactionary." Empirical observation could never justify therapeutic confidence, Bartholow argued, for "experience is fallacious."[61] Only through the physiological method could certainty in therapeutics be attained.

Bartholow was exemplary of those American physicians who were most optimistic about the promise of experimental laboratory science to transform therapeutics and rouse the profession from its gloom. Therapeutics "is an experimental science," he claimed, and some of its facts "are capable of the same kind of experimental proof as are the facts of the biological sciences."[62] In calling for the sort of determinism in therapeutics that Bernard had claimed for physiology, Bartholow was seeking laws of medical practice as certain as those posited by the Enlightenment medical systematists. The empiricism of the Paris clinical school had proved inadequate in effecting positive progress and giving the practitioner assured therapeutic confidence at the bedside, physicians like Bartholow believed. The New Rationalism of therapeutics based upon laboratory knowledge, on the other hand, would generate fixed, unifying therapeutic laws that would in turn revitalize the therapeutist's endeavor. The search for a medical Newton was on again, but this time he was to be a bench man.

— 9 —

Cui Bono?

Bᴇᴛᴡᴇᴇɴ ᴛʜᴇ mid-1860s and the mid-1880s, some American physicians began to articulate an expansive program for reconstructing medicine on the foundation of experimental science. The claim of laboratory science to practical relevance in medical therapeutics did much more than challenge the reign of empiricism: it urged a thoroughgoing rearrangement of the relationships among therapeutic practice, knowledge, and professional identity. As the proponents of the newly laid basis for treatment teased out the implications of physiological therapeutics, they portrayed it as an integral part of a new medical ethos gradually taking shape.

A few practitioners fully gave their hearts and minds over to the new science and its enticing therapeutic promise. Other intellectually prominent physicians, firm in their commitment to clinical empiricism, vocally opposed the new plan's epistemological heresy. The vast majority of American physicians, though, remained ambivalent—but not indifferent. The proposition that experimental science should govern therapeutic practice had fundamental implications for professional identity; the doctor-patient relationship; the professional meanings of the hospital, medical education, and codes of ethics; therapeutic practice; and the very definition of professional orthodoxy. Hence the notion that medical therapeutics should be grounded upon experimental science unavoidably entered into the everyday concerns of practitioners to whom epistemological disputes might otherwise have seemed arcane if not frivolous. Furthermore, the lingering suspicion that too firm an allegiance to science could distract the physician from the care of patients, that the "medical speculator" might be bargaining away moral behavior for expert knowledge, made many practitioners uneasy.

Often the epistemological concerns about experimental therapeutics that some elite physicians explicated—concerns about empiricism versus rationalism, specificity versus universalism, and observation versus experimentation—were distilled into blunter questions: Of what use is it in healing? What difference does it make at the bedside? If these questions were plainer, they were also in some ways harder to answer. The simple fact that knowledge generated in the research laboratory failed to revolutionize actual treatment during these decades sustained critics in their skepticism. At the same time it made the question *Cui bono?* singularly grating to the defenders of experimental science's therapeutic worth, for they were unable to find the compelling evidence they wanted to uphold their bold assertions. However adamantly enthusiasts of experimental physiology and bacteriology foretold the coming revolution in therapeutics, in this period their faith was sustained more by the promise of future relevance than by demonstrated results. That the anticipated therapeutic millennium did not have its advent in their lifetimes was a source of acute disappointment and frustration to them.

Despite the ambivalence toward laboratory science that the overwhelming majority of the profession retained, changes in therapeutic attitude were not confined to a few zealots. The ideals and products of experimental science had a tremendous impact on medical therapeutics in America in the postbellum period despite the fact that their influence was not expressed principally in altered prescribing habits. The pervasiveness of certain changes in language demonstrates that physicians widely shared in the transformation. The declining use of the word *natural* and the rising use of *normal* in its place was but one semantic signal of the changing outlook. The connotations of terms that described epistemological stances in therapeutics began to change at the same time. *Rational* and *empirical* retained their earlier professional connotations, but the methodological meaning of *rational* regained a positive connotation after the 1860s, while that of *empirical* became steadily more negative. Many physicians—not just spokesmen for laboratory science—also began to speak in positive ways about *specific* treatment. And by the 1870s regular physicians were again talking about a *system* of practice as something desirable.

To display the therapeutic permutations experimental science instigated, this chapter first analyzes the blueprint for reform that the laboratory's enthusiasts delineated. The plan they sketched in programmatic statements for restructuring professional identity and practice was bolder than most practitioners were willing to fully accept, but elements of their design are evident in the self-image and practice of the profession as a whole. The forceful protest that experimental science did little to make practitioners better healers—the most common negative expression of physicians' persistent ambivalence—is then

evaluated. Finally, the way American physicians assessed the therapeutic implications of early bacteriology is presented as an exemplar
of both the promise for therapeutics some physicians saw in laboratory
science and the practical, ideological, and emotional objections it elicited from others.

Just as some physicians saw their knowledge and practice to be in
transition between the 1860s and 1880s, so too they correctly perceived
that their professional identity was at a turning point. Because the
alterations in professional identity these decades witnessed entailed a
new assessment of the relationships among knowledge, behavior, and
professional propriety, they were crucial to therapeutic ideology.
Professional identity in medicine was not created anew on the foundation of experimental science in postbellum America, as some writings on "professionalization" tend to suggest, but was instead
transformed; not defined, but redefined.[1]

One key to understanding this transformation is to recognize the
shift that occurred in emphasis from behavior to knowledge as the
basis for professional identity. Instead of regarding practice as the primary support of professional identity, as they had, some physicians
began to place greater stress on their claim to special knowledge. The
practitioner's interactions with patients, correct clinical behavior guided
by experience, and observance of rules for professional etiquette were
gradually subordinated to rigorous biomedical knowledge and its promise of effective action. The defining core of the proper physician's task
became less the *exercise of judgment* and more the expert *application
of knowledge.*

Among the most dramatic consequences of the reconstruction of
therapeutic epistemology and professional identity was a reassessment
of the value of experience. Only with the advent of the New Rationalism was the primacy of experience for the practitioner's therapeutic
ability questioned. The shift from the exercise of judgment to the
application of knowledge as the ideal of the physician's bedside function entailed a new valuation of knowledge over experience. Such an
outlook did not deprecate clinical experience but held it to be insufficient to make a good therapeutist. What was known only by experience, known only empirically, was what remained art in therapeutics.
What was known with certainty and rationally explained was elevated
to the level of the science of therapeutics.[2]

Concurrently the new ideology elevated knowledge about basic
science to unprecedented importance to the practitioner. It became
increasingly imperative that the practitioner know what the normal

state was in order to detect and correct deviations from it. The basic sciences that defined normalcy achieved a new clinical relevance as universalized scientific principles became more important and considerations that fell under the principle of specificity's sway less so. Lacking knowledge of normal biology the physician could practice only empirically, responding to symptoms and lowering or elevating the patient's system without comprehending the underlying abnormality. Extensive knowledge of normal physiological processes, which had been peripheral to the task of restoring the individual patient's natural balance, became a necessary acquirement of the proper therapeutist.

To say only that therapeutics was becoming more "scientific" would be deceptively glib, for the very term *science* used in this way glosses over the actual transformation. To the American disciples of the Paris clinical school, for example, the plan of basing therapeutics on exacting clinical observation was every bit as scientific as the later program of physiological therapeutics was in the eyes of its adherents. A new definition of what constituted therapeutically relevant science in medicine was gaining support, and it in turn demanded of the practitioner new kinds of knowledge.

Experimental science never supplanted clinical observation in the natural historical tradition as a way of therapeutic knowing. For the advocates of experimental therapeutics, however, as for some proponents of experimental laboratory research in biology, experimentation represented a higher order of science than natural history and held greater promise for progress. The shift from *natural* to *normal* in clinical language reflected the movement from natural history to experimentation as the model of medical science. The scientific therapeutist increasingly attended to the kind of norms that experimental laboratory science revealed, giving by comparison less attention to the protean patterns of morbid natural history observed at the bedside.

Faith in experimental therapeutics fundamentally altered the relationship between professional identity and such basic sciences as physiology. So long as the notion prevailed that therapeutics had to be derived from clinical observation, it was possible for a physician ignorant of basic science to be regarded as legitimate by merit of his practical experience. It had been assumed throughout the nineteenth century that knowledge about physiology, for example, was desirable in a regular physician, but knowledge about *practice* was essential to his "profession" of being worthy of public confidence. The elevation of experimental therapeutics to the same plane as the universalized basic sciences and its firm linkage to them gave knowledge about practice a wider definition that now included the basic sciences. Knowledge of the basic laboratory sciences became a component of proper professional identity in a way forestalled during the first two-thirds of the century by the distinctive epistemological category occupied by therapeutics.

Willingness to acknowledge the products and techniques of experimental science as critical to the sound practitioner marked one of the most enduring dividing lines between the old medical ethos and the new. While some physicians urged the new relationship between experimental scientific knowledge and professional identity, others remained committed to clinical empiricism and dismissed laboratory science's claims to therapeutic relevance and to being a component of professional identity. Advising Cincinnati medical graduates in 1880 to "arm yourselves with the weapons of science," a commencement speaker warned that "there are those who will jeer at you . . . The question *cui bono* will be asked time and time again: What is the use of the microscope? What is the use of the thermometer? Why do you study chemistry? Why do you study physics? Didn't our forefathers practice medicine as successfully as we do?" Exemplifying the perceived generational division between those who sought therapeutic guidance in scientific knowledge and those who looked to experience, he noted that the young graduates who put their faith in experimental science would inevitably face ridicule from some of their elders. "The cry is 'he is a young man—he is theoretical!' " He assured the graduates, however, that the old supports of professional identity were giving way to newer ones. "It may be a consolation to you to know that, at the present, it takes more than gray hairs, an owl-like countenance and a gold headed cane to make a successful practitioner. It even takes more than experience!"[3]

The iconography of the ideal physician was being reshaped to sharpen those features most revered in the newer conception of professional identity. The practitioner of "owl-like countenance" whose prestige came from years of experience was less emulated in the new value system than was the man of science. "Something more than the examination of the tongue, the feeling of the pulse, a superficial knowledge of drugs, the treatment of mere symptoms, and the ability to prescribe in the hieroglyphics of a dead language, are now demanded of the educated physician," a Boston physician typically asserted. "He must be able to trace the symptoms to the hidden cause, from a knowledge of chemistry and physiology, without which no rational system of hygiene and therapeutics is possible."[4] An esteemed physician was less often now described as a man of great experience and judgment and more frequently as one of scientific learning. Being an expert in scientific matters, the possession and application of specialized knowledge, was becoming a hallmark of professional identity.

The shift from behavior toward knowledge as the base of professional legitimacy altered the role that intervention with drugs played in defining professional identity. A primary allegiance to scientific knowledge that could dictate abstinence from treatment if that was best for the patient diminished the imperative to therapeutic action. In the newer value system, experimental science was the arbiter of both therapeutic activity and professional morality. Action remained important but was subordinated to the belief that science would decide the most prudent course. Part of the visible control once exercised through drugging was rechanneled into monitoring and understanding the precise course of the patient's deviation from normalcy. The physician preserved the control that conferred professional authority but expressed it more by knowing and less by drugging.[5] One consequence of the diminished role of therapeutic activity in professional identity was that it became more possible to be a nonpracticing physician, a change important for those who moved into the research and experimental science teaching positions created toward the end of the century.

As professional legitimacy came to stem more from an allegiance to science and less from practice, interactions with patients and other practitioners became less critical as a gauge of professional rectitude. The physicians who embraced the ideal of experimental science were less concerned than their forebears had been with setting orthodox practitioners apart from sectarians. During the 1870s and 1880s debate flourished in some regular medical societies about the prohibition against consultation with irregulars. The physicians who most ardently promoted experimental science were often the very ones who opposed rules seeking to sustain professional standards by forbidding association with unorthodox practitioners.[6] It was no longer necessary to rely on rigid rules of professional behavior to distinguish the professionally legitimate physician from the sectarian, they argued. Instead enlightened physicians should look to the test of scientific knowledge to discriminate between the competent practitioner and the quack. "Homoeopathy and allopathy are dreams of a by-gone time," Roberts Bartholow told medical students in an 1872 lecture. Describing the advances in scientific knowledge and asking, "*Cui bono?* What is it all worth?" Bartholow proposed that one consequence of experimental science's rise was to render distinctions among practitioners on the basis of the sectarian dogma or system to which they subscribed nonsensical. The proper physician's primary standard was scientific truth. "Modern science is indifferent to Hippocrates and Hahnemann. If their theories will not bear the bright light of the present, let them wander back into the darkness of the past to which they belong," Bartholow asserted. "The therapeutics of to-day rejects dogmas, and the therapeutics of the future will accept nothing that can not be demonstrated by the tests of science. No longer faith, no longer a blind experience will suffice."[7]

Orthodox therapies lost their significance as emblems of the regular creed that segregated the proper physician from the sectarian. It was no longer necessary to defend regular mainstays and condemn sectarian alternatives by appealing to medical tradition and professional morality. Science would judge all therapeutic practices objectively, confirming the good and unmasking the bad. A primary allegiance to the values of science that transcended—indeed scorned—artificial boundaries among sects made an egalitarian therapeutic ethic possible. The scientific physician was not obliged to intervene out of fear that therapeutic abstinence would link him ethically with the homeopathist, nor did he need to affirm his regularity by prescribing drugs identified with orthodox tradition. He looked to a higher authority, science, for his professional legitimacy and identity.

The shift from behavior to knowledge as the conspicuous support of professional identity also transformed the doctor-patient relationship. In claiming to be an expert in natural science, the physician became less dependent on the authority that derived from his relationships with sick individuals. Changes in therapeutic epistemology further restructured these relationships. Exercise of judgment in discerning each individual's therapeutic needs had been a clear sign of the proper physician, but with the waning of the principle of specificity attention to patient idiosyncrasies became more and more marginal to professional identity. Knowing the normal state that the universalized standards of experimental science defined became more important in treatment than knowing the natural condition that described health for an individual patient. The newly objectified concepts of disease and therapy directed the scientific physician's attention away from the sick individual, and lessened the significance of the doctor-patient relationship as a source of professional legitimacy and an element in therapy.

The declining importance of the principle of specificity also made attention to the social and physical environment secondary. Therapeutic knowledge was to a large extent freed from domination by the individuating characteristics of different environments just as it was from patient idiosyncrasy. The changing medical ideology assured the practitioner that would he but submit his therapeutic decisions to arbitration by the universalized criteria of experimental science, correct treatment would ensue so long as his scientific acumen was sound enough. Therapeutic regionalism, nationalism, classism, moralism, and racism were stripped of much of their earlier justification. These discriminations did not become unimportant, but they lost their significance as cardinal determinants of therapeutic propriety, and attention to them was no longer a salient sign of prudent professional behavior. The free application of knowledge across national, regional, class, and racial boundaries gained unprecedented epistemological and professional legitimacy.

It was for this reason that the ascendancy of the new medical ethos increased, not decreased, the importance of the hospital as an authoritative source of therapeutic knowledge. In making a case for the practical potential of laboratory science and in defending its worth against the more entrenched claims of clinical medicine, the enthusiasts of experimental research often used rhetoric that polarized the laboratory and the clinic. In a limited political sense, of course, these two loci for the pursuit of therapeutic truth were in opposition, as it was only by eroding the hegemony of empirical clinical observation that advocates of laboratory science could secure support for their ideals and methods. It would be a mistake, though, to accept the politically motivated rhetoric of a power struggle at face value in evaluating its intellectual content. The program for therapeutic progress that experimental science informed accorded clinical observation an important place and called for the epistemological changes necessary in order to legitimize the hospital as the heart of therapeutic research.

During the first two-thirds of the nineteenth century the principle of specificity had been the main wellspring of skepticism regarding the pertinence of therapeutic knowledge generated in hospitals to patients outside their walls. The weakening of specificity and the growing commitment to universalism in the decades after the Civil War to a large extent relieved hospital knowledge of its singular status. Just as it became increasingly legitimate to transport therapeutic knowledge produced in one country or region freely to another, it also appeared more and more reasonable to take therapeutic knowledge based on the observation of hospital patients and apply it in private practice. Thus while reductionist laboratory science was beginning to secure its claim as a source of therapeutic authority, the hospital was also gaining a fundamentally new kind of authority as a source of widely applicable therapeutic knowledge. The laboratory did not supplant the clinic; instead, both found in the ideals of experimental science a new foundation of therapeutic legitimacy.

This transformation carried with it a significantly altered attitude toward the hospital as a research institution in therapeutics. The rise of Parisian hospital medicine had failed to make physicians look unreservedly to the hospital for therapeutic instruction because faith in the principle of specificity had rendered therapeutic dictums formulated there suspect for application elsewhere. It was the epistemological transformation experimental science effected that validated the hospital as a leading source of therapeutic knowledge relevant for general medical practice.

Permutations in actual practice between the 1860s and 1880s, described in Chapter 4, reflected those in ideology but were less momentous. The most ardent discussions animated by experimental science centered as much on the promise of change in practice as on its actualization. Still, the sources of guidance practitioners relied on became increasingly rooted in physiological therapeutics. Thousands of postbellum American physicians traveled to German laboratories and clinics to complete their medical training. Even if a young physician had not himself studied in Germany it was more and more likely that his professors had, and a growing proportion of them had been converted to the laboratory's ways. Increasingly, some of these physicians illustrated their teaching with demonstrations on the effects of drugs on animals. Textbooks on practice that emphasized physiological therapeutics, such as those of Bartholow and H. C. Wood, were widely used from the 1870s onward, and journal literature mirrored these teachings.[8]

The Dispensatory of the United States of America itself became a bastion of the physiological method in the mid-1880s. By the time the fifteenth edition (1883) was being prepared, it scarcely reflected the therapeutic orientations of its two original authors: Franklin Bache had been dead for two decades and George B. Wood was nearly eighty. As the preface to that edition noted, "Although [Wood] sympathized with the movement which has resulted in putting therapeutics upon the firm foundation of physiological rationalism, he could not fully apprehend the changes which had occurred in therapeutic methods during the previous decade." His nephew, Horatio C. Wood, whom one reviewer aptly called "the great apostle of Rational Physiological Therapeutics," became senior editor of the work and rewrote it in accord with his disdain for empiricism and belief that physiological experimentation should be the foundation for therapeutic practice.[9]

Although by 1885 the new view of practice had been taken up whole by only a tiny minority, American physicians widely adopted elements of it. The universalization in principle of therapeutic knowledge was expressed as a tendency toward more uniform practice, evident in the growing similarity of prescribing habits in the various regions of the country. Substantial regional variations in the employment of such therapies as venesection and calomel subsided from the 1860s, and the use of the newer drugs never developed strong regional patterns sustained by the principle of specificity. Epidemiological differentials did mean that some broad variations in drug usage endured, notably the more extensive prescription of cinchona bark derivatives in the malarious regions of the South and West. Still, the move to standardization is clear in the practice of hospitals, for example, where the regional differences that persisted, such as those in dietary prescriptions, tended to stem more from economic realities than from medical theory.

Throughout the country the fading imperative of drug intervention to professional identity was expressed at the bedside as a decrease in treatment. Mirroring the shifting emphasis in the clinician's role, from drugging to knowing, the prominence of therapeutic instructions receded in hospital case records. Traditional remedies were given less frequently and in milder doses, and the newer drugs were more often given singly, in contrast to the polypharmacy of the past. The surveillance of patients—for example, monitoring their changing course by recording quantified physiological measurements and the results of chemical tests—became the most striking feature of case records. The tendency to give fewer drugs fittingly accompanied the shift in the foundation of professional identity from behavior to knowledge, many physicians believed, and would improve the profession's standing. "Nothing had so much contributed to elevate the medical profession as the decline of medicine," a Boston observer concluded in 1870.[10]

The deprecation of drugging was supported though not compelled by the persistent belief in the healing power of nature. While it is true that the tradition of clinical empiricism out of which the strong American faith in nature had developed was antagonistic to rational therapeutics based on laboratory science, the notion of the *vis medicatrix naturae* could be comfortably accommodated into the framework defined by physiological therapeutics. Thus a medical professor who in 1881 urged on his students "the importance and utility of the experimental methods of determining therapeutic truths" could assert at the same time that in medical therapeutics "the greatest advance of modern times" was recognition of nature's powers in curing disease. "Aware of this inherent tendency of the organism to revert to its *normal* state," he told his class, "the physician who is well versed in the recent acquisitions of medical science, knows well that all he has to do in mild cases is to watch nature in her work, and to assist her when . . . she is prevented from exercising her curative power."[11] Some devotees of experimental science did offer new explanations for the healing power of nature based on physiological processes that restored a normal state, but most of the physiological therapeutists, like their predecessors, were content to describe nature's healing operations without accounting for them.

Use of the new drugs that came to the fore starting in the 1860s was rationalized in a way that postulated their cooperative relationship with nature. The proponents of physiological therapeutics did not propose to cure self-limited diseases, but they did maintain that the new drugs targeted at specific physiological processes could assist nature in important ways. "Do not mistake the curative processes of nature for the action of drugs, & do not mistake drugging for treatment," one Harvard professor admonished students. He proposed that "drugs do not cure disease, they only modify the physiological action," but that was enough to enable the practitioner who understood the physiological effects of therapies to actively aid the patient.[12] The physician could normalize certain physiological processes rendered abnormal in disease, lightening the burden on nature while trusting her to perform those operations that experimental science had not yet placed within the power of art.

The most striking clinical changes the ideal of physiological therapeutics effected through the 1880s were those in attitude. The shift in the therapeutic conception of disease from a disturbance of the natural balance to a deviation from the normal state altered the categories by which clinical thinking organized therapies. "Very much that has been said about 'phlogistics' and 'anti-phlogistics,' 'stimulants' and 'sedatives,' born of the misconception of physiological conditions, is losing its force," an advocate of rational physiological therapeutics observed in 1874.[13] Such distinctions based on a model of health as balance were viewed as not very useful and were to be eschewed in favor of descriptions that referred more specifically to physiological processes. The physiological therapeutist found it more satisfying to give a febrile patient an antipyretic to normalize temperature, chloral hydrate to encourage sleep, or a cardiac sedative to reduce pulse rate than to elevate or reduce the entire system. Bartholow clearly reflected this opinion when he insisted that readjusting systemic balance in response to observed symptoms was wrongheaded. "The antiphlogistic treatment is neither rational nor scientific," he asserted, and "a blind stimulant treatment, which is the other extreme, is even more mischievous."[14]

Increasingly reductionist criteria for diagnosis and treatment typified the transformation in clinical attitude. Instrumental measurements and chemical tests became important therapeutic guides. Chemical and microscopical analysis of urine was an early instance of the new approach to gathering pertinent signs of physiological disorder that had come into widespread use by the 1860s. Bartholow, for example, voiced a common opinion when he maintained that in patients with pneumonia the reappearance of chlorides in the urine marked the resolution of inflammation. The practitioner could use a simple chemical test of chloride levels to chart the progress of the disease and the patient's therapeutic needs when evidence from physical diagnosis was inconclusive. "Every practical physician should therefore daily test the urine of his cases of pneumonia," Bartholow asserted, "not only for the valuable diagnostic and prognostic indications thereby afforded, but also, to learn the time for critical evacuations which he may hasten, encourage or imitate."[15]

The reliance on evidence such as this fundamentally reorganized the relationships among patient, sign, and physician. Reductionist signs determined by instrumental measurement or chemical tests, such as urine chloride level, were not readily perceptible to patients, much less interpretable by them. Because the patient was unable to say what his or her natural condition was in terms of such signs, the practitioner by necessity depended on normal standards, perceiving the sign vicariously through the mediation of instruments or chemical reagents and using his expert knowledge to interpret it. The patient was alienated from this sort of clinical sign and became unimportant as a reporter about it. That doctor and patient did not have equal access to such signs or comprehension of their meaning does not mean, however, that they did not share a common faith in their importance. Thus in 1880 a rural Louisiana patient could write to a physician, "I have send to you by mail one Bottle of my urine which I dont think that it is all right, I hope that you will examine the same & let me know if there is anything the matter with me."[16] If the resemblance to medieval urinalysis was only superficial, both did share an underlying rationalism and attendant mystification of the clinical sign to the patient.

Above all, the change in therapeutic attitude was exemplified by the greater directedness of treatment. The proselytizers of physiological therapeutics urged that whenever possible the course of therapy should run in a rational channel connecting a drug of known action and a narrowly targeted abnormality. Treatment was increasingly specific to objectively measured signs; it was less a response to symptoms that represented an underlying systemic imbalance and more focused on altering discrete abnormalities in physiological processes. Proponents of physiological therapeutics routinely held up not only new antipyretics such as the salicylates and antipyrine but also older ones like alcohol and quinine as models of the kind of therapy they sought. These drugs normalized a discrete abnormality and were admirably specific. Furthermore, the effects of antipyretic treatment could be monitored vicariously, reduced to numbers and objectified on a graph free from the subjectivity of the patient or physician. The use of drugs rationalized by the principle of physiological antagonism was another commonly cited model for the new therapeutics.

No single drug that emerged during these decades seemed to the advocates of physiological therapeutics to make a stronger case for the New Rationalism than did chloral hydrate. Unlike the therapeutic use of the antipyretics, that of chloral was acclaimed to be fully the product of experimental science, not merely the beneficiary of its support. Its sedative action was first predicted on the basis of knowledge generated in the laboratory and only later confirmed by clinical trials. In 1869 German experimental pharmacologist Oscar Liebreich suggested that since the in vitro treatment of chloral hydrate with a base produced chloroform, a similar reaction should occur in the slightly alkaline human bloodstream. Liebreich maintained that the chloroform liberated thereby would function as a sort of internal anesthetic or hypnotic, inducing sleep. Experiments on animals and subsequent trials on human patients confirmed the predicted effect, though its metabolism was later shown to follow a very different pathway. In American practice chloral hydrate rapidly rose to vogue as a sedative. But it gave the proponents of physiological therapeutics much more than merely another useful drug. "How much soever opinions may clash on the subject of the physiological study of drugs, it is an undeniable fact that some of our most satisfactory knowledge has been obtained by this method of research," Bartholow could declare before a Maryland medical society in 1876. "Every one present is doubtless familiar with that beautiful series of investigations by Liebreich which gave chloral to humanity."[17]

Chloral hydrate represented rational therapeutics par excellence, and it was this aspect of the drug that most appealed to the Americans who regarded experimental science as the proper foundation for therapeutic practice. "Of all the remedies introduced into practice on theoretical grounds, none has been so generally used, or with such satisfactory results, as chloral," one physician observed in 1871. "It was argued, on chemical grounds, that it ought to produce certain effects on the system, and it has wonderfully justified the experiment."[18] Chloral seemed a good harbinger for the fulfillment of experimental science's promise to bring about a therapeutic renaissance, and it was endlessly cited in confirmation of that program's fruitfulness. The portal through which chloral entered practice, one physician argued in the year after it was introduced, was "an admirable illustration of the close alliance between the chemical constitution, the physiological action and the therapeutical use of drugs. This alliance," he predicted, "is becoming every day more apparent, and the time is not far distant when it will be generally recognized by the practising physician, and constantly guide him in the art of prescribing."[19]

What the enthusiasts of experimental science saw as fundamentally new in therapies such as chloral hydrate was the nature of the knowledge that recommended their use. Yet even though these physicians sought dramatic changes in the underpinnings of therapeutic epistemology, their program for reform preserved much of the existing framework of practice. In the reconstruction of therapeutics that became possible in the 1870s and 1880s, the physician's active therapeutic role was retained. If some of the exercise of control was transferred from drugging to surveillance and understanding, the practitioner's ultimate mastery nonetheless endured. Moreover, most of the new drugs, like chloral, ordinarily produced directly observable physiological impressions. The physician might monitor temperature changes produced by antipyretic therapies through the objective means of thermometry, but both the practitioner and the patient's family could still detect directly the reduction in the patient's fever. Much of the architecture of practice was preserved, though often it was rationalized in different ways.

Critics of the emerging order often targeted the epistemological apostasy of physiological therapeutics as its chief evil, but the most common and direct objection to grounding therapeutics upon experimental science was simply that the laboratory offered the practitioner nothing of practical therapeutic value. The form this criticism took was old and well used. It objected not to basing therapeutics on science but to the particular kind of science that was newly claiming therapeutic relevance. This criticism repeated once again the questions, What difference does it make for therapeutic practice? And if it does not improve the physician's ability to heal, why should the practitioner care? The same critique that had been applied to nearly every innovation in medical science's earlier nineteenth-century forms—speculative system building, pathoanatomical investigation, and empirical clinical observation and statistical analysis—was now brought to bear on experimental laboratory science.

Physicians, a New England practitioner had typically asserted in 1834, "must be real utilitarians" when evaluating scientific knowledge and techniques. "With physicians, the *cui bono?* will this make me a better practitioner?—is the only important object."[20] During the ensuing half century, the objection of irrelevance was persistently brought against knowledge and tools that increased understanding but failed

to augment therapeutic power. Even after the diagnostic utility of instruments such as the stethoscope and microscope had become clear,
they were denounced for their therapeutic impotence. "It is quite learned
to understand how to distinguish a cancer cell; but does this distinguishing the cell cure our patient?" one physician asked in 1872. "All
can by training become accustomed to use the microscope so as to
distinguish malignant cells, but who can honestly cure the poor suf-
ferer?"[21] The notion that by temperament and necessity the practitioner's interests must be different from those of the scientist, so evident
in American judgments of Parisian researchers, became even stronger
after midcentury.

As advocacy of basing therapeutics on experimental science mounted
from the 1860s on, so did the charge that whatever the laboratory might
offer basic science it had not contributed much to the practitioner's
ability to heal and was an unlikely source of future practical progress.
Experimentation in the laboratory was ordinarily placed in opposition
to observation at the bedside, with the quest for therapeutic truth at
the bench depicted as not merely irrelevant but self-indulgent. A medical lecturer at the University of Virginia in the late 1880s was typical
of such critics. He told his class that the great progress made in physiology did not imply that therapeutic improvement would ensue. Therapeutics had already been "groping in the dark two decades by studying
the physiological action of drugs on inferior animals." Reflecting the
disdain for the rationalism of experimental therapeutics common among
those who clung to empiricism, he urged his students to take as their
guide clinical observation, not "the recreations of science."[22]

Vivisectional research, the methodological core of the program to
reform therapeutics on the basis of experimental science, provided its
adherents not only concrete scientific products but also a powerful
symbol of therapeutic promise. Animal experimentation was an expression of the newness of the physiological therapeutist's endeavor, for
no one could confuse its methods for discovering therapeutic truth
with those of the clinic.[23] At the same time, the distinctiveness of
vivisectional research made it an eminently vulnerable symbol against
which practitioners committed to an older value system could vent
their dissatisfaction with the changing medical ethos. Animal experimentation remained wholly foreign to the practitioner's routine. Like
the broader origins of the antivivisection movement in desires to preserve an older order and conserve purity, physicians' perception that
vivisection represented the corruption of traditional professional values fueled their criticism. In assailing vivisection they risked violence
to nothing that upheld their self-image but gained a very effective outlet

for voicing resistance to the new, sometimes threatening conceptions of professional identity and morality that were gaining strength.

Detractors charged that whatever might be the value of vivisectional experimentation in elucidating basic physiological principles, it was impotent as a guide to therapeutic activity. The expectation that reasoning from the actions of drugs on laboratory animals to their effects on human patients would yield positive therapeutic progress was illusory. Reviewing a new treatise on the action of medicines in 1878, one physician sneered, "We commend this work to all physicians who are desirous of poisoning guinea pigs, rabbits, pigeons, and frogs."[24] Often critics argued that the evils of such therapeutic rationalism ultimately were visited on the patient. Accusing "the speculative medical experimentalist" of theoretical self-indulgence the practitioner could ill afford, the same reviewer, assailing Bartholow's textbook of therapeutics, commented that "what's death to dogs, cats, rats, rabbits and frogs is often death to the unfortunate human subject."[25]

The practical question of how knowledge should be not just generated but disseminated was also at stake in discussions about experimental therapeutics. Acceptance of its epistemological presuppositions would in principle demand substantial institutional reform. The encroachment of the laboratory on the hegemonic status of the bedside in producing therapeutic knowledge was but the starkest of the envisioned changes. The orientation and priorities of the institutions of medical education—journals, textbooks, and schools—also hung in the balance. Debate over educational reform often prompted physicians to make their objections to the therapeutic pretensions of laboratory science bluntly explicit. Beyond the substantive issues of medical school reform, underlying questions being debated were: What value does experimental science have for the practitioner? Will it make the student a better healer?

One context in which these questions were central was the debate over educational reform at Harvard Medical School. The events at Harvard were hardly typical of American schools, though they presaged changes later enacted more broadly, but they did elicit from the faculty lucid assessments of experimental science's value for the practitioner. When Charles Eliot became president of Harvard in 1869, he sought to transform the medical school into a rigorous professional school modeled after the German ideal of higher education in science. In accordance with Eliot's proposals, the medical school shed its proprietary standing and became an integral part of the university; its two-year program consisting of a single four-month term repeated once was expanded to a graded three-year program of nine-month terms with written examinations; and experimental science gained unprecedented prominence in the curriculum, which emphasized actual laboratory experience for each student. Though the age and training of individual faculty members alone did not determine their attitudes toward the reforms, the younger, German-trained members of the faculty—David Cheever, Calvin Ellis, and James Clark White—did endorse Eliot's program, while Henry Jacob Bigelow and Oliver Wendell Holmes, older faculty who had studied in the Paris hospitals, opposed it.[26]

White, who had been advocating major reforms in the medical school since the mid-1860s, was the staunchest faculty supporter of Eliot's plan. Committed to the value of laboratory medical research since his studies in Germany in the early 1860s, he confidently proclaimed his faith that instruction in experimental science was crucial for the practitioner. White was not a doctrinaire disciple of the laboratory, though, and stressed the importance of clinical education as well. In an introductory address to the medical class in 1870, the message of which he had already described privately to Eliot,[27] White called for the reformation of American medical education to give students a solid grounding in experimental science. "The bedside and the medical lecture-room are no places for you, until you have learned all that physiology will teach, and have made yourselves familiar with chemical reagents and their action upon the normal tissues and fluids of the body," he admonished the students. "You cannot understand therapeutics or venture to produce the physiological action of drugs, until you have studied their toxicological laws and relations of incompatibility."[28] White made clear his belief that empirical clinical observation held only very limited promise. "I would have to dispossess your minds of the too common belief that everything can be learned at the bedside; it is a fatal barrier to individual and national progress in medicine."[29] The student needed experience in the laboratory as well. "I may venture to prophecy that its grandest discoveries are waiting outside the sick room," he asserted, and concluded by endorsing the curricular changes that were to be enacted.[30]

Henry Jacob Bigelow, who was Jacob Bigelow's son and had studied in Paris three decades earlier, was the faculty's most vocal opponent of the position White represented. The two agreed that the ultimate test of educational reform should be its capacity to increase the practitioner's therapeutic power. The medical educator "should never lose sight of the fact that everything in medical instruction is to be made wholly subservient to the prevention and proper treatment of disease," Bigelow maintained. "Therapeutics is the single leading idea, to which no inconsiderable part of modern medical education is secondary, and even tertiary."[31] White held out hope that the graduates of the program he envisioned would contribute to medical knowledge as well as apply it, but he too was willing to submit the proposed reforms to the test of practical utility.[32] Where White and Bigelow diverged was in their assessment of the value of instruction in experimental laboratory science to the practitioner. To White, it was the necessary foundation of therapeutic action; to Bigelow, it was an unjustifiable waste of time.

Several months after the reforms at Harvard were enacted in 1871, Bigelow explained his opposition in an annual address before the Massachusetts Medical Society entitled "Medical Education in America." The primary thrust of his thesis was simple: experimental science was at best peripheral to the task of healing and therefore had no legitimate place in the education of medical practitioners. Reductionism "leads farther and farther from the original object of medical education, which is Therapeutics," Bigelow told his audience. He admitted that subjects such as physiology deserved attention in the didactic curriculum, but he was thoroughly convinced that the laboratory was no place for medical students. He particularly cautioned that the possibility of future practical worth was insufficient justification for including laboratory science in the medical curriculum. "The teacher of the art of healing has no . . . right to employ the time of the ignorant student disproportionately in the pleasant and seductive paths of laboratory experimentation, because some of these may one day lead to Pathology or Therapeutics."[33]

Bigelow's address was much more than a proscription of extensive laboratory training from the medical curriculum. Presented several months too late to forestall reform at Harvard, it was an intellectual and moral protest against the emerging medical ethos and concisely expressed the position of those thinking physicians who resisted the new order. Committed to the older tradition of empirical clinical observation, Bigelow argued on epistemological grounds that experimental physiology had little practical therapeutic value. "A materialism here productive of error is that which leads to the belief that we can so far understand the physiological action of a drug, that we can rely . . . not upon the ultimate condition of the patient, which [it] is well known we can sometimes do, but upon his intermediate machinery." As Elisha Bartlett had done so decisively, Bigelow asserted that therapeutics could not be reduced to physiology. Moreover, experimental laboratory science would train students in dangerous rationalism, distracting them from empirical observation of symptoms, the proper guide for therapeutic action. "The student who expects to influence disease because he understands how a drug passes through the visceral cells will get into a habit of therapeutic reasoning and action very likely to damage the man or woman who owns the viscus." Reflecting the common fear that the New Rationalism would turn therapeutics back to the errors of speculative systems from which his father's generation and his own had extricated it, he told his audience, "The established rules of art are safer teaching than the speculations of science."[34]

Implicit in Bigelow's remarks was an objection to the therapeutic optimism that advocates of physiological therapeutics believed the promise of experimental science warranted. He reiterated his father's point that it was not possible to cut short self-limited diseases. Reasoning from experimental science could foster a false confidence in remedies and excessive drugging. "Experimental physiology," he observed, "leads away from broad and safer therapeutic views, and toward a local and exclusive action of chemistry and cells,—uncertain grounds for students, for whom the result of large and well-attested medical experience is here the safest teaching."[35]

An ardent antivivisectionist, Bigelow denied that this method of research could be justified by its therapeutic yield. He went beyond the criticism that animal experimentation was therapeutically sterile to suggest that it could corrupt the practitioner's character. "My heart sickens," he told the members of the Massachusetts Medical Society, at the "chamber of torture and horrors . . . advertise[d] as a laboratory." Medical students were especially endangered when vivisection was used as a pedagogical tool. "I say it is needless. Nobody should do it. Watch the students at a vivisection. It is the blood and suffering, not the science, that rivets their breathless attention," he stated grimly. "If hospital service makes young students less tender of suffering, vivisection deadens their humanity and begets indifference to it."[36]

Bigelow's remarks were premised on the tacit model of professional identity that had reigned in America during the first two-thirds of the nineteenth century but was being contested at the time he spoke. Behavior and character more than expert knowledge constituted the legitimizing foundation on which the kind of physician he wanted Harvard to train would stand. The exercise of judgment rather than the application of knowledge was the essence of the practitioner's therapeutic task. "The excellence of the practitioner depends far more upon good judgment than great learning," he asserted. "If you fill the mind of the student with Chemistry and Physiology and Drugs, as leading ideas, the chances are that he will apply this collateral, imperfectly applicable knowledge wrongly, and that he will have to forget and disuse much of it before he gets it down to a medical working level." His ideal physician was not an expert in medical science but "a plainer sort of man" who possessed "wide practical experience and sound judgment."[37]

Those physicians who called for physiological therapeutics had only to reaffirm their epistemological beliefs to dismiss Bigelow's central argument that experimental science taught in medical schools would be superfluous to healing. Yet some of them shared Bigelow's fear that medical curriculums might be freighted with scientific instruction without due reference to its therapeutic utility. There was no more devoted acolyte of physiological therapeutics in America during the two decades following the Civil War than Roberts Bartholow, a strident opponent of the epistemological stance Bigelow defended. Like Bigelow, however, Bartholow was disturbed by the possibility that medical schools might seek to make students medical scientists rather than "sound practitioners." Bartholow told his class at the Jefferson Medical College in 1879, "I hold this to be a perversion of the duty of a medical school."[38] The risk that medical schools would teach science for its own sake was especially troubling to therapeutic enthusiasts who feared that such a tendency could discredit their efforts to convince the profession of physiological therapeutics' practical worth. Physicians like Bartholow carefully distinguished the animus of their endeavor—the desire to use experimental science to catalyze a therapeutic renaissance—from that of some scientists who did not practice medicine and who pursued their research unconcerned about its practical applications, but who toward the end of the century increasingly sought to establish a secure place for their work in medical schools.[39]

In soliciting the profession's support, advocates of experimental science often pledged therapeutic products on behalf of the laboratory well beyond anything it was certain it could deliver. The therapeutic promise of the New Rationalism frequently led to disappointment, and nowhere was this more evident than in the emerging field of bacteriology. The main vehicle for therapeutic reconstruction on the basis of knowledge produced in the laboratory before 1885 was clearly physiology, but other branches of laboratory science also took part. Bacteriology offered a distinctively new conduit for medical aspirations. It was especially alluring from a therapeutic perspective, for it seemed at first to resolve complex problems into simple solutions. The reception of bacteriology into American therapeutic thinking between the mid-1860s and the mid-1880s illustrates both the ambiguity of laboratory research's claims to therapeutic relevance and the sources of resistance to the new order.[40]

The notion of treating a patient by destroying the specific, living cause of his or her disease was not new in the 1860s, but it was only then that a substantial number of American physicians began to direct their attention to this possibility. The germ theory had been intensely debated since the 1840s, and by this decade physicians had widely come to think of contagious or infectious diseases as being caused by specific organic particles. While some maintained that these poisons were chemical ferments, increasingly they were conceived of as living germs. A corollary to the germ theory was the suggestion that many diseases might be curable by what was termed *internal antisepsis*, a notion bolstered by success in surgical antisepsis during the 1860s.[41]

In principle devising an effective therapy was simple. "This theory of living germs as the origin of contagious, infectious, or epidemic diseases . . . has an important bearing on the question whether modern science can, by the use of remedies, do anything for the prevention or removal of disease," one physician proposed in 1871.[42] Just as "we can by well-known antiseptics, destroy in the air or elsewhere these parasites, thus preventing their entrance into the human system," he argued, "we can by drugs . . . directly check the zymotic [or germ-induced disease] process in the blood."[43] Hitherto therapeutics had been largely an empirical art fraught with skepticism, he observed, but internal antisepsis grounded upon rationalism would bring therapeutic confidence. "Given these organized germs," Bartholow later observed, "what more rational expedient could be proposed than the use of agents which, whilst not injurious to the tissues, are destructive to these organisms?"[44]

During the 1870s and 1880s, and especially after Robert Koch announced his discovery of the tubercle bacillus in 1882, many of the physicians who urged physiological therapeutics were also exuberant about the therapeutic promise of bacteriology. Like therapy directed by experimental physiology, treatment based on bacteriological knowledge promised to be rational rather than empirical, sustained by laboratory experimentation rather than by clinical observation alone, specific rather than symptomatic, based on a newly objectified concept of disease rather than on a model of imbalance, and universally applicable rather than limited by the principle of specificity. "The study of bacteria," one editorial affirmed in 1885, "possesses a surpassing interest to every physician who is not content merely to plod along in the ancient but obscure, and often dangerous and perplexing, path of empiricism." The author noted that "it has long been the reproach of the medical profession that therapeutics is not an exact science"; but, he maintained, "in the light of the germ theory it might virtually become such."[45]

Bacteriology was not primarily responsible for initiating the move toward specific therapeutics. Experimental physiology did much more to legitimize the idea of "specific" treatment in the decades immediately following the Civil War, dissociating the term from its connotations of quackery. The kind of specific therapy bacteriology implied was somewhat different from that premised upon physiology: in physiological therapeutics treatment was specific to certain physiological processes and abnormalities; the germ theory, on the other hand, suggested the possibility of treatment specific to the living agent that caused disease. The rigid ontological conception of disease informed by early bacteriology and its simple model of etiological specificity supported a sometimes equally simplistic model of disease-specific treatment.

Through the mid-1880s bacteriology's explanatory power was in itself insufficient incentive for most American physicians to consider bacteriological knowledge worthwhile for their therapeutic task. Whether or not its etiological pretensions were true was not really the main issue. For the practitioner a central question by which bacteriology's bid for medical attention should be judged was, What practical difference does it make in healing patients? The question *Cui bono?* was tauntingly asked of bacteriology just as it was of experimental physiology. "A few words to Bacteriology. We all know that it does not cure its cases," a practitioner acidly commented in the late 1880s.[46] "We all aim to be therapeutists. Beautiful diagnoses obtained by scientific methods of examination are very nice, but if they do not cure the case, that is, the treatment based on them, then we are at fault." He concluded that "unless we constantly hold therapeutics before our eyes our profession will become nothing but one of scientific amusement."[47]

The failure of bacteriology rapidly to fulfill what some American enthusiasts had declared to be its therapeutic potential annoyed and frustrated those who believed it should transform practice. The reproach that Koch's discovery of the tubercle bacillus had done nothing to alter treatment, a common one after 1882, was especially vexatious, for that discovery had been the most brilliant emblem of bacteriology's power. "The [tubercle] bac[illus] has made itself the most useful in diagnosis but since Koch discov[ered the] tuber[cle] bacilus no one less has died of tuberculosis," a student ruefully wrote in the same volume in which he copied notes on Koch's lectures in 1885. "Bacteriol has busied itself with simply the simple bacterium & theoretic condition rather than active practical questions."[48] Anxiety over the persistent dearth of effective, safe, bacteria-specific therapeutic agents intensified in subsequent years, especially in the wake of Koch's premature announcement of tuberculin as a specific cure for tuberculosis in 1891. (Vindication did not commence until the production of diphtheria antitoxin in the mid-1890s.) Because the therapeutic promise of early bacteriology seemed so clear and simple, the burden of demonstrating its therapeutic relevance weighed heaviest on the first generation of physicians who placed their faith in laboratory science.[49]

Beyond the objection that bacteriological knowledge did not heal patients, there were deeper reasons that physicians who had been bred with the regular medical values regnant in antebellum America resisted bacteriology's therapeutic pretensions. These reasons clarify why strident opposition, not diffidence, characterized some thinking physicians' broader reception of experimental science in general. The notion that bacteriology should be a basis for therapeutic action embodied much of what had been held illegitimate in therapeutic thought and accountable for the profession's earlier ills. To the minds of physicians committed to clinical empiricism, the rationalism of bacteriological therapeutics threatened to return practice to domination by the sort of simple therapeutic solutions that speculative systems had provided at the start of the century.

Some enthusiasts of bacteriology tellingly chose to underscore their own program's therapeutic promise by explicitly pointing to French teachings as the cause of therapeutic stagnation. It was time, they argued, to move beyond clinical empiricism by embracing the rationalism of therapeutics based on laboratory science.[50] Sharply deviating from the impulse to tear down fixed rules, some physicians sought in bacteriology (as they did in experimental physiology) new rules that would bring a measure of certainty to therapeutics. Practitioners committed to empirical observation, on the other hand, feared that unwarranted therapeutic optimism stemming from bacteriology could blind their brethren to clinical realities and turn the profession back toward the excesses of practice governed by theory.

The simple reasoning that matched treatment to pathogen, which advocates of bacteriological therapeutics urged, ignored the individuating factors deemed so important by the principle of specificity. It directed attention away from careful observation of the idiosyncratic characteristics of patient and environment that practitioners had so long regarded as central to their therapeutic decision making and their identity as proper physicians. Bacteriology implied therapeutic as well as etiological universalism. It not only legitimized disease-specific treatment, it set it up as an ideal.

"Our treatment . . . must be symptomatic," a physician countered in 1884 as part of his protest against basing therapeutic action on knowledge of an unseen germ instead of an observed patient. Calling for attention to the sick individual and not just the objectified bacterium, he urged, "We must tremble lest in the eager hunt for specifics against the bacilli, we lose sight of that most important factor, the predisposition, the soil upon which the bacilli seem to flourish. We may kill the bacilli and at the same time kill our patient, if we disregard this influential agent." Cautioning other physicians against allowing the values of reductionist science to reshape their identity and task, he concluded, "Let the bacilli take care of themselves, let us take care of our patients."[51] Critics believed that bacteriology could divert the profession's energies from what was important in both advancing and applying therapeutic knowledge. Noting that "the craze of the day is the somewhat hypothetical *germ*," one physician asked members of a local medical society in New York in 1883, "Are we 'scientifically' but blindly wasting time, money, material, and all too valuable lives in the minute elucidation of non-essentials?"[52]

In some respects resistance to the new order by professionals committed to an older one followed strikingly similar tacks in the contexts of clinical therapeutics and public health. Both clinicians and sanitarians who held to an older model of professional identity perceived correctly that the confident claims made on behalf of bacteriology tended to minimize the importance of environmental factors in therapy and prophylaxis. To public hygienists, this meant a depreciation of environmental sanitation, an activity central to their professional role. To therapeutists, this (together with the diminished importance of patient idiosyncrasy) meant belittling the principle of specificity and thereby discounting discrimination in assessing therapeutic need, an insignia of the proper physician. Devout sanitarians characteristically were repelled by both bacteriological investigation and vivisectional research, as were some physicians who identified with clinical empiricism.[53]

Physicians who criticized the proposal to ground therapeutics in bacteriology especially feared that domination by theory would oversimplify practice. The complexity of clinical phenomena and the exercise of judgment could not be bypassed by bacteriological reductionism. When practitioner Abraham Jacobi gave the presidential address before the New York Academy of Medicine in 1885 on "bacteriomania," he warned the profession against taking up a single speculative theory as a deus ex machina that would resolve the complex realities of etiology, pathology, and therapeutics. Such a reliance on theory was out of keeping with "the empirical and clinical tendency" that characterized "the American medical mind." Jacobi urged that "Anglo-Saxon medicine has never forgotten that the aim and end of all medical science is the treatment and healing of the sick, and that every special study is but a means to obtain that end." Bacteriomania, he maintained, had been initiated in the speculative German mind and was inappropriate for American medicine. He did, however, single out the German physician Rudolf Virchow for his laudable opposition to bacteriology. "If the bacteriomania of modern time has not been accepted uniformly as the universal gospel of modern pathology," Jacobi observed, "that merit again belongs to a great extent to Virchow."[54]

Virchow's opposition to bacteriology hinged on his fear that its rigid ontology of disease represented a return to the *naturphiloso-phische* or romantic medicine that had reigned in Germany during his youth. Medicine had escaped the domination of speculative theories, Virchow believed, and he denounced bacteriology as a return to their bondage.[55] Had Jacobi elaborated this in his address, it is likely that some of the older members of his audience would have recognized their own misgivings about bacteriology in Virchow's concerns. Physicians who had practiced during the middle third of the nineteenth century had witnessed the campaign waged against speculative medical theories and the systems they upheld. Many of those who had given their allegiance to the epistemological ideals of the Paris clinical school had vigorously participated in the iconoclasm of nineteenth-century American medicine's middle period. Like Virchow, some of them did not see bacteriology as simply a theory to be regarded with calm skepticism until it had been proved or invalidated but rather as one that threatened to return medicine to the speculative errors of the past, undoing what their own labor had won for the profession.

Central to their concern was the fear that bacteriology like experimental physiology would surrender therapeutics back into the grip of rationalism. It seemed to offer the kind of simple, all-explaining theory that could seduce younger physicians to system building, and new talk of creating a rational system greatly disturbed many older practitioners. By reducing the cause of a disease to a specific bacterium, bacteriology appeared to its detractors to endorse a system of pathology every bit as monistic as the products of Enlightenment rationalism. Furthermore, by implying that cure rested in destroying the specific pathogen, early bacteriological therapeutics represented disease-specific treatment that was just as mechanical as the practice by rote depicted in caricatures of early-nineteenth-century systems of practice. Blind adherence to a system grounded in bacteriology, critics believed, could result in the same kind of misdirection in treatment that had stigmatized the followers of Rush, Brown, Cooke, and Broussais. In the case of bacteriology, fears that the New Rationalism of experimental science would lead to speculative systems were aggravated by the discipleship that some enthusiasts proclaimed to the doctrines of a single man, Robert Koch, and to a lesser extent to Louis Pasteur.

Writing to a medical friend in 1884, a North Carolina physician predicted with resignation that his opposition to "the Bacillus craze . . . will be set down to old fogyism."[56] No doubt the judgment of many physicians fulfilled his expectations. Yet it is clear that opposition to the idea of bacteriological therapeutics and to the broader notion that experimental laboratory science should become the foundation for medical therapeutics was not necessarily unthinking resistance to change. Many of those who rejected the therapeutic claims of experimental science did so because they were committed to the idea that a more solidly established tradition of medical science, that of clinical empiricism, was the only solid foundation for therapeutic practice and progress.

Practitioners who remained steadfast in their allegiance to the ideals of the Paris clinical school took upon themselves the task of defending Louis's "barrier against the spirit of system" against the threatened incursions of therapeutic rationalism in the form of experimental physiology and bacteriology, just as they had manned the empiricist barricade against earlier nineteenth-century forms of rationalism. Deploring the influence of experimental science on his students, Stillé complained to his friend Bowditch in 1882, "I find the theses I have to examine are, some of them, full of chemical and physiological speculations instead of clinical facts." He lamented, "Hippocratic-Louisian medicine is at a discount—for the present. But the earth turns!"[57] These older, Paris-trained physicians had fought the battle against rationalism, system, overconfidence, and hyperactivity in therapeutics, and they believed that their victory had uplifted the standing of their profession as well as its practice and validated their generation's efforts. In judging where experimental science was likely to lead therapeutics, they relied on the source of authority they most esteemed, namely, their own experience.

Abbreviations
Used in the Notes

Published Sources

AJMS	*American Journal of the Medical Sciences*
BHM	*Bulletin of the History of Medicine*
BMSJ	*Boston Medical and Surgical Journal*
CHC Report	Commercial Hospital of Cincinnati [name varies], *Annual Report*
CLO	*Cincinnati Lancet and Observer*
JHM	*Journal of the History of Medicine and Allied Sciences*
MGH Report	Massachusetts General Hospital, *Annual Report*
NOMNHG	*New Orleans Medical News and Hospital Gazette*
NOMSJ	*New Orleans Medical and Surgical Journal*
SMSJ	*Southern Medical and Surgical Journal*
WL	*Western Lancet*
WLHR	*Western Lancet and Hospital Reporter*

Manuscript Repositories

AL—State Archives: Maps and Manuscripts Division, State of Alabama Department of Archives and History, Montgomery, Alabama

AL—U. AL Libe.: William Stanley Hoole Special Collections Library, Amelia Gayle Gorgas Library, University of Alabama, University, Alabama

CT—Yale Med. Hist. Libe.: Yale Medical History Library, Yale Medical School, New Haven, Connecticut

CT—Yale U. Libe.: Manuscripts and Archives, Sterling Memorial Library, Yale University, New Haven, Connecticut

DC—LC: Manuscript Division, Library of Congress, Washington, D.C.

DC—National Archives: National Archives and Record Service, Washington, D.C.

FL—U. South FL.: Med. Center Libe.: Medical Center Library, University of South Florida, Tampa, Florida

GA—Emory U. Libe.: Special Collections, Robert W. Woodruff Library for Advanced Studies, Emory University, Atlanta, Georgia

IN—IN U. Libe.: Manuscripts Department, Lilly Library, Indiana University Library, Bloomington, Indiana

KY—Filson: Manuscript Department, Filson Club, Louisville, Kentucky

KY—Transylvania U. Libe.: Special Collections and Archives, Frances Carrick Thomas Library, Transylvania University, Lexington, Kentucky

KY—U. KY Libe.: Special Collections and Archives, King Library, University of Kentucky, Lexington, Kentucky

KY—U. Louisville Med. Libe.: Historical Collection, Kornhauser Health Sciences Library, Health Sciences Center, University of Louisville, Louisville, Kentucky

LA—LA Hist. Center: Louisiana Historical Center, Louisiana State Museum, New Orleans, Louisiana

LA—LSU: Department of Archives and Manuscripts, Library, Louisiana State University, Baton Rouge, Louisiana

LA—Matas: Historical Collection, Rudolph Matas Medical Library, Tulane University, New Orleans, Louisiana

LA—Pharmacy Museum: Historical Museum of Pharmacy, New Orleans, Louisiana

LA—Tulane U. Libe.: Special Collections Division, Howard-Tilton Memorial Library, Tulane University, New Orleans, Louisiana

MA—Countway: Oliver Wendell Holmes Hall, Francis A. Countway Library of Medicine, Harvard Medical School, Boston, Massachusetts

MA—MA Hist. Soc.: Massachusetts Historical Society, Boston, Massachusetts

MD—MD Hist. Soc.: Manuscripts Division, Maryland Historical Society, Baltimore, Maryland

MD—NLM: History of Medicine Division, National Library of Medicine, Bethesda, Maryland

MS—MS State Archives: Manuscript Collection, State of Mississippi Department of Archives and History, Jackson, Mississippi

NC—Duke Med. Libe.: Trent Collection, Duke University Medical Center Library, Durham, North Carolina

NC—Duke U. Libe.: Manuscript Collection, William R. Perkins Library, Duke University, Durham, North Carolina

NC—SHC: Southern Historical Collection, University of North Carolina at Chapel Hill, Chapel Hill, North Carolina

NC—State Archives: North Carolina State Archives, Raleigh, North Carolina

NY—Columbia-Presbyterian: Manuscript Collection, Health Sciences Library, Columbia-Presbyterian Medical Center, New York, New York

NY—NY Acad. Med.: Malloch Rare Book and History of Medicine Room, Library, New York Academy of Medicine, New York, New York

NY—NY Hist. Soc.: Manuscript Department, New-York Historical Society, New York, New York

NY—NY Pub. Libe.: Manuscripts Division, New York Public Library, Astor, Lenox, and Tilden Foundations, New York, New York

OH—Cincinnati Acad. Med.: Academy of Medicine of Cincinnati, Cincinnati, Ohio

OH—Cincinnati Hist. Soc.: Manuscripts Collection, Cincinnati Historical Society, Cincinnati, Ohio

OH—Cincinnati Pub. Libe.: Department of Rare Books and Special Collections, Public Library of Cincinnati and Hamilton County, Cincinnati, Ohio

OH—Dayton Pub. Libe.: Dayton Collection, Dayton and Montgomery County Public Library, Dayton, Ohio

OH—Dittrick: Special Collections, Robert M. Stecher Room, Howard Dittrick Museum of Historical Medicine, Cleveland, Ohio

OH—Hayes: Rutherford B. Hayes Library, Fremont, Ohio

OH—Lloyd Libe.: Lloyd Library, Cincinnati, Ohio

OH—Marietta Coll. Libe.: Archives, Dawes Memorial Library, Marietta College, Marietta, Ohio

OH—Miami U. Libe.: Walter Havinghurst Special Collections Library, Miami University, Oxford, Ohio

OH—Mount Pleasant: Historical Society of Mount Pleasant, Mount Pleasant, Ohio

OH—OH Hist. Soc.: Archives, Ohio Historical Society, Columbus, Ohio

OH—U. Cincinnati, Hist. Hlth. Scis. Libe.: History of the Health Sciences Library and Museum, University of Cincinnati, Cincinnati, Ohio

OH—U. Cincinnati Libe.: Special Collections Department, University Library, University of Cincinnati, Cincinnati, Ohio

OH—Western Reserve: Western Reserve Historical Society, Cleveland, Ohio

PA—College of Physicians, Phila.: Historical Collection, Library, College of Physicians of Philadelphia, Philadelphia, Pennsylvania

PA—U. PA Archives: University Archives, University of Pennsylvania, Philadelphia, Pennsylvania

PA—U. PA Libe.: Special Collections, Van Pelt Library, University of Pennsylvania, Philadelphia, Pennsylvania

SC—Med. U. SC, Main Libe.: South Carolina Room, Main Library, Medical University of South Carolina, Charleston, South Carolina

SC—South Caroliniana Libe.: Manuscripts Division, South Caroliniana Library, University of South Carolina, Columbia, South Carolina

SC—Waring: Waring Historical Library, Medical University of South Carolina, Charleston, South Carolina

TN—TN State Libe.: Manuscripts Section, Tennessee State Library and Archives, Nashville, Tennessee

TN—Vanderbilt Med. Libe.: History of Medicine Collection, Health Sciences Library, Vanderbilt University, Nashville, Tennessee

TX—U. TX Libe.: Barker Texas History Center, Library, University of Texas at Austin, Austin, Texas

VA—U. VA Libe.: Manuscripts Department, Alderman Library, University of Virginia, Charlottesville, Virginia

N.B.: Citations of manuscript sources in the notes follow a partially standardized format rather than adhering precisely to the diverse cataloging conventions used by the various repositories. The guiding rule has been to be brief but to provide sufficient description so that the reader has a clear idea of the nature of the source and the researcher has the information needed to locate it. In citations of manuscripts other than correspondence, square brackets are used only to identify information that is uncertain.

Notes

Introduction

1. Charles E. Rosenberg, "The Therapeutic Revolution: Medicine, Meaning, and Social Change in Nineteenth-Century America," *Pespectives in Biology and Medicine*, 20 (1977): 485.

2. Several historians have recently made use of American practice records to describe therapeutic behavior. See David L. Cowen, Louis D. King, and Nicholas G. Lordi, "Nineteenth Century Drug Therapy: Computer Analysis of the 1854 Prescription File of a Burlington Pharmacy," *Journal of the Medical Society of New Jersey*, 78 (1981): 758–761; J. Worth Estes, "Therapeutic Practice in Colonial New England," in *Medicine in Colonial Massachusetts, 1620–1820*, ed. Philip Cash, Eric H. Christianson, and J. Worth Estes (Boston: Colonial Society of Massachusetts, 1980), pp. 289–383; Regina Markell Morantz and Sue Zschoche, "Professionalism, Feminism, and Gender Roles: A Comparative Study of Nineteenth-Century Medical Therapeutics," *Journal of American History*, 63 (1980): 568–588; and Martin S. Pernick, *A Calculus of Suffering: Pain, Professionalism, and Anesthesia in Nineteenth-Century America* (New York: Columbia University Press, 1985).

3. The decision to exclude surgical therapeutics was by no means arbitrary. At least through the 1860s the mechanical aspects of surgical therapeutics (though not its medical ones) held an epistemological status fundamentally different from that occupied by *medical* therapeutics. Surgical therapeutics was not governed by the principle of specificity in the same way as was medical therapeutics (see Chapter 3); instead, some surgical precepts derived from one type of patient and environment could be transferred and applied relatively freely to a different context. Accordingly, many of the generalizations I make are inapplicable to the mechanical manipulations that were important in surgical, dental, and obstetrical therapeutics, and these therefore require a separate analysis.

4. Erwin H. Ackerknecht, "A Plea for a 'Behaviorist' Approach in Writing the History of Medicine,"*BHM*, 22 (1967): 211–214.

1. Intervention and Identity

1. N. West, "Commencement Address," *CLO*, 38 (1877): 317.

2. Pierre Louis to James Jackson, Sr., Paris, 22 May 1833, James Jackson Papers, MA—Countway. Tocqueville's comment appears in his section "Why

the Americans Are More Concerned with the Applications than with the Theory of Science," in *Democracy in America*, ed. J. P. Mayer, trans. George Lawrence (Garden City, New York: Doubleday, 1969; first pub. 1835), p. 461.

3. James Jackson, *A Memoir of James Jackson, Jr., M.D., with Extracts from His Letters to His Father; and Medical Cases, Collected by Him* (Boston, 1835), p. 55.

4. Several such letters are pasted into the Louisiana physician George Colmer's Record Book, vol. 1, LA—Tulane U. Libe. For example, on 20 April 1869 Uriah Duck sent his son to Colmer with a note saying, "'i am verry bad of and i send to you for some medical aide if you will be kind enoughe to send me some medisine and directions to youse it i will be much oblige to you and if i get able to work a gaine i will settel withe you for your troubel and medisines."

5. S., "Medical Improvement," *BMSJ*, 9 (1833–34): 203.

6. My thinking about the professional identity of American physicians has been shaped especially by Barbara Gutmann Rosenkrantz, "The Search for Professional Order in 19th-Century American Medicine," in *Sickness and Health in America: Readings in the History of Medicine and Public Health*, ed. Ronald L. Numbers and Judith Walzer Leavitt, 2nd ed. (Madison: University of Wisconsin Press, forthcoming).

7. S., "Medical Improvement," p. 327.

8. "Health of the Country," *New Orleans Medical Journal*, 1 (1844–45): 247; and see H. V. Wooten, Address before the Alabama State Medical Association at Its First Regular Session in Selma, 9 March 1848, Hardy Vickers Wooten Papers, AL—State Archives.

9. J. C. Nott to Colonel Beck, Mobile, 7 January 1862, Samuel Hollingsworth Stout Papers, NC—Duke U. Libe.

10. James Jackson, Sr., to James Jackson, Jr., Waltham, Massachusetts, 16 June 1832, Jackson Papers.

11. John Ware, "Success in the Medical Profession," *BMSJ*, 43 (1850–51): 498.

12. Ibid., p. 503.

13. J. M. Bonner to Mother, New Orleans, 5 May 1860, Samuel C. Bonner and Family Papers, LA—LSU; and see Joseph Milligan to Joseph A. S. Milligan, Augusta, [Georgia], 4 June 1846, Milligan Family Papers, NC—SHC.

14. Report of the Committee of Ethics, Minutes of the Meeting of the Hamilton County Medical Association, Madisonville, 29 March 1853, in William C. Langdon, Record Book, 1853–1900, OH—Cincinnati Hist. Soc.; and see William L. Broyles, "The Life of a Physician" (M.D. thesis, University of Nashville, 1857), TN—Vanderbilt Med. Libe.; Thomas M. Logan, *The Ethics of Medicine. An Anniversary Address, Delivered Third April, 1844, before the Medico-Chirurgical Society of Louisiana* (New Orleans, 1844), p. 7; and Medical Ethics, Minutes of the Medical Society for the Sixteenth District, Ohio, 1824–30, OH—Western Reserve.

15. Calvin Pease, "Address to the Medical Graduates in the University of Vermont, June 4, 1856," *BMSJ*, 55 (1856–57): 127; "The Medical Profession," *WLHR*, 8 (1848): 125–128; Tho[ma]s D. Mitchell, *The Good Physician: Being an Introductory to the Course of Lectures on Materia Medica and Therapeutics in the Medical Department of Transylvania University, for the Session 1842–3* (Lexington, 1842), p. 7.

16. See, for example, Henry Edwin Morril, "The Formation of Medical Character" (M.D. thesis, University of Pennsylvania, 1840), PA—U. PA Libe.

17. Daniel Drake, Valedictory Address to Graduates of the Louisville Medical Institute, Third Session, 10 March 1840, Drake Manuscripts, OH— U. Cincinnati, Hist. Hlth. Scis. Libe.

18. Henry C. Clark, "The Science of Medicine" (M.D. thesis, University of Pennsylvania, 1853), PA—U. PA Libe. See Milton N. Taylor, "Moral Responsibilities of a Physician" (M.D. thesis, Washington University, Baltimore, n.d.), Joseph M. Toner Papers, DC—LC; George D. Shadburne, "The Study of Medicine" (M.D. thesis, Transylvania University, 1839), KY—Transylvania U. Libe.; and Ja[me]s Norcom to Benjamin Rush Norcom, Edenton, North Carolina, 22 January 1833, Dr. James Norcom and Family Papers, NC—State Archives.

19. Max Neuburger, *The Doctrine of the Healing Power of Nature throughout the Course of Time*, trans. Linn J. Boyd (New York: New York Homeopathic Medical College, 1933; first pub. 1926), remains the best general history of the concept of the healing power of nature. On this idea in nineteenth-century America, see John Harley Warner, " 'The Nature-Trusting Heresy': American Physicians and the Concept of the Healing Power of Nature in the 1850's and 1860's," *Perspectives in American History*, 11 (1977–78): 291–324.

20. John Austin, Notes Taken on Lectures Given by Benjamin Rush, 1809, LA—Matas. And see John Y. Kennedy, Notes Taken on Lectures Given by Benjamin Rush, 1801–11, OH—Dittrick, and P. Washington Little, Notes Taken on Lectures Given by Benjamin Rush on Physiology and Pathology, 1805–06, P. Washington Little Papers, NC—Duke Med. Libe.

21. Benjamin Huger, Notes Taken on Lectures on Materia Medica Given by Nathaniel Chapman, 1816, SC—Waring; and see Samuel Barrington, Notes Taken on Lectures on the Practice of Medicine Given by Nathaniel Chapman, Professor of the Institutes and Practice of Physic, University of Pennsylvania, 1818–19, 1820–21, 1821–22, MD—NLM.

22. Remarks of John P. Harrison at meeting of 1 March 1849, Hamilton County Medical Club, Minutes of Meetings, 21 May 1842–4 April 1850, MD— NLM.

23. Alex[ander] McBride, "A Chemico-Pathological Classification of Fevers, and Hints at Treatment Based Thereon," *CLO*, 25 (1864): 23.

24. Bennet Dowler, "Speculative and Practical Researches on the Supposed Duality, Unity, and Antagonism of Nature and Art in the Cure of Diseases," *NOMSJ*, 15 (1858): 789.

25. George C. Shattuck, "The Medical Profession and Society," *Medical Communications of the Massachusetts Medical Society*, 10 (1866): 421.

26. C. B. Coventry, *Nature and Art in the Cure of Disease. Read before the Medical Society of the County of Oneida, July, 1859* (Utica, 1859), quotations on pp. 3, 4, and 7.

27. Samuel Murphey, Notes Taken on Lectures Given by Nathaniel Chapman, 1830, vol. 1, PA—U. PA Archives.

28. Bennet Dowler, "Medication? or Non-Medication? That Is the Question," *NOMSJ*, 17 (1860): 661.

29. "[Review of] John Forbes, *Homoeopathy, Allopathy, and 'Young Physic'* (1846)," *WL*, 5 (1846–47): 198.

30. Bennet Dowler, "Critical and Speculative Researches on the Fundamental Principles of Subjective Science in Connection with Medical and Experimental Investigations, with Remarks on the Present State of Medicine," *NOMSJ*, 15 (1858): 46.

31. "Medical Essays.—No. I," *BMSJ*, 19 (1838–39): 174; C. Grant, "The

Fallacy of a Supposed Vis Medicatrix Naturae," *WLHR*, 11 (1850): 351. And see John Dickson, "On the Vis Medicatrix Naturae," *AJMS*, 15 (1834–35): 116–120; W. Fletcher Holmes, "The Vis Medicatrix Naturae," *Charleston Medical Journal and Review*, 5 (1850): 311–312, 314; and S. Watkins Vaughan, Jr., "A Thesis on the '*Vis Medicatrix Naturae*'," *Atlanta Medical and Surgical Journal*, 4 (1858–59): 261–268. On the perception of decline, see Chapter 2.

32. "[Review of] *Brief Expositions of Rational Medicine* . . . by Jacob Bigelow," *Medical Journal of North Carolina*, 2 (1859): 359.

33. Whitfield J. Bell, Jr., "Medicine in Boston and Philadelphia: Comparisons and Contrasts, 1750–1820," in *Medicine in Colonial Massachusetts 1620–1820*, ed. Philip Cash, Eric H. Christianson, and J. Worth Estes (Boston: Colonial Society of Massachusetts, 1980), pp. 170–181; and in the same volume, C. Helen Brock, "The Influence of Europe on Colonial Massachusetts Medicine," pp. 107–113. On Holyoke, see James Jackson to Ellen (Dwight) Twisleton, [Boston], 1 July 1860, in James Jackson Putnam, *A Memoir of James Jackson* (Boston and New York: Houghton Mifflin, 1905), p. 397.

34. James Jackson, Jr., Notes Taken on Lectures Given by James Jackson, Sr., Boston, 1826–1827, lecture of 10 January 1827, MA—Countway.

35. John Call Dalton, Notes Taken on Lectures Given by James Jackson, 1816–17, vol. 1, lecture of 13 January 1817, MA—Countway.

36. Ibid., lecture of 20 December 1816.

37. H. I. Bowditch, Notes Taken on Lectures Given by James Jackson, Boston, 1831–32, lecture on therapeutics, MA—Countway.

38. David Humphreys Storer, Notes Taken on Lectures Given by James Jackson on the Theory and Practice of Medicine, 1824–25, lecture of 11 December 1824, MA—Countway. And see Aaron Cornish, Extracts Taken from Lectures Given by James Jackson, Boston, 1818–19, MD—NLM; Abel Lawrence Peirson, Notes Taken on Lectures Given by James Jackson on the Theory and Practice of Physic, Boston, 1814–16, 4 vols., MA—Countway; and Jonathan Greely Stevenson, Notes Taken on Lectures Given by James Jackson on the Theory and Practice of Physic, 1817–19, 2 vols., MA—Countway.

39. James Jackson, Sr., to James Jackson, Jr., Boston, 27 January 1833, Jackson Papers; and see Elisha Bartlett, Notes Taken on Lectures Given by James Jackson on the Theory and Practice of Physic, 1824–25, lecture of 18 November 1825, Elisha Bartlett Papers, CT—Yale U. Libe.

40. Ibid., 20 March 1833.

41. On the Paris clinical school, see Erwin H. Ackerknecht, *Medicine at the Paris Hospital, 1794–1848* (Baltimore: Johns Hopkins Press, 1967).

42. Vincent Y. Bowditch, *Life and Correspondence of Henry Ingersoll Bowditch*, vol. 2 (Boston and New York: Houghton Mifflin; Cambridge, Massachusetts: Riverside Press, 1902), p. 286.

43. For example, see Jackson, Jr., Notes Taken on Lectures Given by James Jackson, Sr., and idem, Notes Taken on Clinical Lectures Given by James Jackson, Sr., 1830–31, MA—Countway.

44. James Jackson, Jr., to James Jackson, Sr., Paris, 26 June 1831, Jackson Papers.

45. Ibid., Paris, 6 November 1831. The published letter is in Jackson, *Memoir of James Jackson, Jr.*, pp. 86–88.

46. James Jackson, Jr., to James Jackson, Sr., Paris, 18 March 1832, Jackson Papers. The comment on Jackson, Jr.'s, relation to Louis was made in Francis Boott to James Jackson, Sr., London, 3–4 February 1834, Jackson Papers; and see Jackson, Jr., to Jackson, Sr., Paris, 27 June 1833, and Paris, 13 July 1833,

Jackson Papers; and Jackson, Jr., to [Abel Lawrence] Peirson, Paris, 29 August 1833, MA—Countway.

47. James Jackson, Jr., to James Jackson, Sr., Havre, 25 April 1832, Jackson Papers.

48. James Jackson, Jr., to James Jackson, Sr., Paris, 22 February 1833, Jackson Papers.

49. James Jackson, Jr., to James Jackson, Sr., Paris, 16 January 1833, in Jackson, *Memoir of James Jackson, Jr.*, pp. 173–175.

50. James Jackson, Jr., to James Jackson, Sr., Paris, 16 January 1833, Jackson Papers.

51. James Jackson, Jr., to James Jackson, Sr., Paris, 24 November 1832, in Jackson, *Memoir of James Jackson, Jr.*, p. 162.

52. James Jackson, Jr., to James Jackson, Sr., Paris, 24 November 1832, Jackson Papers. Resolving the tension between the physician's dual role as (in Jackson, Jr.'s, words) "doctor" and "scientific man" may have been peculiarly difficult in America. Walter Artelt's study contrasting the expressions of Parisian skepticism in the United States with those in Austria is particularly suggestive. In Vienna, Artelt asserts, Joseph Dietl became by his own estimation a *Naturwissenschaftler*, whereas Bigelow, like the Americans who studied with Louis, preserved his commitment to therapeutic action and his identity as an *Artz* ("Louis' amerikanische Schüler und die Krise der Therapie," *Sudhoffs Archiv für Geschichte der Medizin und der Naturwissenschaften*, 42 [1958]: 291–301).

53. James Jackson, Sr., to James Jackson, Jr., Boston, 20 March 1833, Jackson Papers.

54. Ibid., 20 March 1833; and see ibid., 27 January 1833.

55. James Jackson, Jr., to James Jackson, Sr., Paris, 14 May 1833, Jackson Papers; and see ibid., Paris, 6 May 1833.

56. Jackson, *Memoir of James Jackson, Jr.*, p. 72. On the return voyage, see James Jackson, Sr., to James Jackson, Jr., Waltham, Massachusetts, 15 August 1833, and Jackson, Jr., to Jackson, Sr., Ship George Washington off Sandy Hook, 23 August [1833], Jackson Papers.

57. On Bigelow's recollections of his early practice, see George E. Ellis, *Memoir of Jacob Bigelow, M.D., LL.D.* (Cambridge, Massachusetts, 1880), p. 27. And for Bigelow's early conservatism in therapy, see his "Phthisis Pulmonalis" (M.D. thesis, University of Pennsylvania, 1810), PA—U. PA Libe.

58. [Jacob Bigelow], "Preface," *The Pharmacopoeia of the United States of America. 1820* (Boston, 1820), especially pp. 20–26. "Retrenchment" was a leading theme of Bigelow's preface and remained a feature of his medical teachings. He told students in a lecture in 1852, "One half perhaps of the Medicinal agents now used, or a quarter or rather an eighth might well be relied on to the exclusion of all others. Materia medica is very much encumbered by the number of its substances" (Horatio R. Storer, Notes Taken on Lectures Given by Jacob Bigelow on Materia Medica, Harvard Medical School, 1852–53, lecture of 6 November 1852, MA—Countway).

59. B[enjamin] E. C[otting], " 'Nature in Disease'—A Review," *BMSJ*, 51 (1854–55): 330. James Jackson commented on the address's lack of originality in his *Another Letter to a Young Physician: To Which Are Appended Some Other Medical Papers* (Boston, 1861), pp. 47–48.

60. Jacob Bigelow, "Self-Limited Diseases," *Medical Communications of the Massachusetts Medical Society*, 5 (address of 27 May 1835) (1830–36): 322.

61. Ibid., p. 343.

62. Oliver Wendell Holmes, *Currents and Counter Currents in Medical Science, an Address Delivered before the Massachusetts Medical Society, at the Annual Meeting, May 30, 1860* (Boston, 1860), p. 15.

63. Holmes, *Currents and Counter Currents*, p. 16.

64. Ibid., p. 14. For example, see Oliver Wendell Holmes, *Homeopathy, and Its Kindred Delusions: Two Lectures Delivered before the Boston Society for the Diffusion of Useful Knowledge* (Boston, 1842).

65. Holmes, *Currents and Counter Currents*, p. 31. And see his development of this theme in *Elsie Venner: A Romance of Destiny* (Boston, 1861).

66. Jacob Bigelow, Case Books, 2 vols., 20 December 1838–29 February 1839, MA—Countway; Henry Ingersoll Bowditch, Medical Records, 102 vols., 1839–91, MA—Countway; Oliver Wendell Holmes, Case Books, 2 vols., 1844–48, MA—Countway; James Jackson, Alms House Case Book No. 1, Boston, 1810–11, MA—Countway; James Jackson, Case Books, Massachusetts General Hospital, 1825–26, MA—Countway. The case record books of the medical wards of the Massachusetts General Hospital are deposited in MA—Countway.

67. A fuller explication of these figures and their provenance is given in Chapter 4.

68. George Cheyne Shattuck, Diary Notes on Patients, 1832, Notes Taken at the Massachusetts General Hospital on Clinical Lectures Given by James Jackson, lecture of 23 December 1832, MA—Countway.

69. Massachusetts General Hospital, Medical Case Records, vols. 48 and 50 (1832).

70. John Ware, Clinical Lectures at the Massachusetts General Hospital, 1830 and 1835, lecture of 1830, Ware Papers, MA—Countway. The case was that of a woman admitted 19 July 1830, Massachusetts General Hospital, Medical Case Records, vol. 38.

71. On Viennese therapeutic nihilism, see H. Buess, "Zur Frage des therapeutischen Nihilismus in 19. Jahrhundert," *Schweizerische Medizinische Wochenschrift*, 87 (1957): 444–447; Erna Lesky, "Von den Ursprungen des therapeutischen Nihilismus," *Sudhoffs Archiv für Geschichte der Medizin und der Naturwissenschaften*, 44 (1960): 1–20; and Lloyd G. Stevenson, "Joseph Dietl, William Osler and the Definition of Therapeutic Nihilism," in *Festschrift für Erna Lesky zum 70. Geburtstag*, ed. Kurt Ganzinger, Manfred Skopec, and Helmut Wyklicky (Vienna: Hollinck, 1981), pp. 149–152.

72. A. Flint to James Jackson, New York, 31 August 1862, Jackson Papers (MA—MA Hist. Soc.). Typical expressions of resentment against the Boston medical elite are "Atlanta Medical College," *Atlanta Medical and Surgical Journal*, 2 (1856–57): 756, and N. S. Davis, "Nature and Art. Their Relative Influence in the Management of Diseases. Are They Antagonistic or Co-Operative? An Essay Read to the Chicago Medical Society, Oct. 19th, 1860," *Chicago Medical Examiner*, 2 (1861): 130.

73. Holmes, *Currents and Counter Currents*, pp. 37–38.

74. Henry Jacob Bigelow, *Medical Education in America: Being the Annual Address Read before the Massachusetts Medical Society, June 7 1871* (Cambridge, Mass., 1871), p. 34; and see John T. Morse, Jr., *Life and Letters of Oliver Wendell Holmes*, vol. 2 (Cambridge, Massachusetts, 1896), p. 23.

75. "Dr. Holmes's Address," *NOMNHG*, 7 (1860–61): 786; italics added. The resolution was printed on the verso of the title page to Holmes, *Currents and Counter Currents*.

76. *A System of Medical Etiquette, Rules and Regulations, As Adopted*

by the *Medical Association of North Eastern Kentucky* (Maysville, 1839), p. 8.

77. Samuel D. Gross to Benjamin P. Aydelott, Philadelphia, 25 January 1862, Benjamin Parkman Aydelott Papers, OH—Cincinnati Hist. Soc. Gross noted that the term "conservative medicine" was Austin Flint's; see, for example, Austin Flint, "Conservative Medicine," *North American Medico-Chirurgical Review*, 5 (1861): 1038–59.

78. Eleanor M. Tilton, *Amiable Autocrat: A Biography of Dr. Oliver Wendell Holmes* (New York: Henry Schuman, 1947), pp. 421–422.

79. Jackson, *Another Letter to a Young Physician*, pp. v-vi.

80. Ibid., pp. 6–7.

81. Ibid., p. vii.

82. Ibid., p. 80.

83. Henry Ingersoll Bowditch to James Jackson, Sr., Florence, 16 May 1834, and ibid., Paris, 13 July 1834; and James Jackson, Jr., to James Jackson, Sr., Paris, 16 January 1833, Jackson Papers (MA—Countway). And see Henry Ingersoll Bowditch, Notes Taken on Clinical Lectures Given by Pierre Louis, 1832–33; To which Is Added His "Resume" of Four Years' Previous Observation, MA—Countway.

84. Henry Ingersoll Bowditch, Introductory to the Course on Clinical Medicine, Course of 1861–62, lecture of 28 November 1861, MA—Countway.

85. Bowditch, *Life and Correspondence of Henry Ingersoll Bowditch*, vol. 2, p. 261.

86. Henry Ingersoll Bowditch, Outline of Course of Lectures for Winter 1860–61, MA—Countway.

2. Epistemology, Social Change, and the Reorganization of Knowledge

1. On the perception of decline in the professions, see Daniel H. Calhoun, *Professional Lives in America: Structure and Aspiration, 1750–1850* (Cambridge, Massachusetts: Harvard University Press, 1965), pp. 178–197. On medical licensing, see Joseph F. Kett, *The Formation of the American Medical Profession: The Role of Institutions, 1780–1860* (New Haven and London: Yale University Press, 1968), pp. 1–96, 181–184; and Richard Harrison Shryock, *Medical Licensing in America, 1650–1965* (Baltimore: Johns Hopkins Press, 1967). Of an ample literature describing sectarian assaults, among the most useful works are Alex Berman, "The Impact of the Nineteenth Century Botanico-Medical Movement on American Pharmacy and Medicine" (Ph.D. diss., University of Wisconsin—Madison, 1954); Harris L. Coulter, *Divided Legacy. A History of the Schism in Medical Thought*, vol. 3, *Science and Ethics in American Medicine: 1800–1914* (Washington, D.C.: McGrath Publishing Co., 1973); Martin Kaufman, *Homeopathy in America: The Rise and Fall of a Medical Heresy* (Baltimore and London: Johns Hopkins Press, 1971); and William G. Rothstein, *American Physicians in the Nineteenth Century: From Sects to Science* (Baltimore and London: Johns Hopkins University Press, 1972), pp. 125–174, 217–246.

2. Alfred Stillé to [George Cheyne] Shattuck, Philadelphia, 5 October 1857, MA—Countway.

3. The most useful survey of antebellum medical schools remains William Frederick Norwood, *Medical Education in the United States before the Civil*

War (Philadelphia: University of Pennsylvania Press, 1944); on the content and diversity of training, see Ronald L. Numbers, ed., *The Education of American Physicians: Historical Essays* (Berkeley, Los Angeles, and London: University of California Press, 1980).

4. On medical societies, see James G. Burrow, *AMA: Voice of American Medicine* (Baltimore: Johns Hopkins Press, 1963); Ronald L. Numbers, "Public Protection and Self-Interest: Medical Societies in Wisconsin," in *Wisconsin Medicine: Historical Perspectives*, ed. Ronald L. Numbers and Judith Walzer Leavitt (Madison: University of Wisconsin Press, 1981), pp. 75–104; and Rothstein, *American Physicians*, pp. 63–121. On the use of institutional reform as a means of uplifting the profession as a whole in one region, see John Harley Warner, "A Southern Medical Reform: The Meaning of the Antebellum Argument for Southern Medical Education," *BHM*, 57 (1983): 364–381. Little attention has been given to cultural participation as a means for physicians in the United States to improve their standing; see John Harley Warner, "Essay Review of Ian Inkster and Jack Morrell, eds., *Metropolis and Province: Science in British Culture, 1780–1850* (1983)," *Transactions and Studies of the College of Physicians of Philadelphia*, s. 5, 5 (1983): 377–384.

5. A useful survey of epistemological changes in American medicine and the tensions between rationalism and empiricism enduring in medicine from ancient times is Richard H. Shryock, "Empiricism versus Rationalism in American Medicine, 1650–1950," *Proceedings of the American Antiquarian Society*, n.s. 79 (1969): 99–150. On the social animus of epistemological change, see John Harley Warner, "The Selective Transport of Medical Knowledge: Antebellum American Physicians and Parisian Medical Therapeutics," *BHM*, 59 (1985): 213–231. Of a large literature on the French medical empiricism that was a resource for Americans, see Erwin H. Ackerknecht, *Medicine at the Paris Hospital 1794–1848* (Baltimore: Johns Hopkins Press, 1967), and George Rosen, "The Philosophy of Ideology and the Emergence of Modern Medicine in France," *BHM*, 20 (1946): 328-339.

6. A brief introduction to the system-making impulse is Lester S. King, *The Medical World of the Eighteenth Century* (Chicago: University of Chicago Press, 1958).

7. "[Review of] Brief Expositions of Rational Medicine," *Medical Journal of North Carolina*, 2 (1859): 360.

8. For example, see "Dunglison's General Therapeutics," *BMSJ*, 15 (1836–37): 144.

9. Ro[bert] W. Haxall, "Medical Systems," *Stethoscope*, 5 (1855): 245 and 246.

10. Jerome Cochran, "Rationalism and Empiricism: The Laws and Limitations of Scientific Investigation," *Nashville Journal of Medicine and Surgery*, 18 (1860): 215.

11. Jacob Bigelow, *Brief Expositions of Rational Medicine: To Which Is Prefixed the Paradise of Doctors, a Fable* (Boston, 1858), p. 48.

12. Ibid., pp. 56–57.

13. William Octavius Eversfield, Notes Taken on Lectures Given by James L. Cabell, 1859–60, lecture of 4 March 1860, William Octavius Eversfield Notebooks, VA—U. VA Libe.

14. Alfred Boyd, "Finale of Twenty Years Study and Practice of Medicine" (M.D. thesis, Medical College of the State of South Carolina, 1856), SC—Med. U. SC, Main Libe.; and see S. E. Chaillé, Lectures Given on Physiology, Medical College, New Orleans, 1867, vol. 1, LA—Matas.

15. "[Review of] John Forbes, *Homoeopathy, Allopathy, and Young Physic* (1846)," *WL*, 5 (1847): 211.

16. Samuel A. Cartwright to Rezin Thompson, New Orleans, 15 June 1856, reproduced in "Letter from Dr. Cartwright," *Nashville Journal of Medicine and Surgery*, 11 (1856): 213.

17. E. H. Barton, *An Address, before the Louisiana State Medical Society* (New Orleans, 1851), p. 7.

18. J. Y. Henry, "Medical Systems" (M.D. thesis, Transylvania University, 1843), KY—Transylvania U. Libe.

19. On Sydenham and empiricism, see Kenneth Dewhurst, *Thomas Sydenham (1624–1688): His Life and Original Writings* (Berkeley: University of California Press, 1966).

20. "[Review of] John Forbes," p. 199.

21. "Medical Ethics, Adopted by This Society from the 'Central Medical Society of Georgia,' " 1829, in Minutes of the Medical Society, for the Sixteenth Medical District, Ohio, 1824–30, OH—Western Reserve.

22. Report of the Committee on Ethics, Miami Medical Association Minutes, Madisonville, 29 March 1853, in William C. Langdon, Record Book, 1853–1900, OH—Cincinnati Hist. Soc.

23. James V. Ingham, "An Essay on Empiricism" (M.D. thesis, University of Pennsylvania, 1866), PA—U. PA Libe.

24. Bigelow, *Rational Medicine*, p. 290; also see pp. 103–105.

25. Lundsford P. Yandell, Notes Taken on Lectures Given by Charles Caldwell, Transylvania University, Lexington, Introductory Lecture of 7 November 1825, Daniel Drake Papers, Emmet Field Horine Collection, KY—U. KY Libe.; George B. McKnight, Notes Taken on Lectures Given by David Hosack on the Theory and Practice of Physic and Clinical Medicine, New York, 1814–16, Joseph M. Toner Papers, DC—LC. And see Benjamin S. Downing, Notes Taken on Lectures Given by Joseph Mather Smith on the Theory and Practice of Medicine, College of Physicians and Surgeons at the University of the State of New York, 1826, NY—Columbia-Presbyterian.

26. On Cooke's career, see "Dr. John Esten Cooke," *Church Review and Ecclesiastical Register*, 9 (1856): 226–243.

27. John Esten Cooke, *Treatise of Pathology and Therapeutics*, vol. 1 (Lexington, Kentucky, 1828), pp. iii–iv.

28. Elisha B. Stedman, "The Theory of Broussais" (M.D. thesis, Transylvania University, 1833), KY—Transylvania U. Libe.

29. Lundsford Pitts Yandell, Diary, 1824–43, Yandell Family Papers, entry for 24 June 1836, KY—Filson; "Dr. John Esten Cooke."

30. [Leonidas M. Lawson], "Thoughts on Bilious Disease," *WL*, 1 (1842–43): 385.

31. Edward T. Jones, "The Influence of Names on the Progress of Medical Philosophy" (M.D. thesis, Transylvania University, 1843), KY—Transylvania U. Libe. Similar Transylvania theses include J. Y. Henry, "Medical Systems" (1843), and John W. Williams, "Systems of Medicine" (1842).

32. J. Y. Bassett to Marguerite Bassett, Paris, 28 August 1836, J. Y. Bassett Papers, AL—State Archives. And see Erwin H. Ackerknecht, "Broussais or a Forgotten Medical Revolution," *BHM*, 27 (1953): 320–343.

33. F. J. V. Broussais, *History of Phlegmasiae, or Chronic Inflammations, Founded on Clinical Experience and Pathological Anatomy, Exhibiting a View of the Different Varieties of and Complications of These Diseases, with Their Various Methods of Treatment*, trans. from 4th French ed. by Isaac

Hayes and R. Egelsfeld Griffith, vol. 2 (Philadelphia, 1831), p. 10, and see p. xx.

34. Edward H. Barton, *The Application of Physiological Medicine to the Diseases of Louisiana* (Philadelphia, 1832), pp. 1 and 3.

35. Ibid., p. 38.

36. Ibid., p. 45.

37. B. Burgh Smith, "Country Fever" (M.D. thesis, Medical College of the State of South Carolina, 1836), SC—Med. U. SC, Main Libe.

38. James Jackson, Jr., to James Jackson, Sr., Paris, 13 November 1832, Jackson Papers, MA—Countway. Pierre Louis assailed Broussais's medical doctrines most forcibly in his *Examen de l'examen de M. Broussais relativement a la phthisie et a l'affection typhoide* (Paris, 1834), which he dedicated to the memory of James Jackson, Jr.

39. B. B. Smith, "What of Theory!" (M.D. thesis, University of Nashville, 1857), TN—Vanderbilt Med. Libe.

40. Stedman, "Theory of Broussais."

41. Elisha Bartlett, *An Essay on the Philosophy of Medical Science* (Philadelphia, 1844), pp. 201 and 290. Louis's disciples clearly recognized in Bartlett's book the empirical indictment of medical systems their mentor preached. Alfred Stillé, a Philadelphia student of Louis, wrote to G. C. Shattuck after reading the treatise that Bartlett's views were "those of my own medical creed, & of yours, & of all of us who have been brought up in the school of . . . Louis" (Philadelphia, 24 October 1844, Shattuck Papers, vol. 18, MA—MA Hist. Soc.). And see Elisha Bartlett to James Jackson, Baltimore, 23 December 1844, Jackson Papers; James Jackson to Elisha Bartlett, Boston, 25 January 1844, Bartlett Papers, CT—Yale U. Libe.; and P. C. A. Louis to H. I. Bowditch, Paris, 23 March 1846, MA—Countway.

42. Bartlett, *Philosophy of Medical Science*, p. 205.

43. "[Review of] John Forbes," pp. 191, 201, and 208; and see Hamilton County Medical Club, Minutes of Meetings, 21 May 1842–4 April 1850, meeting of 7 October 1847, MD—NLM.

44. [L. M.] L[awson], "Letter from Prof. Bartlett" (Transylvania University, 17 January 1849), *WLHR*, 9 (1849): 195.

45. P. C. A. Louis to H. I. Bowditch, Paris, 5 February 1840, MA—Countway.

46. Erwin H. Ackerknecht, "Elisha Bartlett and the Philosophy of the Paris Clinical School," *BHM*, 24 (1950): 60.

47. John C. Cardwell, Notes Taken on Lectures Given by James Conquest Gross, Transylvania University Medical Department, Lexington, Kentucky, 1843–44, Drake Papers, Horine Collection.

48. "Medical Systems and Habits," *WL*, 1 (1842–43): 235.

49. George Washington Bowen, Notes Taken on Lectures Given by Charles D. Williams on the Institutes and Practice of Homoeopathy, Cleveland Institute of Homoeopathy, 1851–52, OH—Western Reserve.

50. See, for example, John Walker Diary, King and Queen County, Virginia, 1826–49, vol. 2, entries for 12 August 1834 and 28 March 1835, NC—SHC.

51. On homeopathy as a system, see for example Bartlett, *Philosophy of Medical Science*, pp. 189–200, and E. D. F[enner], "[Review of] Homoeopathy, Allopathy, and 'Young Physic,' by John Forbes (Phila., 1846)," *NOMSJ*, 2 (1845–46): 760–761.

52. David G. Weems, "The Vis Medicatrix Natura in Man" (M.D. thesis, Washington University of Baltimore, 1846), Toner Papers. And see James Lakey,

Diary, vol. 5, 25 March 1853–15 December 1853, entry for 1 April 1853, James Lakey Papers, OH—Cincinnati Hist. Soc.

53. "Medical Delusions," *WL*, 1 (1842–43): 477.

54. Thomas Henderson, "Cases of Pulmonary Consumption, with Observations," *BMSJ*, 5 (1831–32): 121.

55. John A. Lyle, "Exclusive Systems of Medicine" (M.D. thesis, Transylvania University, 1841), KY—Transylvania U. Libe.

56. *Annual Circular of the Medical Department of the University of Louisiana, Session of 1859–1860* (New Orleans, 1859), p. 7. On the emphasis on clinical education, see Dale Cary Smith, "The Emergence of Organized Clinical Instruction in the Nineteenth Century American Cities of Boston, New York, and Philadelphia" (Ph.D. diss., University of Minnesota, 1979).

57. Medical College of Ohio, Faculty Minutes, 1831–52, meeting of 18 August 1831, OH—U. Cincinnati Libe.

58. Baltimore Almshouse Medical Reports, 1833–37, Case Notes of Dr. James H. Miller, entry for 1 February 1834, MD—MD Hist. Soc.

59. B[enjamin] E. C[otting], " 'Rational Medicine'—A Review," *BMSJ*, 59 (1858–59): 189.

60. "[Review of] *Brief Exposition of Rational Medicine* . . . By Jacob Bigelow," *Charleston Medical Journal and Review*, 14 (1859): 97.

61. "[Review of] Brief Expositions of Rational Medicine" (*Medical Journal of North Carolina*), pp. 359–360.

62. B[ennet] Dowler, "[Review of] *Brief Expositions of Rational Medicine*: By Jacob Bigelow," *NOMSJ*, 16 (1859): 900.

63. George K. G. Todd, "Young Physic" (M.D. thesis, Transylvania University, 1848), KY—Transylvania U. Libe.

64. This theme was strong in French medicine from the late eighteenth century on, as in the writings of Phillipe Pinel and Pierre-Jean-Georges Cabanis. American physicians' expressions of it were certainly informed by prevalent conventions in American oratory as well. Appeals for the sweeping away of artificial encumbrances and a return to an earlier, purer way were endemic in the American culture of the second quarter of the nineteenth century. One historian has suggested, for example, that a restoration theme—that is, calls to restore the purity of an idealized ancestral way characterized by independence, simplicity, self-assurance, and stability—was the single element that all Jacksonians held in common (Marvin Meyers, *The Jacksonian Persuasion: Politics and Belief* [Stanford: Stanford University Press, 1960; first pub. 1957]). In their epistemological arguments, Americans drew upon these prevalent rhetorical forms to reinforce their calls for the demolition of rationalistic systems and restoration of a less artificial, purer, Hippocratic observation of nature.

65. James Jackson, *Another Letter to a Young Physician: To Which Are Appended Some Other Medical Papers* (Boston, 1861), quotations from pp. 3–4 and 91.

66. "A System of Rational Therapeutics," *BMSJ*, 87 (1872): 13.

67. "Poole's Physiological Therapeutics," *BMSJ*, 101 (1879): 276; italics added.

3. The Principle of Specificity

1. John B. Rice, Notes Taken on Lectures Given by Alonzo B. Palmer on Materia Medica and Therapeutics, University of Michigan College of Medicine

and Surgery, Ann Arbor, Michigan, 1855, OH—Hayes; and see Notes Taken on Lectures Given by David Hosack on the Theory and Practice of Physic, College of Physicians and Surgeons, New York, [ca. 1810–20], PA—College of Physicians, Phila.

2. For example, see Henry W. DeSaussure, Notes Taken on Lectures Given by Eli Geddings on the Theory and Practice of Medicine, Charleston, South Carolina, 1866–67, lecture of 15 November 1866, SC—Waring. The variables of person and place taken into account in therapeutic decision making are discussed in Ronald L. Numbers and John Harley Warner, "The Maturation of American Medical Science," in *Scientific Colonialism, 1800–1930: A Cross-Cultural Comparison*, ed. Nathan Reingold and Marc Rothenberg (Washington, D.C.: Smithsonian Institution Press, forthcoming); Martin S. Pernick, *A Calculus of Suffering: Pain, Professionalism, and Anesthesia in Nineteenth-Century America* (New York: Columbia University Press, 1985); Charles E. Rosenberg, "The Therapeutic Revolution: Medicine, Meaning, and Social Change in Nineteenth-Century America," *Perspectives in Biology and Medicine*, 20 (1977): 485–506; and John Harley Warner, "The Idea of Southern Medical Distinctiveness: Medical Knowledge and Practice in the Old South," in *Science and Medicine in the Old South*, ed. Ronald L. Numbers and Todd L. Savitt, forthcoming.

3. The medical aspects of surgical therapeutics, such as the control of postoperative inflammation and administration of anesthetics, and the medical aspects of, for example, midwifery, were of course subject to the limitations the principle of specificity imposed.

4. David W. Cheever, "The Value and the Fallacy of Statistics in the Observation of Disease," *BMSJ*, 63 (1860–61): 483 and 514.

5. F. J. V. Broussais, *On Irritation and Insanity, a Work wherein the Relations of the Physical with the Moral Conditions of Man, Are Established on the Basis of Physiological Medicine*, trans. Thomas Cooper (Columbia, South Carolina, 1831), p. xx.

6. "Editorial and Miscellaneous," *Virginia Medical and Surgical Journal*, 3 (1854): 86.

7. Ja[me]s C. Billingslea, "An Appeal on Behalf of Southern Medical Colleges and Southern Medical Literature," *SMSJ*, n.s. 12 (1856): 400.

8. For example, Notes Taken on Lectures Given by Professor Freeman, Eclectic Medical College, Cincinnati, 1853–54, Ashton Mss., IN—IN U. Libe.; George Washington Bowen, Notes Taken on Lectures Given by Charles D. Williams on the Institutes and Practice of Homoeopathy, Institute of Homoeopathy, 1851–52, OH—Western Reserve; Frances Janney, Notes Taken on Lectures Given on Clinical Medicine, Boston University School of Medicine, 1876–77, OH—OH Hist. Soc.; Henry Noah Martin, Notes of Indications Taken at the Homeopathic Medical College, 1864–65, MD—NLM.

9. Samuel Brown to Orlando Brown, Lexington, Kentucky, 20 January 1821, Orlando Brown Papers, KY—Filson.

10. W. B. Woodbridge, "The Medical Student" (M.D. thesis, University of Nashville, 1857), TN—Vanderbilt Med. Libe.

11. John Austin, Notes Taken on Lectures Given by Benjamin Rush, University of Pennsylvania, 1809, LA—Matas.

12. Andrew Stone, "Remarks on Diseases of the West.—No. I" (letter to the editor, Crown Point, Indiana, 12 December 1845), *BMSJ*, 33 (1845–46): 476–477.

13. John Ware, "Success in the Medical Profession," *BMSJ*, 43 (1850–51):

501; and see Thomas J. Griffith, Notes Taken on Lectures Given by Professor Armor, University of Michigan Department of Medicine and Surgery, 10 October 1865–15 March 1866, lecture of 14 December 1865, Griffith Mss., IN—IN U. Libe.; and Samuel Murphey, Notes Taken on Lectures Given by Nathaniel Chapman, University of Pennsylvania, 1830, PA—U. PA Archives. On the history of the notion of disease as a specific entity, see Owsei Temkin, "The Scientific Approach to Disease: Specific Entity and Individual Sickness," in *Scientific Change: Historical Studies in the Intellectual, Social and Technical Conditions for Scientific Discovery and Technical Invention from Antiquity to the Present*, ed. A. C. Crombie (New York: Basic Books, 1963), pp. 629–647; and see Knud Faber, "Nosography in Modern Internal Medicine," *Annals of Medical History*, 4 (1922): 1–63.

14. James R. R. Horne, "Specifics in Medicine" (M.D. thesis, University of Nashville, 1857), TN—Vanderbilt Med. Libe.

15. W[illia]m A. Booth, "Quinine: The Importance of Understanding, and a Theory Relating to, Its Modus Operandi," *NOMNHG*, 6 (1859–60): 251. The many disease-specific patent medicines hawked during the nineteenth-century epitomized the mountebankian notion that a specific drug could cure a particular disease.

16. James Somers, Jr., "Intermittent Fever" (M.D. thesis, University of Nashville, 1858), TN—Vanderbilt Med. Libe.

17. Thomas Fairfax Keller, Notes Taken on Lectures Given by Daniel Drake on Pathology and Practice, 1847, lecture on yellow fever, AL—State Archives.

18. [John P.] H[arrison], "Notices of Empiricism," *WLHR*, 8 (1848): 122; italics added.

19. John A. Lyle, "Exclusive Systems of Medicine" (M.D. thesis, Transylvania University, 1841), KY—Transylvania U. Libe.

20. "The American Pharmaceutical Association," *BMSJ*, 58 (1858): 404.

21. Cheever, "The Value and the Fallacy of Statistics," p. 498.

22. D. G. Kolb, "The Disadvantages of Therapeutics" (M.D. thesis, Medical College of the State of South Carolina, 1859), SC—Med. U. SC, Main Libe.; and see Cincinnati Medical Society, Minutes, 9 October 1874–20 February 1877, comments of C. P. Judkins at meeting of 1 December 1874, OH—Cincinnati Acad. Med.; and G. W. Scranton, Resident Student, Case Book, Charity Hospital, New Orleans, Louisiana, 1873–74, LA—Matas.

23. Jacob Townsend Gilford, Notes Taken on Lectures Given by David Hosack, n.d., NY—NY Hist. Soc. On the persistence of the concept of temperament, see John S. Haller, Jr., *American Medicine in Transition, 1840–1910* (Urbana, Chicago, and London: University of Illinois Press, 1981), pp. 3–35.

24. Lewens Dixon Gray, "The Province and Purpose of Medical Science" (M.D. thesis, University of Pennsylvania, 1844), PA—U. PA Libe.

25. See, for example, L. P. Yandell, Jr., Lecture Notes, University of Louisville, Department of Medicine, [personal copy of his notes, probably 1870s], Yandell Family Papers, KY—U. Louisville Med. Libe. On perceptions of the biomedical singularity of blacks, see Kenneth Kiple and Virginia Himmelsteib King, *Another Dimension to the Black Diaspora: Diet, Disease, and Racism* (Cambridge: Cambridge University Press, 1981); Todd L. Savitt, *Medicine and Slavery: The Diseases and Health Care of Blacks in Antebellum Virginia* (Urbana, Chicago, and London: University of Illinois Press, 1978); and William Stanton, *The Leopard's Spots: Scientific Attitudes toward Race in America, 1815–1859* (Chicago and London: University of Chicago Press, 1960). The

resonances of these ideas in later American thinking, as in the biological themes that fed the eugenics movement and immigration restriction, are manifest.

26. R. B. Berry, "Circumstances Modifying the Effects of Medicines" (M.D. thesis, University of Pennsylvania, 1855), PA—U. PA Libe.

27. George L. Houze, "Inflammation" (M.D. thesis, Transylvania University, 1848), KY—Transylvania U. Libe. And on blacks, see Gamma, "Effects of Mercury on the Constitution of Negroes," *BMSJ*, 11 (1835): 256.

28. Luther V. Bell, "On Diet," *BMSJ*, 13 (1835–36): pp. 267 and 302.

29. "Effects of Breathing Impure Air," *BMSJ*, 6 (1832): 14.

30. Anonymous, Notes Taken on Lectures Given by Benjamin Dudley, 1830, LA—Matas.

31. "[Review of] *A Treatise on the Science and Practice of Medicine* . . . By Alonzo B. Palmer," *BMSJ*, 106 (1882): 541.

32. See Chapter 6.

33. Daniel D. Slanson, Notes Taken on Lectures of Professor Webster, Geneva College, Introductory Lecture, 1846, Medical Daybook, 1846–77, Daniel D. Slanson Papers, LA—LSU; and see Lundsford P. Yandell, Notes Taken on Lectures Given by Professor Richardson, Transylvania University, Introductory in the Chapel, 9 November 1825, KY—U. KY Libe.

34. Baltimore Almshouse Medical Reports, 1833–37, Case Notes of Dr. James H. Miller, Report on Clinical Instruction, 1 February 1834, MD—MD Hist. Soc. And see James Lawrence Cabell to [Joseph C. Cabell], Baltimore Almshouse, 13 December 1834, and Cabell to Uncle, Baltimore Almshouse, 22 February 1835, James Lawrence Cabell Papers, VA—U. VA Libe.

35. Gilford, Notes Taken on Lectures Given by Hosack; and see Benjamin S. Downing, Notes Taken on Lectures Given by Joseph Mather Smith on the Theory and Practice of Medicine, College of Physicians and Surgeons at the University of the State of New York, 1826, NY—Columbia-Presbyterian.

36. Robert Peter, Notes Taken on Lectures Given by Benjamin Dudley on Surgery, Transylvania University, 1834 (front cover marked: "Condensed from the copy common among the students, Dec. 1834"), KY—Transylvania U. Libe. On neurasthenia, see Charles E. Rosenberg, "George M. Beard and American Nervousness," in idem, *No Other Gods: On Science and American Social Thought* (Baltimore and London: Johns Hopkins University Press, 1976), pp. 98–108.

37. Houze, "Inflammation."

38. W. Taylor, "Changeability of Disease," *Proceedings of the Medical Association of the State of Alabama, at Its Sixth Annual Meeting, Begun and Held in the City of Selma, Dec. 13–15, 1852, with an Appendix and List of Members* (Mobile, 1853), p. 79.

39. See, for example, G. Volney Dorsey, "Epidemics of Miami County Ohio," *WL*, 13 (1852): 605; and P. H. Lewis, "Medical History of Alabama," *NOMSJ*, 3 (1846–47): 692. On the tradition out of which this thinking came, see Gilbert Chinard, "The American Philosophical Society and the Early History of Forestry in America," *Proceedings of the American Philosophical Society*, 89 (1945): 44–89; and Clarence J. Glacken, *Traces on the Rhodian Shore: Nature and Culture in Western Thought from Ancient Times to the End of the Eighteenth Century* (Berkeley and Los Angeles: University of California Press, 1967), pp. 501–713.

40. "Medical Schools, No. 1," *NOMNHG*, 3 (1856–57): 678.

41. John Leonard Riddell, Notes Taken on Lectures Given by Dr. Smith, Medical College of Ohio, 1834–35, vol. 26, John Leonard Riddell Manuscript Volumes, LA—Tulane U. Libe.

42. Joseph Jones, Lectures on Physiology and Pathology, University of Nashville, 1866–67, Joseph Jones Papers, vol. 7, LA—LSU. The scorbutic taint was similarly understood by physicians to be a modifier of various pathological conditions as often as it was the constituent core of a disease entity.

43. John Henry Fitts, Notes Taken on Lectures Given by Dr. Mitchell, Jefferson Medical College, n.d., NC—Duke Med. Libe.

44. "Epidemical and Local Influences upon Disease," *Atlanta Medical and Surgical Journal*, 1 (1855–56): 495; and see Samuel A. Cartwright, "The One Dose Cure of Camp Dysentery," Natchez, n.d., Samuel A. Cartwright and Family Papers, LA—LSU; and William Octavius Eversfield, Notes Taken on Lectures Given on Surgical Pathology, University of Virginia, 1859–60, lecture in April 1860, William Octavius Eversfield Notebooks, VA—U. VA Libe.

45. H., "Introductory Lectures," *WL*, 7 (1848): 91–103 (lecture of O. W. Holmes), p. 96.

46. A. B. Shipman, "Medical Practice at the West" (Indiana Medical College, Laporte, 20 January 1849), *BMSJ*, 40 (1849): 162–163.

47. Montgomery W. Boyd, "The Influence of Climate" (M.D. thesis, Transylvania University, 1843), KY—Transylvania U. Libe.

48. Fitts, Notes Taken on Lectures Given by Mitchell; John George Metcalfe, Notes Taken on Lectures Given by James Jackson on Cases at the Massachusetts General Hospital, Boston, 1825–26, vol. 2, lecture 46, MA—Countway.

49. George B. McKnight, Notes Taken on Lectures Given by David Hosack on the Theory and Practice of Physic and Clinical Medicine, College of Physicians and Surgeons, New York, 1814–16, Joseph M. Toner Papers, DC—LC.

50. Gilford, Notes Taken on Lectures Given by Hosack.

51. Buckner Hill, Notes Taken on Lectures Given by David Hosack, 1824, Buckner Hill Notebooks, NC—State Archives.

52. This analysis of the animus and expression of the case for regional medical particularity draws heavily on Warner, "The Idea of Southern Medical Distinctiveness," and John Harley Warner, "A Southern Medical Reform: The Meaning of the Antebellum Argument for Southern Medical Education," *BHM*, 57 (1983): 364–381.

53. Jeremiah Butt, Jr., "The Influence of Climate" (M.D. thesis, Medical College of the State of South Carolina, 1835), SC—Med. U. SC, Main Libe.; and see Lewis Byrum Mitchell, "Biliary Derangements" (M.D. thesis, University of Nashville, 1858), TN—Vanderbilt U. Libe.

54. Benjamin Huger, Notes Taken on Lectures Given by Nathaniel Chapman on Materia Medica, University of Pennsylvania, 1816, SC—Waring; and see James P. Miller, Notes Taken on Lectures Given by Benjamin Rush, University of Pennsylvania, 1811–12, NC—Duke U. Libe.

55. Lundsford Pitts Yandell, Diary, 1824–43, KY—Filson.

56. Samuel Prescott Hildreth, "Meteorological Journal of the Weather, Flowering of Plants, Ripening of Fruits etc. and Continuation of a Medical Journal, or a History of the Diseases Which Prevailed in Marietta & Vicinity," typescript vols. for 1831–37, and manuscript vols. for 1838–54, OH—Marietta. Hildreth kept meteorological records earlier as well, but only those after 1830 survive. And see Job Clark, Meteorological Journal, Ravenna, Ohio, 1841–58, Job Clark Papers, CT—Yale U. Libe.; George Colmer, Daily Journal, 1842–78,

LA—Tulane U. Libe.; Physician's Visiting List, 1857 (with weather observations at the end of the volume), vol. 6, Milligan Family Papers, NC—SHC; and R. F. McGuire, Diary, Monroe, Louisiana, 1818–52, LA—LSU.

57. Case History Books, Medical Wards, Massachusetts General Hospital, vols. 84-90, 1838, MA—Countway.

58. Baltimore Almshouse Medical Reports, entry for 1 July 1833; Commercial Hospital of Cincinnati, Medical Staff Minute Book, 1861–91, meeting of 1 March 1870, OH—U. Cincinnati Libe.

59. Minutes of the Ohio State Medical Society, 1846–59, resolution at meeting in Dayton, 7 June 1853, OH—Dittrick; Baltimore Pathological Society, Minutes, vol. 1, 1853–58, meeting of 23 October 1855, NC—Duke U. Libe.; H. W. DeSaussure, "Report of the Meteorological and Sanitary Condition of Charleston, for the Year 1857–8, Read before the Medical Society of South Carolina," *Charleston Medical Journal and Review*, 14 (1859): 290.

60. Samuel A. Cartwright, "Address, Delivered before the Medical Convention, in the City of Jackson, January 13, 1846," *NOMSJ*, 2 (1845–46): 730.

61. Daniel Drake, *A Systematic Treatise, Historical, Etiological, and Practical, on the Principal Diseases of the Interior Valley of North America, as They Appear in the Caucasian, African, Indian, and Esquimaux Varieties of Its Population* (Cincinnati, 1854). See Daniel Drake to Samuel Hildreth, Cincinnati, 3 April 1827, and ibid., 17 June 1838, Samuel Prescott Hildreth Papers, OH—Marietta Coll. Libe. Numerous letters from Drake soliciting meteorological observations (for example, Daniel Drake to Professor Day [Yale College], Cincinnati, 9 April 1811) are deposited in the Daniel Drake Papers, Emmet Field Horine Collection, KY—U. KY Libe.

62. John Y. Bassett, "Report on the Topography, Climate and Diseases of Madison County, Ala.," *Southern Medical Reports*, 1 (1849): 256–281, and idem, "On the Climate and Diseases of Huntsville, Ala., and Its Vicinity, for the Year 1850," *Southern Medical Reports*, 2 (1850): 315–323.

63. E. D. Fenner to John Y. Bassett, New Orleans, 24 October 1849, John Young Bassett Papers, NC—SHC; and in the same collection, see Fenner's requests for meteorological information from Bassett in his letters of 8 August 1849 and 18 September 1849.

64. S. L. Grier, "The Negro and His Diseases," *NOMSJ*, 9 (1852–53): 763. Practitioners often traced the ways their own experiences had led them to this realization; for example, see J. H. Bernard, "Pneumonia" (M.D. thesis, University of Nashville, 1857), TN—Vanderbilt Med. Libe.

65. Much of this discussion is based on Warner, "A Southern Medical Reform"; on the political context of regional medical education, see also John Duffy, "Sectional Conflict and Medical Education in Louisiana," *Journal of Southern History*, 23 (1957): 286–306. The argument for regional medical education was not, of course, entirely curtailed by the Civil War; see, for example, L. L. Todd, "Natural Forces," address delivered at the Medical College of Indiana, 6 October 1880, IN—IN U. Libe. The course of the argument for distinctively southern medical education in the postbellum South is discussed briefly in John Harley Warner, "Medical Education," in *Encyclopedia of Southern Culture*, ed. William Ferris and Charles Wilson (Chapel Hill: University of North Carolina Press, forthcoming).

66. "Northern Schools, and Southern Students," *New Orleans Medical Journal*, 1 (1844–45): 122; italics in original.

67. William W. Cozart, "The Place where Southern Students Should Ac-

quire Their Medical Knowledge" (M.D. thesis, Medical College of the State of South Carolina, 1856), SC—Med. U. SC, Main Libe.

68. E. D. Fenner, *Introductory Lecture, Delivered at the Opening of the New Orleans School of Medicine, on the 17th November, 1856* (New Orleans, 1856), p. 23.

69. This analysis is elaborated in Warner, "The Idea of Southern Medical Distinctiveness," and idem, "A Southern Medical Reform."

4. Therapeutic Change

1. Typical of this sort is C. A. Hentz, Medical Diary, Quincy, Florida, November 1858–August 1862, which recorded, as a note on the volume's cover states, "interesting cases" (vol. 14, Hentz Family Papers, NC—SHC).

2. One practitioner set his new case book aside for a decade after filling a few pages, repentantly recording in it on 21 November 1875, "Some years have elapsed since this book has been opened—Constant occupation is my excuse for the negligence—Henceforth as time permits I shall continue to fill its pages with my observations" (Joseph Goodwin Rogers, Case Book, 3 July 1864–79, Rogers Manuscripts, IN—IN U. Libe.). Another physician who had recorded the course of his practice for five years acerbically scrawled, "Here I lay aside a book that has cost me more trouble to keep than it was worth" (C. H. Jordan, Daybook, North Carolina, 1849–54, NC—State Archives).

3. Beyond stylistic variations in record keeping, fundamental asymmetries among physicians' practices further forestall meaningful quantitative comparison of their recorded activities. In the antebellum lower South, for example, physicians who treated slaves on large plantations often made entries for the treatment (and fees) for a group of patients as a block rather than for individuals. Examples of records from practices largely devoted to slaves are Alonzo Snyder, Record Book, 1848–55, Alonzo Snyder Papers, LA—LSU; and Walter Wade, Plantation Diary, Mississippi, 1834–54, 2 vols., MS—State Archives. Entries in Wade's book typically record the charges for "Visit & prescript[ion] for 23 Negroes" or medical treatment "round Negro quarter."

4. Especially useful in identifying the expectations of treatment is Charles E. Rosenberg, "The Therapeutic Revolution: Medicine, Meaning, and Social Change in Nineteenth-Century America," *Perspectives in Biology and Medicine*, 20 (1977): 485–506. Other sketches of the broad movements in nineteenth-century therapeutics are Erwin H. Ackerknecht, *Therapeutics from the Primitives to the 20th Century* (New York: Hafner Press, 1973), pp. 94–125; Alex Berman, "The Heroic Approach in 19th-Century Therapeutics," *Bulletin of the American Society of Hospital Pharmacists*, 11 (1954): 320–327; William G. Rothstein, *American Physicians in the Nineteenth Century: From Sects to Science* (Baltimore and London: Johns Hopkins University Press, 1982), pp. 41–62, 177–197; and John Harley Warner, " 'The Nature-Trusting Heresy': American Physicians and the Concept of the Healing Power of Nature in the 1850's and 1860's," *Perspectives in American History*, 11 (1977–78): 291–324.

5. A useful introduction to etiological thinking is Charles E. Rosenberg, "The Cause of Cholera: Aspects of Etiological Thought in 19th-Century America," *BHM*, 34 (1960): 331-354.

6. The sample population and the sampling techniques employed are described in notes 33 and 37.

7. All examples and quotations in the text not otherwise identified are

drawn from either the cases sampled for quantitative analysis (see note 37) or from others (male and female) recorded in the medical case history books described in note 33. I have elected throughout strictly to respect patient confidentiality even though the archives did not formally insist on it, and I would encourage other historians to do likewise so that scholars will continue to enjoy the free access to patient records that I have been granted.

8. Georges Canguilhem's writings, while they do not explicitly analyze the natural in contradistinction to the normal, are of special heuristic value through their close explication of the relationship between concepts of normality and those of abnormality in nineteenth-century biomedical thought. See "Le normal et la pathologique," in *La connaissance de la vie* (Paris: J. Vrin, 1980; first pub. 1952), pp. 155–169; "La question de la normalité dans l'histoire de la pensée biologique," in *Idéologie et rationalité dans l'histoire des sciences de la vie* (Paris: J. Vrin, 1981; first pub. 1977), pp. 121–139; and *On the Normal and the Pathological*, trans. Carolyn R. Fawcett (Dordrecht, Holland, and Boston: D. Reidel, 1978; first pub. 1966). My attention to the "natural history" of words such as *natural* and *normal* has been substantially informed by Donald Fleming, "Attitude: The History of a Concept," *Perspectives in American History*, 1 (1967): 287–365.

9. The evidence supporting the efficacy of regular therapies was conclusive, one physician argued. "It will require more logic than man can command to convince the practitioner that he does not know, as the result of *principles* and *observations*, the effects of blood-letting, of opium, of tartar emetic, of mercury, and numerous other agents and means belonging to the materia medica. These agents are well known to produce particular effects, under given circumstances; and these results are sufficiently certain to constitute a *science*" ("[Review of] John Forbes, *Homoeopathy, Allopathy, and Young Physic* (1846)," *WL*, 5 (1847): 211).

10. In conformity with the principle of specificity, such an attitude forestalled the mechanical application of rules of practice. "No special rule should be laid down by a Physician as to how many ounces of blood should be abstracted in any disease," a Philadelphia student wrote in his thesis. "He should not bleed for ounces but for effect" (Henry W. Doss, "Venesection" [M.D. thesis, University of Pennsylvania, 1858], PA—U. PA Libe.).

11. This included to a large extent a tacit belief in the principle of specificity. Advising her sister on how to prepare for the approaching cholera, a Louisiana woman wrote, "Take a dose of calomel (your habitual quantity)" (Rachel O'Conner to Mary C. Weeks, Louisiana, 7 November 1832, David Weeks and Family Papers, LA—LSU); and see James Melvin to Audley Clark Britton, Eutaw, [Louisiana?], 8 December 1862, Audley Clark Britton and Family Papers, LA—LSU; and Sallie Roach to Dr. Raine, n.p., 21 September 1875, John R. Raine Papers, NC—Duke U. Libe. Of the large literature on self-help medicine, particularly useful is *Medicine without Doctors: Home Health Care in American History*, ed. Guenter B. Risse, Ronald L. Numbers, and Judith Walzer Leavitt (New York: Science History Publications, 1977).

12. For example, no single remedy dominated the practice of William Dawson Dorris, who practiced in the vicinity of Nashville, Tennessee, and who itemized most of the drugs he prescribed. Between 1840 and 1844, Dorris venesected on only 3.2 percent of his professional visits (14 venesections/432 visits in sample), cupped on 1.4 percent, and gave morphia on 6.0 percent, mercury on 12.5 percent, and tartar emetic on 2.1 percent (Ledgers, 3 vols., 1836–56, FL—U. South FL, Med. Center Libe.). Nor did any particular therapy

dominate the prescriptions that John Harney Davis, a Charleston, South Carolina, practitioner, made between 1827 and 1843. He venesected on 1.7 percent of his visits (15 venesections/881 visits in sample) and gave calomel in 7.6 percent, quinine or cinchona bark in 11.5 percent, and opium in 7.6 percent (Account Book, 1827–43, Charleston, SC—South Caroliniana Libe.). While the records of these physicians seem relatively complete, it is of course impossible to know what was not recorded. Larger relative frequencies of use for both opiates and mercurials were not uncommon. In the account book of a Baltimore druggist for 1834, for example, opiates were given in 19.1 percent (49 instances/257 cases) of the prescriptions sampled, and mercury in 25.7 percent (Stewart Account Book, 1834–37, MD—Hist. Soc.). If any group of drugs did dominate treatment, it was the cinchona bark derivatives used as antiperiodics in malarious regions. For example, when Daniel D. Slanson practiced in New York in 1852–54 and thereafter in Detroit, quinine was not particularly prominent in his treatments, but after he moved to Louisiana in 1866 he used it in approximately half of his prescriptions (Medical Daybook, 1846–77, 2 vols., LA—LSU); and see Ellis Malone, Medical Daybook, North Carolina, 1865–68, NC—Duke U. Libe.

13. A list follows of representative daybooks that were analyzed to determine the frequency of venesection. Given in parentheses is the period from which each sample was taken, followed by a fraction whose numerator is the number of venesections recorded and whose denominator is the number of entries in the sample. The samples represent varying proportions of the total number of entries, never under 10 percent and in some instances encompassing the entire source. Care was taken to select a representative seasonal cross section of each physician's practice to avoid skewing the sample by unduly stressing hot or cold months. John Angie Hyde, Daybooks, Freeport, [Massachusetts], 1804–25, vol. 1, 1804–07, vol. 2, 1822–25 (1822–25, 64/2,384), MA—Countway; Dr. George Hughes Parker Papers, Daybook, New Market, Frederick County, Maryland, 1 April 1819–23 September 1820 (1819–20, 50/238; 1821, 26/254), MD—MD Hist. Soc.; James Foster, Medical Record Books, Simpson County, Kentucky, 1826 (1826, 8/1,091), LA—LSU; Edward Young Kemper, Daybooks, 8 vols., volume begins in Waynesville, 1811, thereafter Cincinnati, 1811–17 (1811–17, 39/1,015), OH—Cincinnati Hist. Soc.; Isaac Parker, Ledger, Mount Pleasant, Ohio, 1811–32 (1811–19, 25/335), OH—Mount Pleasant; Anonymous, Ledger, Hagerstown, Maryland, 2 October 1835–6 June 1838 (1835–38, 26/487), NY—NY Hist. Soc.

14. These are the percentages of the debt entries, that is a physician's entries in his record book of the services rendered (including travel) and drugs prescribed to a patient, in which venesection appeared. Ordinarily a practitioner made a separate entry in his ledger each time he visited a patient, though it is not possible to determine this with certainty. Some record books are sufficiently detailed and regular to support an estimate of the number of visits (debt entries) made per case (and therefore the proportion of *cases* in which venesection was used) on the basis of the dates of entries and the specification of patient name and ailment (rather than merely the name of the head of the household who was billed). Often only one visit was made in a case, though repeated visits were also common. The physician engaged in a country practice where distance between patients was a dominant consideration in ordering his routine tended to make fewer visits per case than a physician practicing in an urban area, further complicating meaningful comparison.

15. A partial list of the private practice ledgers (beyond those identified

elsewhere in the notes) on which this generalization is based is in John Harley Warner, "The Therapeutic Perspective: Medical Knowledge, Practice, and Professional Identity, 1820–1885" (Ph.D. diss., Harvard University, 1984).

16. For example, Francis Jones Smith, Medical Account Books, Hillsborough, North Carolina, 1838–73, Mary Ruffin Smith Papers, NC—SHC; William B. Rowland, Account Books, 6 vols., Rowlandsville, Maryland, 1834–83, vol. for 1866–83, MD—MD Hist. Soc.; Edward W. Magann, Ledger, [Indiana], 12 September 1860–27 May 1897, IN—IN U. Libe.; Robert H. Ryland, Daybooks, vol. 1, 1849–56, vol. 2, 1856–83, Robert H. Ryland Papers, LA—LSU.

17. Some, of course, venesected at a relatively steady level. For example, Benjamin and Benjamin West Robinson, Account Books, Vermont and North Carolina, 1805–63, vol. 5, 1825–27, and vol. 12, 1836–37, both in Fayetteville, North Carolina (1825–27, 50/910 = 5.5 percent; 1836–37, 25/448 = 5.6 percent), NC—SHC; Henry M. Sneed, Ledger, [Tennessee], 1837–51 (1837–39, 13/482 = 2.7 percent; 1840–45, 10/327 = 3.1 percent), Sneed Family Papers, TN—TN State Libe.

18. Edwin W. Cowles, Book of Visits, Cleveland, 19 July 1832–November 1833; idem, Brest, Michigan, 1838; and Blackwood and Cowles Practice of Medicine, October 1848–March 1851, OH—Dittrick.

19. Hyde, Daybooks (1804, 44/497; 1822–25, 64/2,384).

20. Henry Marshall Turner, Record Book, 2 vols., Montgomery County, North Carolina, 1822–29 and 1848–58 (1825–29, 33/762; 1848–52, 17/591), Harnett County Papers, NC—SHC.

21. Rowland, Account Books (1835–38, 60/356; 1841–47, 38/328; 1853–55, 38/286; 1863–67, 14/135; 1866–83 [mainly 1870s], 20/326). The number of Rowland's visits per case diminished as he grew older, falling from 2.3 to 1.6. The proportions of *cases* in which Rowland bled for the above groups of years are, respectively, 38.2, 26.0, 24.9, 15.6, and 10.9 percent.

22. For an example of the prominence of opiates in the 1840s, see Samuel Holt, Ledger, Montgomery, Alabama, 1847–48, Dr. Samuel Holt Papers, AL—State Archives. A study of a Burlington, New Jersey, pharmacy's prescription records for 1854 reveals that of all drugs, opium in various forms was the most frequently prescribed (David L. Cowen, Louis D. King, and Nicholas G. Lordi, "Nineteenth Century Drug Therapy: Computer Analysis of the 1854 Prescription File of a Burlington Pharmacy," *Journal of the Medical Society of New Jersey*, 78 (1981): 760). It is likely that the pharmacy was typical in this respect. In the same year opium was the drug most often indicated in the prescription book of a Charleston, South Carolina, pharmacy, where it was called for in 42.9 percent of the prescriptions; this was also the case in 1862, when it was given in 44.4 percent of the prescriptions. A decade later, in 1872, it was an ingredient in only 28.3 percent (Prescription Books, 19 vols., 1853–72, Pankin Drug Store Records, Charleston, South Carolina, NC—SHC, samples from vol. 6, November 1853–June 1855, vol. 17, Jan 1860–August 1862, and vol. 24, June 1871–June 1872). This is consistent with the frequencies from New Orleans pharmacies from the same period given in note 30.

23. Demand for quinine escalated accordingly. "The druggists say that they have never before sold so much of this article [quinine] as they have this season," a Georgian wrote to his physician son in 1846, adding in a later letter that the quantity of quinine sold was "incredible" (Joseph Milligan to Joe [Joseph A. S. Milligan], Augusta, 10 September and 24 September 1846, Milligan Family Papers, NC—SHC). And see Erwin H. Ackerknecht, *Malaria in the Upper Mississippi Valley, 1760–1900* (Baltimore: Johns Hopkins Press, 1945),

pp. 98–115; and Dale C. Smith, "Quinine and Fever: The Development of the Effective Dosage," *JHM*, 31 (1976): 343–367

24. Prescription Book, Second North Carolina Military Hospital, Petersburg, Virginia, 18 August–25 September 1864, Confederate Hospital Records, NC—SHC. These records were kept by day, not by patient, and no diagnoses were recorded. The sample of 511 entries includes all new drug prescriptions but not the direction to continue the previous course of treatment, which often is ambiguous. Quinine appeared in 8.6 percent of the prescriptions and iron compounds in 4.3 percent. On alcohol use see also the extensive use of brandy and whiskey in Union Post Hospital, Columbus, Kentucky, Prescription Book, 1863–64, KY—Filson; Edward Kershner, Naval Case Book, 1862–64, Edward Kershner Papers, NC—Duke U. Libe.; and Prescription Book, Pettigrew Hospital, Raleigh, North Carolina, 1865, Ernest Haywood Collection, NC—SHC.

25. Confederate States of America, "General Prescription Book. No. 2," [Virginia], 1864–65, VA—U. VA Libe. The sample of 112 cases (not entries), taken from 29 June 1864 to 1 November 1865, represents only about one-twentieth of the cases entered in this volume. Successive days of a patient's history were entered together, and diagnoses were given in about three-fourths of the cases. Note that percentages of drug use for this source are by case and are not comparable with the ones for the Petersburg hospital, which are by prescription.

26. For example, see Field Hospital Register, Confederate States of America, 1862, Robert D. Barbour Collection, NC—State Archives; Invoices of Lynchburg, Virginia, Hospital, in Confederate States of America Archives, Army, NC—Duke U. Libe.; List of Medicines Received since 1 January 1864, U.S.S. Niagara, New York Harbor, 15 January 1864, Samuel Warren Abbott Letterbook, 1862–77, DC—LC; Requisition for Medicines, 1863, Oak Ridge, Mississippi, Jno. B. Rice, and Invoice of Medicine Issued to Jno. B. Rice, 4 November 1863, John B. Rice Papers, OH—Hayes; and List of Supplies, Way Side Hospital, Columbia, South Carolina, 1862–65, SC—South Caroliniana Libe. A systematic comparison of the medical practice of northern and southern medical officers during the Civil War would be of considerable interest, and ample materials survive to support such a study.

27. Dover's powder was included in 0.4 percent of all prescriptions, laudanum in 10.8 percent, morphia in 22.7 percent, and opium powder in 6.1 percent.

28. At the Petersburg hospital 5.5 percent of all prescriptions contained blue mass, 1.8 percent compound cathartic pills, and 1.4 percent simple calomel; at the other hospital, calomel alone was prescribed for 12 percent of the patients and 16 percent were given blue mass, a milder mercurial purgative.

29. This use of venesection primarily as a palliative was obvious in the practice of John Knox, a Kentucky physician, by the late 1840s. In his exceptionally detailed case history book, bleeding with the lancet is recorded as being used only in direct response to severe pain. Typically, in 1848 Knox instructed one family that after he left the patient was "to be bled if the pain returned" (15 January 1848). The effects produced by venesection repeatedly confirmed his expectations. For example, visiting a woman with pain in her breast and back, Knox first administered "some P[ain] killer without any effect," then applied a blister for the pain, which made her "no better," and then tried an opiate. The patient remained in such acute pain that she could not lie down, at which point Knox entered into his case record, "I bled her & after a little while I opened the orifice again & took more blood—blood very bad—

she gets considerable relief from the bleeding" (23 March 1848). John Knox, Medical Case Books, [Kentucky], 2 vols., 1847–55, KY—U. KY Libe.

30. The therapies of heroic medicine nevertheless retained a place in private practice at least through the 1880s, with the near exception of venesection. Mercury, for example, remained an important agent in some physicians' practices, though calomel (containing 85 percent mercury by weight) was in part supplanted by milder preparations. The records of New Orleans pharmacies illustrate this. At E. G. Wunderlich's Pharmacy, 22.4 percent of the prescriptions filled in 1866 contained mercury (43 mercurial prescriptions/ 192 sampled), 17.7 percent in 1868 (53/300), and 16.0 percent in 1870 (66/413); for these years calomel appeared in, respectively, 12.5 percent, 9.3 percent, and 7.5 percent of the prescriptions. At Ferrers Pharmacy 13.8 percent of the prescriptions in 1875 contained mercury (30/217) as did 7.8 percent in 1879 (8/ 103). In 1886–87 8.3 percent (27/326) of the prescriptions filled at Llados Pharmacy contained mercury, and 10.3 percent (12/117) of those at S. Frank's Pharmacy in 1890. Opiates appeared in these records in 34.4 percent of the prescriptions for 1866, 21.7 percent for 1868, 23.7 percent for 1870, 23.5 percent for 1875, 15.5 percent for 1878, 14.7 percent for 1886–87, and 18.0 percent for 1890. The corresponding proportions for cinchona bark derivatives in these years were, respectively, 31.8, 25.0, 18.6, 18.4, 24.3, 17.2, and 18.0. The Llados records are in LA—LA Hist. Center; all others are in LA—Pharmacy Museum.

31. The quotation appears in the Minutes of the Union District Medical Association, Oxford, Ohio, 1880–96 (internally dated 1881), OH—Miami U. Libe.

32. The most useful studies of the history of medical instrumentation are Audrey B. Davis, *Medicine and Its Technology: An Introduction to the History of Medical Instrumentation* (Westport, Connecticut, and London: Greenwood Press, 1981); and Stanley Joel Reiser, *Medicine and the Reign of Technology* (Cambridge: Cambridge University Press, 1978).

33. The MGH records, deposited in MA—Countway, include 384 volumes of medical case history books for the years from 1823 to 1885. Of these, 127 are from the West Wing, opened in 1847, and the remaining 257 are from the wards that became the East Wing. While the wards were segregated by gender, the record books were not. Surgical case histories are preserved in a separate set of books. The Commercial Hospital records, deposited in OH—U. Cincinnati, Hist. Hlth. Scis. Libe., include fifty-one volumes of male medical case records for the years 1837–81 (including several volumes containing some female medical entries during the early 1860s) and an additional twenty volumes of female medical records for 1840–81. There are no nineteenth-century medical case history books dated after 1881 for this hospital. Surgical records were kept in separate volumes, which also survive.

34. See the circular letter by James Jackson and John C. Warren, Boston, 20 August 1810, in N. I. Bowditch, *A History of the Massachusetts General Hospital* (Boston, 1851), pp. 3–9. The *MGH Report* for 1833 typically characterized the hospital's patient population as "generally from among the industrious and prudent classes" (p. 2).

35. Charles E. Rosenberg, "And Heal the Sick: Hospital and Patient in 19th Century America," in *The Medicine Show: Patients, Physicians and the Perplexities of the Health Revolution in Modern Society*, ed. Patricia Branca (New York: Science History Publications, 1977), pp. 121–140. Information on the institutional history of the hospital has been culled chiefly from the *MGH Reports*, especially those for 1836, 1838, and 1848.

36. On the duties of the resident physician, see *MGH Report*, 1850, p. 1; *MGH Report*, 1864, p. 5; and James Clark White, *Sketches from My Life, 1833–1913* (Cambridge, Massachusetts: Riverside Press, 1914), p. 72.

37. The sample represents 10 percent of admissions by year to each hospital's male medical wards, with the exception that for the comparatively small MGH, twenty-five cases annually were sampled if fewer than 250 male patients were admitted to the medical wards during the course of the year. This yielded a sample of 1,762 cases for the MGH (1823–85) and 2,023 cases for the Commercial Hospital of Cincinnati (1837–81). Cases were evenly sampled from throughout each calendar year's admissions to reflect the actual seasonal distribution of admissions. Sixty variables were recorded from each of these cases for computer analysis.

38. James Jackson outlined the hospital trustees' admission policies in "The Massachusetts Hospital," *BMSJ*, 3 (1830–31): 194–195; and see *MGH Report*, 1839, p. 4, and *MGH Report*, 1859, p. 15. In the period from 1839 to 1841, not atypical years, the hospital turned away about one-third of all those who applied for the free beds (*MGH Report*, 1841, p. 4). The trustees regularly reported the proportion of the total patient population who were paying; see, for example, *MGH Report*, 1839, p. 28, showing that 53 percent of the patients were paying.

39. The mean duration of stay of sampled MGH patients from the 1820s to the 1880s was, by decade, 29.2, 25.6, 27.0, 31.2, 28.4, 30.8, and 24.9 days. On the perceived excesses in the duration of stay, especially of the free patients, see *MGH Report*, 1835, p. 4, *MGH Report*, 1842, p. 7, and *MGH Report*, 1855, p. 5. The phrase "comfortable home" was used in *MGH Report*, 1859, p. 15, to describe the goal of malingerers. On the patient population, see *MGH Report*, 1823, p. 4, and *MGH Report*, 1885, p. 27. On the "magnificent" facilities of the MGH, see E[rasmus] D[arwin] F[enner] to the Editors, Boston, 15 May 1846, *NOMSJ*, 3 (1846–47): 201–202.

40. The distribution of sampled MGH patients by occupational category is given by decade in Warner, "The Therapeutic Perspective," Table 2. The mean age of these patients was, by decade from the 1820s to the 1880s, 29.9, 29.8, 29.3, 30.2, 32.4, 33.0, and 34.2 years.

41. Stephan Thernstrom calculated the figure for Boston using the 1880 census data and the same classification of occupations that, with modifications, has been applied to the sample of MGH patients. Out of the 68 percent of Boston's male labor force that was blue collar in 1880, 36 percent was skilled manual, 17 percent semiskilled and service, and 15 percent unskilled labor (*The Other Bostonians: Poverty and Progress in the American Metropolis, 1880–1930* [Cambridge, Massachusetts: Harvard University Press, 1973], pp. 50, 289–292). The breakdown of the 83 percent of sampled MGH patients who were blue collar is given in Warner, "The Therapeutic Perspective," Table 2. On the MGH patient population in the 1870s and 1880s, see Morris J. Vogel, *The Invention of the Modern Hospital: Boston, 1870–1930* (Chicago: University of Chicago Press, 1980), pp. 1–28.

42. The nativity of sampled MGH patients is broken down by decade in Warner, "The Therapeutic Perspective," Table 1. In 1850 45 percent of the city's male workers were foreign born, compared with 67 percent of the sampled MGH patients admitted in the 1850s. In 1880 the figure for Boston was 41 percent; the corresponding figure for the hospital for the period 1880–1885 was 52 percent. The Boston proportions are from Thernstrom, *The Other Bostonians*, p. 113.

43. The relative frequency of selected diagnoses and diagnostic categories for sampled MGH patients is given in Warner, "The Therapeutic Perspective," Table 3.

44. The outcome of sampled patients' stay in the Commercial Hospital of Cincinnati is analyzed by decade in ibid., Table 4. The most common diagnoses of male medical patients who died at the MGH were typhoid fever and pulmonary diseases, especially tuberculosis. Together typhoid and tuberculosis made up about 40 percent of the diagnoses cited for patients who died from the 1830s through 1850s, a figure that declined to about 25 percent (a decrease in proportion due to the declining frequency of both diagnoses) in the next three decades. These diseases were leading causes of adult mortality in the Boston community as well. During the 1830s and 1840s the categories "typhus" (which encompassed typhoid fever) and "consumption" (ordinarily identified with tuberculosis in its most common, pulmonary form) together accounted for about one-fifth of the deaths in Boston. On the sources of statistics for Boston, see Robert Gutman, "Birth and Death Registration in Massachusetts," *Milbank Memorial Fund Quarterly*, 36 (1958): 58–74, 373–402, 37 (1959): 297–326, 386–417.

45. Even though some differences between native-born and Irish-born patients are discernible, no noticeable differences in treatment were found. The populations of native-born, Irish-born, and all foreign-born patients were compared by decade for such indices of treatment as opium and calomel dosages, frequencies of quinine and alcohol prescriptions, number of times treatment was changed during the first five days in the hospital, and total number of treatments given. While no distinctive correlation between treatment and ethnicity was discovered, this finding must be qualified by the fact that in some instances the number of cases in each subpopulation (for example, Irish-born who were given alcohol in the 1840s) was so small that meaningful conclusions cannot be drawn from the data.

46. The most useful studies of the transformation of the hospital in late-nineteenth-century America are Charles E. Rosenberg, "Inward Vision & Outward Glance: The Shaping of the American Hospital, 1880–1914," *BHM*, 53 (1979): 346–391; David Rosner, *A Once Charitable Enterprise: Hospitals and Health Care in Brooklyn and New York, 1885–1915* (Cambridge: Cambridge University Press, 1982); and Vogel, *The Invention of the Modern Hospital*.

47. The history of the Commercial Hospital of Cincinnati is summarized in Arch I. Carson, compiler, *Register of Internes of the Cincinnati Hospital (Formerly Commercial Hospital) 1830–1900* (Cincinnati: The Society of Internes, 1900), p. 5. On the hospital's early organization, see Daniel Drake to Samuel P. Hildreth, Cincinnati, 1 January 1819, Hildreth Papers, OH—Marietta; and Drake to Governor Brown, Cincinnati, 25 November 1821, Drake Papers, Emmet Field Horine Collection, KY—U. KY Libe. John B. Harrison described the hospital's patient population, then numbering around 1,500 annually, in "Hospital Cases, with Reflections," *WL*, 1 (1842–43): 1.

48. The reorganization bills of 1861 and 1868 were printed in the *CHC Report*, 1865–66, pp. 506–511, and *CHC Report*, 1869, p. 53. The rules and regulations governing the hospital, including those delineating admissions policies, were regularly printed in the hospital's annual report, as in *CHC Report*, 1865–66, pp. 512–533.

49. The CHC's board of trustees' vote to disallow connections between the hospital staff and the medical college was recorded in Cincinnati Hospital,

Board of Trustees Minutes, 1869–80, entry for 26 December 1873 (although the rule had been in effect since 1 October 1871), OH—U. Cincinnati Libe. For its part the Medical College of Ohio saw its association with the CHC as one of its strongest lures in recruiting students; see, for example, *Annual Announcement of the Medical College of Ohio, for the Session 1847–8* (Cincinnati, [1848]), p. 5; and Medical College of Ohio, Board of Trustees Minutes, 1838–60, OH—U. Cincinnati Libe.

50. "The Western Christian Advocate and Medical Politics," *WLHR*, 12 (1851): 462. The rules governing the medical staff were printed in the *CHC Report*, 1866–67, pp. 89–91. On concern about the irregular visits of attending physicians, see Commercial Hospital of Cincinnati, Board of Trustees, Minutes, 1861–69, entry for 24 May 1862, OH—U. Cincinnati Libe.

51. The quotations are from, respectively, Medical College of Ohio, Faculty Minutes, February 1822–February 1831, entry for 6 November 1829 (which records the "Rules for the House Surgeon of the Commercial Hospital and Lunatic Asylum of Ohio"), OH—U. Cincinnati Libe., and the *CHC Report*, 1865–66, p. 520. The rules for the resident physician were further codified in the Medical College of Ohio, Faculty Minutes, entry for 21 April 1834.

52. George C. Shattuck, Jr., Diary, entry for Cincinnati, 3–21 May 1834, Shattuck Papers, MA—MA Hist. Soc.

53. *CHC Report*, 1865–66, p. 465; and see *MGH Report*, 1841, p. 4, and *MGH Report*, 1846, p. 459. Admissions figures are recorded in John P. Harrison, "Introductory to a Course of Clinical Instruction. Delivered Nov. 3d, 1847, in the Cincinnati Hospital and Lunatic Asylum of Cincinnati," *WL*, 7 (1848): 14; and in *Annual Catalogue of the Officers & Students of the Medical College of Ohio. Session 1840–1841* (Cincinnati, 1841), p. 16.

54. Commercial Hospital of Cincinnati, Board of Trustees, Minutes, 1861–69, entry for 15 May 1861.

55. *CHC Report*, 1869–70, p. 51, described the new building.

56. Daily Record, Commercial Hospital, April 1867–April 1881, entries for 11 June 1867, 12 September 1868, December 1869, and June 1873, OH—U. Cincinnati, Hist. Hlth. Scis. Libe. Reports on patient fighting and theft abounded in the case records, as in the note on a patient in 1847: "Eloped—having stolen a small sum of money (45 cts) from a dying man."

57. Daily Record, Commercial Hospital, entries for November 1878 and 24 December 1878. Further complaints against the resident staff, including a reprimand from the hospital's board of trustees, were recorded in the same volume in January 1879. Discipline for patients who violated the rules could be severe. A day after one man was admitted for intermittent fever in 1847, for example, the case record noted that he "was caught smoking in the ward today and was by the steward of the house sent to the cells for 48 hours—put on bread and water."

58. Unless otherwise specified, all subsequent statistics concerning the CHC patient population refer to the sampled cases drawn from the male medical wards. On the case records and sampling procedures, see notes 33 and 37.

59. The occupational structure of sampled CHC patients is given by decade in Warner, "The Therapeutic Perspective," Table 5. Competition among Cincinnati's hospitals for the care of sick mariners became aggressive; see H. M. Jones [superintendent, CHC] to John W. Woodworth [supervising surgeon, Marine Hospital Service], Cincinnati, 22 July 1871; F. P. Anderson [medical officer of the Good Samaritan Hospital] to John S. Billings [assistant surgeon, U.S.

Army], Cincinnati, 3 April [1872]; and Billings to Woodworth, 10 June 1872, all in Incoming Correspondence, Cincinnati, 1869, 1872–76, 1880–81, Marine Hospital Service Records, Record Group 90, DC—National Archives.

60. The nativity of sampled CHC patients is broken down by decade in Warner, "The Therapeutic Perspective," Table 6. A separate record book, Paupers Admitted to the Hospital, 1860–66, OH—U. Cincinnati, Hist. Hlth. Scis. Libe., noted the nativity and occupation of pauper patients, many of them immigrants. Nativity was scantily recorded in the CHC records before the 1860s, so comparisons based upon it are only valid for the last three decades of this study. Indices of patient attention (total number of treatments, and number of times treatment was changed during the first five days in the hospital), doses of two key drugs (mercury and opium), and relative frequencies of use of alcohol and quinine were compared for Irish, German, and native-born patients for these decades, but no substantial differences were found among them. As at the MGH, the commonality of hospital patients overwhelmed ethnicity as a determinant of treatment. From the 1830s to the 1880s, the mean age of sampled CHC patients by decade was 31.3, 31.6, 30.7, 33.1, 34.6, and 36.1 years.

61. The relative frequencies of selected diagnoses and diagnostic groups for sampled CHC patients are given by decade in Warner, "The Therapeutic Perspective," Table 7.

62. The proportions of sampled CHC patients whose hospital stays had various outcomes are presented in Warner, "The Therapeutic Perspective," Table 8. The leading diagnoses of patients who died at the CHC were gastrointestinal disorders and pulmonary diseases, especially tuberculosis, but it is not possible to determine disease-specific mortality rates with any reliability. Irregularity in the recording of diagnosis in the case books (diagnosis was noted for only 13.6 percent of the patients sampled from the 1860s, compared to 84.1 percent from the 1870s) is chiefly responsible for this. A much smaller proportion of the CHC patients who died were diagnosed as having typhoid fever than of those at the MGH, a phenomenon that may reflect record keeping and diagnostic refinement more than actual differences between the two populations. The mean duration of time that sampled patients stayed in the CHC was, by decade from the 1830s to the 1880s, 19.3, 20.4, 16.5, 15.0, 17.3, and 19.1 days.

63. At both hospitals, heroic depletive therapies such as venesection, calomel, and tartar emetic, if the patient received them at all, were by and large prescribed soon after admission. During the 1840s and 1850s at the CHC, for example, in 75.0 percent and 92.2 percent respectively of cases in which these drugs were administered, their use was noted within the first four days.

64. The changing mean doses of mercury in all forms closely parallel those for calomel. The index of mercury dosage employed here is the amount of mercury in grains (contained in whatever mercurial drug was prescribed) given on the first day mercury was used. For all cases, including those in which no mercurial was used, the mean values at the CHC were for the 1830s—12.7 grains, 1840s—4.0, 1850s—5.1, 1860s—0.9, 1870s—0.2, and 1880s—0.1. Calculated for only those cases in which some mercurial was prescribed, the mean values were for the 1830s—17.8 grains of mercury, 1840s—7.6, 1850s—8.1, 1860s—4.0, 1870s—3.4, and 1880s—2.9.

65. This contrast was not unremarked at the time. Calomel, Jacob Bigelow commented in an 1841 lecture at Harvard, "has been recommended in fevers

generally, and is now much used in intermittents of the South and West in doses which *we* rarely give in common cases; but there is not sufficient evidence of its utility, and it is not used here—in chronic diseases of the liver" (Samuel Kneeland, Jr., Notes Taken on Lectures Given by Dr. Bigelow on Materia Medica, vol. 6, 6 January 1841–18 February 1841, MA—Countway).

66. James Jackson emphasized the importance of cathartics shortly before the opening of the MGH. "The operation of cathartics is a very depletory process," he told his students, "and, next to blood-letting, they constitute the most important part of the antiphlogistic treatment" (Jonathan Greely Stevenson, Notes Taken on Lectures Given by James Jackson on the Theory and Practice of Physic, Boston, 1817–19, vol. 2, MA—Countway). Jackson later noted that in typhoid fever, even though mercurial cathartics had been widely used at the MGH when it opened in the 1820s, the "faith in them was lessening from year to year; and they have been given up almost entirely in typhoid fever, since 1830" ("Report on Typhoid Fever," *BMSJ*, 19 (1839): 53). Jackson was correct in saying that the MGH's physicians (of whom he was one) used mercurials much less frequently in treating patients with typhoid fever after 1830; mercurials were prescribed for 70.0 percent of the sampled patients who had typhoid fever in the 1820s but for only 30.4 percent in the 1830s. Still, his perception that mercury had been "given up almost entirely in typhoid fever, since 1830" is scarcely borne out by the fact that nearly a third of the sampled patients admitted with typhoid in the 1830s were dosed with mercury. In fact, mercurials continued to be given to more than a tenth of the sampled typhoid patients at the MGH through the 1860s (1840s—23.4 percent, 1850s—13.9 percent, 1860s—14.8 percent).

67. A very small proportion of the calomel used was prescribed in syphilis as an alterative, that is, as a drug that altered the entire physiological order of the body in a way that precluded the continued existence of the original disease. Such constitutional treatment essentially sought to cure syphilis through the therapeutic effects of mercury poisoning. Because the admissions policies of the MGH discriminated against patients with venereal diseases, the syphilitic population of the medical wards was small.

68. When the agents of heroic depletion were used at the MGH, generally they were initially prescribed during the first few days after the patient's admission. During the height of depletive practice, from the 1820s through the 1840s, in between 62.2 percent and 86.7 percent (by decade) of the cases in which tartar emetic, venesection, or mercurials were prescribed, they were first given within four days of the patient's admission. The declining reliance of MGH physicians on mercury, shown by reduced frequency of use, can be seen as well in the timing of the introduction of mercurials into cases. When these therapies were prescribed in the decades from the 1820s to the 1860s (the subpopulation size for the 1870s and 1880s is too small to support generalizations), they were first used during the initial four days in, respectively, 74.5, 74.0, 65.1, 58.3, and 48.9 percent of the cases. (The frequencies with which twenty-six selected treatments were used for the first time within the first one, two, three, four, five to seven, eight to fourteen, fifteen to twenty-one, and twenty-two or later days of each case were tabulated for both the MGH and the CHC).

69. The mean amount of mercury given on the first day mercury was used, calculated for all sampled MGH cases, was for the 1820s—3.0 grains, 1830s—2.1, 1840s—1.2, 1850s—1.1, 1860s—0.6, 1870s—0.2, and 1880s—0.1.

For only those cases in which some mercurial was used, the values were for the 1820s—5.0 grains, 1830s—4.1, 1840s—3.0, 1850s—4.0, 1860s—3.4, 1870s—3.8, and 1880s—2.5.

70. In quotations pharmaceutical symbols that appear in the case histories have been converted into conventional English, such as ounces, drachms, and scruples. Roman numerals have also been transcribed as Arabic numerals when doing so would unclutter the text.

71. On the animus and meaning of this therapeutic event, see John Harley Warner, "Professional Power, Sectarian Conflict, and Orthodox Identity in Mid-Nineteenth-Century American Medicine: Therapeutic Change at the Commercial Hospital in Cincinnati," *Journal of American History*, forthcoming.

72. Among the MGH patients who were venesected while the practice was popular, pain was reported as a prominent feature of their condition in over three-fourths of the cases (1820s—93.3 percent, 1830s—77.8 percent, 1840s—93.3 percent).

73. When asked why he bled patients with pneumonia though theory opposed the practice used to cure, James Jackson replied bluntly, "I bleed to diminish agony" ([Walter] Channing's remarks in Z. B. Adams, "Extracts from the Records of the Norfolk District Medical Society of Massachusetts," *BMSJ*, 76 [1867]: 514). Henry Ingersoll Bowditch's lecture on the palliative value of venesection to students in the MGH is recorded in his Clinical Course of Lectures, No. 2, 1862–63, MA—Countway.

74. "The lancet lies year after year unused in my pocket," Henry Ingersoll Bowditch informed his students at the MGH in 1861, "but as I felt compelled to use it a few years ago in this hospital to relieve horrible symptoms and pain in acute pleurisy . . . I feel that I may be obliged to use it again" (Introductory to the Course of Clinical Medicine, Course of 1861–62, lecture of 28 November 1861, MA—Countway).

75. At the CHC, the mean volumes of blood let per venesection for the 1830s through the 1860s, calculated using the first venesection of those cases in which it was practiced, are by decade 22.0, 12.6, 11.7, and 3.0 ounces. The corresponding values at the MGH were in the 1820s—18.4 ounces, 1830s—13.2, 1840s—11.4, 1850s—12.6, and 1860s—18.7. The high mean for the 1860s at the MGH represents only three exceptionally desperate cases.

76. Explaining the diagnostic value of venesection, one Tennessee student wrote in his thesis, "We can often determine whether or not some Local pain is caused by inflamation or not, by placing the Patient in the Erect posture, and opening a vein, for if he bear the loss of much Blood, you may be assured that Inflamation is present" (Benjamin M. Alford, "Blood-letting and Its Therapeutic Effects" [M.D. thesis, University of Nashville, 1856], TN—Vanderbilt Med. Libe.).

77. Even Broussais's classic treatment by gum arabic and leeches could be prescribed for reasons other than the Broussaisian ambition of reducing gastrointestinal irritation, however. For example, Jackson indicated in his private record of MGH cases that he had ordered gum arabic and leeches for one victim of typhus fever, but made it clear that he prescribed the leeches to reduce pain, not inflammation (James Jackson, Case Book, 1825–1826, MA—Countway).

78. Walter Gilman Curtis, Notes Taken on Lectures Given by John Ware and Jacob Bigelow, Massachusetts Medical College, Boston, [ca. 1847–53], lecture by Ware, Walter Gilman Curtis Papers, vol. 2, NC—SHC. Opium, a Michigan medical professor typically told his class in 1866, is "one of the *essentials*

of the materia med[ica] and the most *used* of any other" (Thomas J. Griffith, Notes Taken on Lectures Given by Professor Armor, University of Michigan Department of Medicine and Surgery, 10 October 1865–15 May 1866, lecture of 5 February 1866, IN—IN U. Libe.).

79. By 1873 a New Orleans professor could recommend chloral hydrate to his class as "a powerful sedative & to a certain extent an anodyne," noting that "there are not the bad effects following use of Chloral that always succeed taking opium—This is one of the reasons why Chloral is so often prescribed instead of opium—Statistics show the quantity of chloral used at the present day to be *perfectly enormous*" (G. W. Scranton, Resident Student, Notes Taken at the Charity Hospital, New Orleans, Louisiana, 1873–74, LA—Matas).

80. MGH physicians' growing reliance on Dover's powder in the 1840s and 1850s is further illustrated by the fact that concurrently with using it more frequently, they also tended to have recourse to it sooner after a patient's admission. In 60.0 percent of the cases in which Dover's powder was given in the 1830s, it was prescribed only after the fourth day of the case. In the 1840s, fifties, and sixties, that proportion diminished to 34.5, 32.7, and 18.6 percent of the cases respectively.

81. An increasing proportion of patients who received morphia during their hospital stays were never given any other form of opium: 3.6 percent of admitted patients in the 1850s, 5.8 percent in the 1860s, 12.9 percent in the 1870s, and 14.0 percent in the 1880s. Conversely, the proportion of those who received crude opium but no morphia decreased: it was 49.4 percent in the 1850s, 39.1 percent in the 1860s, 30.1 percent in the 1870s, and 15.3 percent in the 1880s.

82. When prescribed, opium tended to be given in increasingly large doses. While the frequencies with which laudanum and Dover's powder were given had dropped by the 1860s to, respectively, only 5.8 and 3.7 percent of all cases, prescriptions of opium powder remained high by comparison. Reflecting the shift to more potent forms of opium compounds, the proportion of cases in which some mild compound such as Dover's powder, laudanum, or paregoric was given in which powdered opium was *not* given dropped from between 64.8 percent and 70.0 percent between the 1830s and the 1850s to 42.3 percent in the 1860s.

83. In his lectures at the CHC in 1850, for example, Leonidas M. Lawson, one of the attending physicians, told his students that calomel "is generally given for its local influences as in affections of the stomach bowels and Liver but in some diseases its Constitutional effects are desired. In fevers, we may wish either its Local or Constitutional affects and our use of the article must be regulated according to our desires." Still, he cautioned that it was not essential to produce mercury poisoning in febrile patients to effect a cure. "It is not necessary that we Ptyalise to cure a case of fever. This used to be the practice but is now abandoned" (William W. Dawson, Notes Taken on Lectures Given at the Medical College of Ohio and at the Commercial Hospital, 1849–50, lectures given by Lawson on 10 and 11 February 1850, OH—Cincinnati Hist. Soc.).

84. On opiate addiction in nineteenth-century America, see David T. Courtwright, *Dark Paradise: Opiate Addiction in America before 1945* (Cambridge and London: Harvard University Press, 1982).

85. The one circumstance in which alcohol was clearly used as a stimulant prior to 1850 was in patients prostrated by their diseases and plainly in decline. Physicians often gave brandy or wine as last-ditch efforts to save a dying patient

by aggressively rousing his enfeebled system. This practice continued through the 1880s, leading one MGH physician in 1878 to try a more direct approach: subcutaneously injecting two drachms of brandy into a moribund patient (who did not recover).

86. In the report for 1857 the superintendent stated that the problem of extravagance had existed for several years and demanded that it "must receive the earnest attention of the Trustees" (*MGH Report*, 1857, p. 5). In the following year the expenditure at the MGH for wine and spirits, earlier subsumed under the general term "medicines," began to be itemized separately. Medicines (including alcohol) represented 9.3 percent of the annual budget in that year; 12.9 percent of the expenditures for medicine and alcohol together went for alcohol. "It is to be hoped that the rigid system, recently introduced, of recording the delivery of all stores, medicines, and liquors, as well as the daily diet of the patients,—a system which checks, to a great extent, any waste or improper use,—will ensure, during the coming year, as great economy as is consistent with the comfort and welfare of the sick," the resident physician stated (*MGH Report*, 1858, pp. 9, 17). In 1866 45.9 percent of all money the hospital paid for drugs was spent on wines and spirits (*MGH Report*, 1866, p. 4; in the *MGH Report*, 1873, p. 14, the proportion given was 49.2 percent). J. C. White related one case in which an MGH physician refused to acquiesce to trustees' pressure in *Sketches*, pp. 72–73.

87. Quotations on the 1867 incident are taken respectively from Commercial Hospital of Cincinnati, Medical Staff, Minute Book, 1861–68, meeting of 6 March 1867, OH—U. Cincinnati Libe.; Minutes of the Meetings of the Cincinnati Hospital Board of Trustees, 2 January 1867–2 June 1869, meeting of 3 April 1867, OH—U. Cincinnati, Hist. Hlth. Scis. Libe.; and Commercial Hospital of Cincinnati, Medical Staff, Minute Book, 1861–91, meeting of 8 April 1867. The comparison of expenditures at the MGH and the CHC appears in *CHC Report*, 1865–66, p. 465. In 1867 medicines, instruments, and alcohol together represented 10.2 percent of the hospital's annual budget for the male wards (*CHC Report*, 1867–68, p. 22). Probably prompted by the trustees' concern, the annual reports began to itemize the amounts paid for each kind of alcoholic beverage; in 1868–69 40.5 percent of the hospital's annual budget for drugs, medicines, and alcohol was spent on beverage alcohol (*CHC Report*, 1868–69, p. 19). In 1869–70, when the figure was 34.1 percent, the hospital purchased 19 gallons of brandy, 25 gallons of catawba wine, 12 gallons of claret wine, 22 gallons of sherry wine, 21 gallons of madeira wine, 26 gallons of port wine, 3 gallons of sherry and rhine wine, 888 dozen bottles of ale, and 159 gallons of whiskey (*CHC Report*, 1869–70, pp. 25–26).

88. The lower cost of cinchonidia sulphate made it especially appealing to large public charities. A clinical lecturer at the Louisville Hospital told his students bluntly, "We use this remedy because it is cheaper than quinine" (A. A. Marrett, Notes Taken on Lectures Given by L. P. Yandell, Jr., on Clinical Medicine, Louisville City Hospital and the Medical University of Louisville, 1873–74, KY—Louisville Med. Libe.). The extent to which cinchonidia sulphate was substituted for quinine was much greater in institutions where the prevalence of periodic fevers was high, necessitating the use of large quantities of costly cinchona bark derivatives. For example, in the medical wards of the Charity Hospital of New Orleans, where the bulk of the patients were admitted with intermittent fevers, cinchonidia sulphate had almost entirely supplanted quinine by the 1880s (Charity Hospital Case Books, 1882–84, 4 vols., LA—LSU).

89. Cinchonidia sulphate first appears in the sampled cases from the MGH in 1878, and between that year and 1885 it was prescribed to only 2.8 percent of the admitted male medical patients.

90. This was not true in the 1880s at the CHC, however, an exception attributable to the predominance of cinchonidia sulphate use in that decade. The points at which the largest proportion of the quinine prescribed was used in nonmalarial cases came in the 1860s and 1870s at the MGH (respectively 89.1 percent and 89.9 percent of the cases in which quinine was given) and (with the exception of the 1880s) in the 1860s at the CHC (45.5 percent); see Warner, "The Therapeutic Perspective," Table 15.

91. One student attending a medical lecture on cinchona bark derivatives in Cincinnati in the 1860s copied into his notebook, "In *small doses* they are Tonic in *larger doses Stimulants* and still *larger* [produce] Symptoms analogous to Delirium Tremens. Its great *use* is where there is *general* Debility, Aenemic condition" (Thomas J. Griffith, Notes Taken on Lectures Given by E. B. Stevens on Materia Medica, Miami Medical College, Cincinnati, Ohio, lecture of 23 October 1866, Griffith Mss., IN—IN U. Libe.).

92. The mean dose of quinine given at the CHC on the first day it was used was for the 1830s—11.1 grains, 1840s—16.9, 1850s—16.1, 1860s—16.7, 1870s—17.6, and 1880s—15.8.

93. The mean dose of quinine given at the MGH on the first day it was used in a case was for the 1820s—12.0 grains, 1830s—14.5, 1840s—4.6, 1850s—5.9, 1860s—6.8, 1870s—7.4, and 1880s—12.2. The high figures for the 1820s and 1830s reflect the fact that although quinine was infrequently prescribed during these decades (5.7 percent and 8.4 percent respectively of the cases admitted), compared with later years a very large proportion (49.0 percent in the 1820s) of that used was prescribed in sizable doses for cases exhibiting malarial signs and/or symptoms. Even though the 1840s marked the introduction of still larger doses of quinine in treating intermittent fever, by then very little of that prescribed at the MGH was in fact used as an antiperiodic (20.6 percent in the 1840s, with the proportion diminishing to a low point in the 1870s of 10.1 percent). The small mean doses given from the 1840s through the 1870s, contrasted with those of the 1820s and 1830s, reflect quinine's tonic use. The gradually enlarging mean doses prescribed after the 1840s indicate the increasingly aggressive use of stimulants at the MGH, and the inordinately elevated mean dose given in the 1880s represents not only quinine's use as a stimulant but also its use in massive doses as an antiperiodic.

94. At the MGH quantified pulse was recorded in the 1820s in 91.4 percent of the cases, 1830s—92.8 percent, 1840s—84.7, 1850s—80.1, 1860s—83.9, 1870s—71.3, and 1880s—82.0. The corresponding proportions for the CHC were in the 1830s 12.7 percent of the cases, 1840s—18.9 percent, 1850s—40.6, 1860s—70.8, 1870s—49.4, and 1880s—63.3.

95. Quantified respiration was recorded at the MGH in (seriatim between the 1820s and 1880s) 4.0, 12.4, 12.1, 16.7, 22.3, 22.6, and 78.8 percent of cases. At the CHC respiration was first recorded quantitatively in the 1840s in 0.4 percent of the cases, in the 1850s—2.1 percent, 1860s—9.5, 1870s—18.7, and 1880s—38.5.

96. Quantified temperature was given at the MGH in 9.9 percent of the cases in the 1860s, 42.2 percent in the 1870s, and 82.0 percent in the 1880s; and at the CHC in 10.3 percent of the cases in the 1860s, 38.4 percent in the 1870s, and 65.1 percent in the 1880s.

97. For example, a sketch of the "abnormal elements in the blood" made

by a microscopic examination was pasted into the record of a patient admitted in 1868 with intermittent fever, and the history of a patient who entered with empyema in 1876 included a report on the examination of his blood using Louis-Charles Malassez's method for counting the number of blood cells.

98. Because the salicylates were used at both institutions largely to treat patients with rheumatism, the fact that rheumatism was more common among the MGH patient population in the 1870s (13.0 percent) and 1880s (16.7 percent) than among the CHC's inmates (9.3 percent and 13.2 percent) accounts in part for the drugs' greater use at the Boston hospital.

5. Attitudes toward Change

1. "Editorial and Miscellaneous," *NOMNHG*, 2 (1855–56): 139.

2. "The Fifteenth Volume of the New Series of the Southern Medical and Surgical Journal," *SMSJ*, 15 (1859): 65; and see David W. Cheever, "An Introductory Lecture Delivered before the Medical Class of Harvard University, Oct. 2, 1871," *BMSJ*, 85 (1871): 209.

3. Z. Collins McElroy, "Conditions of Organic Life, with a Glimpse of the Coming Science of Life and Medicine," *CLO*, 34 (1874): 451.

4. "Progress versus Conservatism," *BMSJ*, 100 (1879): 830.

5. "The Relations of the Medical Profession to Modern Education," *BMSJ*, 84 (1870): 79.

6. David Rice, "Necessity of Medication in Disease," *BMSJ*, 73 (1865–66): 269.

7. W. Taylor, "Changeability of Disease," in *Proceedings of the Medical Association of the State of Alabama, at Its Sixth Annual Meeting, Begun and Held in the City of Selma, Dec. 13–15, 1852, with an Appendix and List of Members* (Mobile, 1853), p. 73; W[illia]m B. Johnson, "Report on the Diseases Which Prevailed in the Village of Marion, Perry Co., Alabama, from the Year 1842, to the Close of the Year 1848," *NOMSJ*, 6 (1849): 451.

8. [William Wood Gerhard], "Epidemic Tendencies of Different Seasons," *BMSJ*, 22 (1840): 78. And see Hamilton County Medical Club, Minutes of Meetings, 21 May 1842–5 April 1850, remarks of William Judkins at meeting of 2 July 1846, MD—NLM; Richard H. Lymer, "Epidemic Influence" (M.D. thesis, University of Pennsylvania, 1866), PA—U. PA Libe.; Samuel L. McKeehan, "Nosology" (M.D. thesis, Washington Medical College, Baltimore, Maryland, 1829), DC—LC.

9. "While modern medicine admits of improvements," a New York physician correctly stated, "it cannot admit of revolutions" (E. W. Spafford, "Remarks on the Treatment of Pneumonia," *Georgia Medical and Surgical Encyclopedia*, 1 [1860]: 241). I refer here to the *process* of change without disputing the use of the term *revolution* to describe the net change between the early and late nineteenth century.

10. C. E. Lavender, "On the Topography, Climate, and Diseases of Selma, Alabama. Read before the Alabama Medical Association, on the 7th and 8th March, 1849," *NOMSJ*, 6 (1849–50): 343–344.

11. G. Volney Dorsey, "Epidemics of Miami County Ohio," *WL*, 13 (1852): 605 and 606.

12. Robert Southgate, "An Essay on Bloodletting, Read before the Medical Association of the State of Georgia, at Their Annual Meeting, Held at Rome, April 11th, 1860," *SMSJ*, 16 (1860): 581.

13. I. Bernard Cohen, *The Newtonian Revolution: With Illustrations of*

the Transformation of Scientific Ideas (Cambridge: Cambridge University Press, 1980), p. 39.

14. John M. Richardson, Diary, 1 February 1853–16 June 1854, Lincoln County, North Carolina, NC—SHC; and see Charles Arnould Hentz, *Autobiography*, 1894, Hentz Family Papers, NC—SHC; and the log of medical reading kept during apprenticeship in Thomas H. Wade, Journal, Richland, Mississippi, 1850–52, LA—Matas.

15. Jefferson Howard DeVotie to James H. DeVotie, Headquarters, 7th Battalion, South Carolina Volunteers, 23 February 1863, James H. DeVotie Papers, NC—Duke U. Libe.

16. Elias Benson Thompson to Mary Eleanor Thompson, Bellevue, Alabama, 9 August 1867, Benson-Thompson Family Papers, NC—Duke U. Libe.

17. Willi Armblin to Ruffin Thomson, n.p., [1867], Ruffin Thomson Papers, NC—SHC; and see G. F. Manning to John Y. Bassett, Philadelphia, 9 May 1835, AL—State Archives.

18. "Editorial," *WL*, 15 (1854): 123.

19. William Octavius Eversfield, Notes Taken on Lectures Given by James C. Cabell on Special Pathology, 1859–60, William Octavius Eversfield Notebooks, VA—U. VA Libe.

20. Simon Baruch, Notes Taken on Lectures Given by Eli Geddings on the Institutes and Practice of Medicine, Medical College of South Carolina, 1860–61, GA—Emory U. Libe.

21. See, for example, George B. Wood and Franklin Bache, *The Dispensatory of the United States of America*, 9th ed. (Philadelphia, 1851). The *Dispensatory* was a commentary on the *Pharmacopoeia (The Pharmacopoeia of the United States of America by Authority of the National Medical Convention, Held at Washington, A.D. 1850* [Philadelphia, 1851]).

22. In addition to the examples cited below, see Daniel Drake to Jared Mansfield, Philadelphia, 25 January 1816, Jared Mansfield Papers, OH—OH Hist. Soc.; G. Volney Dorsey to Maj. James M. Dorsey, Cincinnati, 30 January 1835, Goodwin Volney Dorsey Papers, OH—OH Hist. Soc.; Jno. B. Elliott to Habersham Elliott, Charleston, 27 January 1867, Habersham Elliott Papers, NC—SHC; Matthew Gayle to W. B. Crawford, Philadelphia, 19 February 1843, Sarah Ann and William B. Crawford Papers, AL—U. AL Libe.; T. L. Janis to Thomas Settle, Baltimore, 3 November 1867, Thomas Lee Settle Papers, NC—Duke U. Libe.; James D. Maxwell, Memorandum Book, Bloomington, Indiana, 1836–44, entry for 2 November 1843, IN—IN U. Libe.; and Sith S. to J. E. Hawkins, Louisville, Kentucky, 23 May 1878, J. E. Hawkins Papers, LA—LSU.

23. Jefferson Howard DeVotie to James H. DeVotie, New Orleans, 8 December 1861 (and see letter of 1 December 1861), 2 February 1862, 16 February 1862, 26 February 1862, and 4 March 1862 (and see letters of 15 December 1861, 22 December 1861, 13 January 1862, and 15 February 1862), DeVotie Papers.

24. G. Volney Dorsey to Maj. James M. Dorsey, Cincinnati, 19 February 1836, Dorsey Papers.

25. See, for example, University of Pennsylvania, Minutes of the Medical Faculty, vol. 3, 1829–45, entry for 1 January 1836, PA—U. PA Archives.

26. Proceedings of the Faculty of the Medical College of Louisiana, May 1835–February 1847, entry for 15 March 1845, LA—Matas. Instances of the rejection of M.D. degree candidates on the basis of their examinations are readily found in Cincinnati College of Medicine and Surgery, Faculty Minutes, 1851–68, OH—Cincinnati U. Libe.; Proceedings of the Faculty of the Medical

College of Louisiana, 1835–1904, LA—Matas; Miami Medical College, Faculty Minutes, 1852–81, OH—U. Cincinnati Libe.; Medical College of Ohio, Faculty Minutes, 1831–52, OH—U. Cincinnati Libe.; University of Pennsylvania, Minutes of the Medical School Faculty, 1829–73, PA—U. PA Archives; Rutgers Medical College, Minutes of the Board of Professors, December 1826–October 1827, NY—NY Hist. Soc.; and Transylvania University, Medical Department, Minute Book, 1819–49, KY—Transylvania U. Libe.

27. Cincinnati College of Medicine and Surgery, Board of Trustees Minutes, 1851–89, entry for 15 February 1854.

28. Lundsford Pitts Yandell, Diary, 1824–43, entry for Craggy Bluffs, 19 April 1825, Yandell Family Papers, KY—Filson.

29. For example, Samuel Clark, "Medical Science in the United States" (M.D. thesis, University of Pennsylvania, 1820), PA—U. PA Libe.; and [Josiah Clark Nott] to James M. Gage, n.p., [1837], James M. Gage Papers, NC—SHC.

30. The conservative as well as the change-promoting influences of sectarianism on the regular profession are examined in John Harley Warner, "Medical Sectary, Therapeutic Conflict, and the Shaping of Orthodox Professional Identity in Antebellum America," in *Medical Fringe and Medical Orthodoxy*, ed. William F. Bynum and Roy Porter (London: Croom Helm, forthcoming).

31. Burton Randall to Alexander Randall , New Orleans, 6 February 1831, Randall Family Papers, VA—U. VA Libe.; and see Nathaniel E. McClelland to William L. McClelland, Lexington, Kentucky, 30 January 1831, McClelland and Family Papers, NC—SHC; and William D. Somers to "My Dear Wife," Memphis, 9 July 1865, William D. Somers Papers, NC—Duke U. Libe. See also William Barlow and David O. Powell, "To Find a Stand: New England Physicians on the Western and Southern Frontiers, 1790–1840," *BHM*, 54 (1980): 386–401.

32. Burton Randall to Alexander Randall, Williams Port, Maryland, 7 September 1828, Randall Family Papers.

33. C. G. Comegys to Diathea [M. Tiffin], Cincinnati, 13 January 1851, Matthew Scott Cook Papers, OH—Western Reserve.

34. William H. Thomson to Hannah L. Thomson, Hinds County, Mississippi, 12 July 1835, Ruffin Thomson Papers. "This country is overrun with half educated physicians," Alfred Stillé complained in a letter to George Cheyne Shattuck, "besides whole brigades of quacks, and the chances of earning one's meat & drink are just about in proportion to one's disregard of truth, honor, and modesty" (Philadelphia, 6 August 1844, Shattuck Papers, vol. 18, MA—MA Hist. Soc.).

35. "Letters from Saml. D. Holt, M.D., upon Some Points of General Pathology. Letter No. 15," *SMSJ*, n.s. 12 (1856): 594.

36. Job Clark, Medical Diary and Notes of Cases, November 1836–November 1837, Ravenna, Ohio, entry for 23 November 1836, Job Clark Papers, CT—Yale U. Libe.; and see Joseph Milligan to Joseph A. S. Milligan, Augusta, [Georgia], 9 July 1846, Milligan Family Papers, NC—SHC.

37. "[Review of] Oliver Wendell Holmes, Currents and Counter Currents in Medical Science," *Charleston Medical Journal and Review*, 15 (1860): 777.

38. E. D. F[enner], "Review of Homoeopathy, Allopathy, and 'Young Physic,' by John Forbes, . . . (Phila., 1846)," *NOMSJ*, 2 (1845–46): 760 and 761; and see R. P. Little, Diary, commenced 28 November 1842, P. Washington Little Papers, NC—Duke Med. Libe.; and Notes Taken on Lectures Given by George B. Wood on Practice, University of Pennsylvania, 1858–59, PA—U. PA Archives.

39. Samuel A. Cartwright to John Francis Hamtramck Claiborne, Comments on the Character of Major General John A. Quitman, 1859, John Francis Hamtramck Claiborne Papers, NC—SHC.

40. Harris L. Coulter has traced this process in the instance of regular assimilation of compounds used by homeopathists in *Homoeopathic Influences in Nineteenth-Century Allopathic Therapeutics* (St. Louis: Formur, 1977; first pub. 1973).

41. Alfred Boyd, "Finale of Twenty Years Study and Practice of Medicine" (M.D. thesis, Medical College of the State of South Carolina, 1856), SC—Med. U. SC, Main Libe.

42. J. R. Black, "The Benefactions of Homeopathy," *Cincinnati Lancet and Clinic*, 8 (1882): 214.

43. Minutes, Cuyahoga County Medical Society, 1881–83, entry for 4 July 1882, OH—Dittrick.

44. C. G. Comegys to Scott Cook, Cincinnati, 7 January 1851, Cook Papers.

45. William Henry Holcombe, Diary and Notes, 1855–57, entry for 4 April 1855, NC—SHC.

46. Ibid., entry for 3 March 1855.

47. For typical charges, see the accusations brought against an orthodox society member for consulting with steamers and practicing homeopathy in Minutes of the Miami Medical Association, in William C. Langdon, Record Book, 1853–1900, entry for 4 July 1854, OH—Cincinnati Hist. Soc.

48. Minutes of the Faculty of the Medical College of the State of South Carolina, 1873–83, entry for 30 October 1874, SC—Waring; and see Medical College of Ohio, Faculty Minutes, 1831–52, entries for 17 and 27 December 1845; and Miami Medical College, Faculty Minutes, 1852–81, entry for 2 February 1867.

49. "Death Caused by Homoeopathic Pills," *WL*, 1 (1842–43): 93. One confirmation of this sort of observation is the striking frequency with which calomel appeared in prescriptions written at the Eclectic Medical Institute in Cincinnati despite eclectic rhetoric denouncing calomel as allopathic poison (Eclectic Medical Institute, Cincinnati, Prescription Book, 1849, OH—Lloyd).

50. Cuyahoga County Medical Society, Minutes, 1881–83, entry for 4 July 1882. And see Theosur Blatchform to John W. Francis, Troy, 27 July 1842, John W. Francis Papers, NY—NY Pub. Libe.; Edward E. Jenkins to "Dear Father," Paris, 6 June 1854, John Jenkins Papers, SC—South Caroliniana Libe.; and C. W. Short to J. C. Short, Mayfield, Kentucky, 21 September 1855, Short Family Papers, OH—Cincinnati Hist. Soc.

51. James Otis Moore to Lizzie Moore, Williamsburg, [Virginia?], 12 April 1864, James Otis Moore Papers, NC—Duke U. Libe.; and see letters from various camps dated 18 June 1864, 2 July 1864, 10 July 1864, and 17 March 1865. On a similar circumstance, see S. G. Jerrard to George Washburn, Camp Seward, Virginia, 1 November 1862, Simon G. Jerrard Papers, LA—LSU.

52. Minutes of the Union District Medical Association, 1867–80, meeting at Connersville, Indiana, 29 October 1868, OH—Miami U. Libe.

53. The physician John Leonard Riddell was by no means unique in having both orthodox and sectarian medical friends, though his tactic of playing the prejudices of each group against the other—criticizing either the regulars or the sectarian reformers depending on whom he was talking to—may have been more unusual; see letters copied into John Leonard Riddell, Notebooks, 21 vols., especially vol. 5, 10 August 1832–7 September 1832, Worthington, Ohio; and vol. 9, 25 July 1833–17 December 1833, Worthington, Ohio, John Leonard

Riddell Manuscript Volumes, LA—Tulane U. Libe.; and J. L. Riddell to S. P. Hildreth, Worthington, Ohio, 15 January 1833, Samuel P. Hildreth Papers, OH—Marietta Coll. Libe. And see James Lakey, Diary, vol. 2, 15 November 1849–13 January 1851, entry for 20 November 1849, and vol. 5, 21 March 1853–15 December 1853, entries for 28 May and 7 August 1853, James Lakey Papers, OH—Cincinnati Hist. Soc.

54. James Jackson to Edward B[rooks] Peirson, Boston, 4 August 1857, MA—Countway.

55. Burdon Randall to Alexander Randall, Williams Port, [Maryland], 26 August 1828, Randall Family Papers; and see Ja[me]s Norcom to Benjamin Rush Norcom, [North Carolina], 4 March 1834, Dr. James Norcom and Family Papers, NC—State Archives.

56. Sam[ue]l A. Cartwright, "Synopsis of Medical Etiquette, Presented to the Natchez Medical Society," New Orleans Medical Journal, 1 (1844–45): 103.

57. The long and acrimonious trial before the Richmond Academy of Medicine in the mid-1870s of a member who had told a patient that the treatment an earlier physician had adopted was "all wrong" illustrates this. A collection of letters on the trial, including charges, countercharges, and committee reports, is deposited in the Charles Macgill Papers, NC—Duke U. Libe. And see "Patronage of Quackery," WL, 1 (1842–43): 190.

58. Thomas M. McIntosh to Emma McIntosh, Atlanta, 14 November 1876, Thomas M. McIntosh Papers, NC—Duke U. Libe.; and see [John B. Rice] to "Dear Brother," Young's Point, Louisiana, 19 April 1863, John B. Rice Papers, OH—Hayes.

6. Attitudes toward Foreign Knowledge

1. Elisha Bartlett, Notes Taken on Lectures Given by James Jackson on the Theory and Practice of Physic, 1824–25, lecture of 11 December 1824, Elisha Bartlett Papers, CT—Yale U. Libe. Among the most useful analyses of the Paris clinical school are Erwin H. Ackerknecht, Medicine at the Paris Hospital, 1794–1848 (Baltimore: Johns Hopkins Press, 1967); William Coleman, Death Is a Social Disease: Public Health and Political Economy in Early Industrial France (Madison: University of Wisconsin Press, 1982), esp. pp. 3–33; and Michel Foucault, The Birth of the Clinic: An Archaeology of Medical Perception, trans. A. M. Sheridan Smith (New York: Pantheon Books, 1973; first pub. Paris, 1963).

2. Of an extensive literature on American physicians and the Paris clinical school, see Russell M. Jones, "American Doctors and the Parisian Medical World, 1830–1840," BHM, 47 (1973): 40–65, 177–204; idem, "American Doctors in Paris, 1820–1861: A Statistical Profile," JHM, 25 (1970): 59–81; idem, "An American Medical Student in Paris, 1831–1832," Harvard Library Bulletin, 15 (1967): 59–81; and idem, "Introduction," in The Parisian Education of an American Surgeon: Letters of Jonathan Mason Warren (1832–1835) (Philadelphia: American Philosophical Society, 1978), pp. 1–69.

3. Courtney J. Clark, Notes Taken on Lectures Given by Charles Caldwell, Medical Institute of Louisville, Kentucky 1841–42, Courtney J. Clark Papers, NC—Duke U. Libe. The selectivity with which Americans took up Parisian medicine is analyzed in John Harley Warner, "The Selective Transport of Medical Knowledge: Antebellum American Physicians and Parisian Medical Therapeutics," BHM, 59 (1985): 213–231.

4. R. T. Dismukes, Notes Taken on Lectures Given by B. W. Dudley on Anatomy and Surgery, Medical Department of Transylvania University, Lexington, Kentucky, 1838–39, NC—Duke U. Libe.

5. Clark, Notes Taken on Lectures Given by Caldwell.

6. See Gilbert Chinard, "Eighteenth Century Theories on America As a Human Habitat," *Proceedings of the American Philosophical Society*, 91 (1947): 27–57; Antonello Gerbi, *The Dispute of the New World: The History of a Polemic, 1750–1900*, trans. by Jeremy Moyle (Pittsburgh: University of Pittsburgh Press, 1973; first pub. Milan and Naples, 1955); and George Rosen, "Political Order and Human Health in Jeffersonian Thought," *BHM*, 26 (1952): 32–44.

7. James Rackliffe, Notes Taken on Lectures Given by Benjamin S. Barton, Philadelphia, lecture of 1 November 1815, NC—Duke Med. Libe.

8. Lawrence Jefferson Trotti, Notebook, bound with catalog from Transylvania University, 1828, KY—Transylvania U. Libe.

9. Alex[ander] McBride, "A Chemico-Pathological Classification of Fevers, and Hints at Treatment Based Thereon," *CLO*, 25 (1864): 23.

10. Edward Keller, Diary as a Student at South Carolina College and Notes Taken on Lectures Given by Lieber, Geddings, and Laborde, 1849–59, quotation from "Remarks and Lectures of Dr. Laborde for the Sopho[mo]re Class of 1854 Concerning Physiology," SC—South Caroliniana Libe.

11. "[Review of] William Stokes (Dublin), Lectures on the Theory and Practice of Physic, & John Bell (Phila.), Phila., 1846," *WL*, 1 (1842–43): 354; and see Robert Battey to Mary Battey, Paris, 23 February 1860, Robert Battey Papers, GA—Emory U. Libe.

12. "Dr. Paine's Reply to H. I. B[owditch], No. V," *BMSJ*, 23 (1840–41): 271; and see William Wood Gerhard to James Jackson, Sr., Philadelphia, 11 July 1834, James Jackson Papers, MA—Countway.

13. "Foreign Hospitals" (extract from lecture of Professor Henry H. Smith, University of Pennsylvania), *NOMSJ*, 13 (1856–57): 242–243.

14. Robert Peter to Frank [Frances] Peter, Paris, 22 June 1839, Catherine (Peter) and Howard Evans Papers, KY—U. KY Libe.

15. John P. Caffey, "A Thesis on Calomel in Southern Fevers" (M.D. thesis, Medical College of the State of South Carolina, 1839), SC—Med. U. SC, Main Libe.

16. "Scientific and Practical Medicine," *Virginia Medical Journal*, 12 (1859): 344. Americans did take up the new drugs (such as quinine and morphine) generated by François Magendie and other French experimentalists, but this did not alter their judgment of Parisian *clinicians'* performance. On early experimental pharmacology in Paris during this period, see John. E. Lesch, *Science and Medicine in France: The Emergence of Experimental Physiology, 1790–1855* (Cambridge, Massachusetts, and London: Harvard University Press, 1984).

17. James Lawrence Cabell to Joseph C. Cabell, Paris, 28 January 1837, James Lawrence Cabell Papers, VA—U. VA Libe.

18. "Modern Practice of Medicine," *BMSJ*, 12 (1835): 351 and 352.

19. "Andral's Medical Clinic," *WL*, 2 (1843–44): 148.

20. P. H. Lewis, "Reply to Doctor W. M. Boling's Review of Doctor Lewis' Medical History of Alabama, with Some New Facts and Remarks, in Relation to the Diagnosis and Identity of the Fevers of the State," *NOMSJ*, 4 (1847–48): 639.

21. Z., [to the author of "Essays on Medical Improvement"], "Medical Improvement—No. VII," *BMSJ*, 9 (1834): 194.

22. John Ware, "Success in the Medical Profession," *BMSJ*, 43 (1850–51): 499 and 509.

23. See, for example, D. D. Slade to George Lord, Cambridge, 21 November 1845, George Lord Papers, NC—Duke U. Libe.

24. Eugène Sue, *The Mysteries of Paris*, vol. 3 (London, 1846; first pub. Paris, 1843), pp. 291, 292, 295, 300, 301, 303, 304, and 307. On Sue (who came from a medical family) and the animus of his social reformism, see Nora Atkinson, *Eugène Sue et le roman-feuilleton* (Nemours: André Lesot, 1929); Charles Arlo Isetts, "Eugène Sue: A Writer for the People" (Ph.D. diss., Miami University, 1974); and John Moody, *Les idées sociales d'Eugène Sue* (Paris: Presses Universitaires de France, 1938).

25. O. W. Holmes, "Experiments in Medicine," *BMSJ*, 30 (1844): 201–203.

26. A. Stillé to G. C. Shattuck, Philadelphia, 24 October 1844, Shattuck Papers, vol. 18, MA—MA Hist. Soc.

27. The quotations are from James Jackson, Sr., to James Jackson, Jr., Waltham, Massachusetts, 12 June 1833 and 20 June 1833, Jackson Papers. And see, for example, Ashbel Smith to James Jackson, Jr., Salisbury, North Carolina, 21 February 1834, MA—Countway; and A. Stillé to G. C. Shattuck, Philadelphia, 9 October 1842, Shattuck Papers, vol. 17. On the plan suggested by Louis, see James Jackson, Jr., to James Jackson., Sr., Havre, 25 April 1832, Jackson Papers.

28. "Foreign Correspondence" (Paris, January 1857), *Nashville Journal of Medicine and Surgery*, 12 (1857): 304; and on Parisian brutality see Henry Bronson, Diary, 20 November 1839–26 May 1840, entry for Paris, 9 March 1840, CT—Yale U. Libe., and Auguste Shurtleff, Journal of a Trip to Europe, 1850–52, vol. 1, entry for Paris, 20 January 1851, MA—Countway.

29. Benjamin J. Hicks to John Y. Bassett, Paris, 31 July 1837, John Young Bassett Papers, AL—State Archives; and see Robert Peter to Frank [Frances] Peter, Paris, 27 June 1839, Evans Papers.

30. "Notice of Lisfranc's Clinics," *SMSJ*, 1 (1836–37): 372. Describing the way patients at one Parisian medical clinic were "*passed* around the room for us to examine," one American student noted that "the French seem to take this sort of thing very calmly and undergoe, what to an American, would be very repulsive" (Stephen Henry Bronson to Dr. and Mrs. Henry Bronson, Paris, 18 December 1867, Bronson Papers, CT—Yale Med. Hist. Libe.).

31. William B. Crawford to Margaret [sister], Paris, 14 February 1833, Sarah Ann (Gayle) Papers, NC—Duke U. Libe.

32. George C. Shattuck, Journal, 1833, entry for 5 March 1833, MA—Countway; and see C. G. Comegys to Scott Cook, Cincinnati, 25 March 1852, Matthew Scott Cook Papers, OH—Western Reserve.

33. See for example E. D. Fenner, "London Correspondence," (8 July 1859) *NOMNHG*, 6 (1859–60): 535–536; Senex, "Foreign Practice, As Applied to the Diseases of This Country," *BMSJ*, 8 (1833): 220–221; Thomas T. Wall, "Nature and Art in the Cure of Disease,"*NOMSJ*, 17 (1860): 178.

34. L. M. Lawson, "Foreign Correspondence," (London, June 1845) *WL*, 4 (1845–46): 150–151.

35. Ware, "Success in the Medical Profession," quotations from pp. 509, 510, and 520.

36. "[Review of] William Stokes," p. 355; and see Benjamin S. Downing, Notes Taken on Lectures Given by Joseph Mather Smith on the Theory and

Practice of Medicine, College of Physicians and Surgeons at the University of the State of New York, 1826, NY—Columbia-Presbyterian.

37. Joseph T. Webb to Rutherford B. Hayes, London, 15 November 1870, Joseph Webb Papers, OH—Hayes.

38. See [Charles T. Jackson to Charles Brown], Paris, 13 May 1831, Charles Thomas Jackson Papers, DC—LC, on the contrast between London and Paris. And see Edward E. Jenkins to John Jenkins, Paris, 12 August 1853, John Jenkins Papers, SC—South Caroliniana Libe.; and Ashbel Smith to "Dear Father," Paris, 31 January 1832, Ashbel Smith Papers, TX—U. TX Libe.

39. See, for example, Henry K. Oliver, Jr., "The Vienna Hospitals," *BMSJ*, 57 (1857–58): 49–58, 71–77; and Alfred Stillé to Geo[rge] C. Shattuck, Vienna, 15 January 1851, and Philadelphia, 28 September 1851, Shattuck Papers, vol. 22.

40. Joseph T. Webb to Jim [James D. Webb], Paris, 21 March 1868, Webb Papers.

41. Joseph T. Webb to Rutherford B. Hayes, Vienna, 12 May 1868, Webb Papers.

42. Joseph T. Webb to Lu[cy], Vienna, 11 October 1868, Webb Papers; and see John Singleton Copley Greene to James Jackson Putnam, Vienna, 5 March 1872, MA—Countway; and J. W. Humrichouse to C. W. Humrichouse, Vienna, 15 April 1877, Ridgley Papers, MD—MD Hist. Soc.

43. W[illia]m P. Thornton, "Letters to the Editors of the Lancet and Observer" (Vienna, 25 February 1859), *CLO*, 20 (1859): 238; and see "Skoda of Vienna," *SMSJ*, 15 (1859): 69–70; and James C. White to Henry I. Bowditch, Belfast, Maine, 27 August 1857, H. I. Bowditch, Collection of Autograph Letters and Portraits, MA—Countway.

44. J. R. Black, "Remarks on the Semiology and Therapeutics of Chronic Diseases," *Cincinnati Lancet and Clinic*, n.s. 7 (1881): 110–111.

45. J. T. Webb to Maria Webb, Berlin, 1 August 1866, Webb Papers.

46. Patrick A. O'Connell, "A Letter from Vienna," *BMSJ*, 86 (1872): 214 and 215.

47. James Jackson, Jr., to James Jackson, Sr., Paris, 27 February 1832, in James Jackson, *A Memoir of James Jackson, Jr., M.D., with Extracts from His Letters to His Father: and Medical Cases, Collected by Him* (Boston, 1835), p. 123. On the numerical method, see M. Bariéty, "Louis et la méthode numérique," *Clio Medica*, 7 (1972): 177–183; Alfred Jay Bollet, "Pierre Louis: The Numerical Method and the Foundation of Quantitative Medicine," *AJMS*, 266 (1973): 92–101; James H. Cassedy, *American Medicine and Statistical Thinking, 1800–1860* (Cambridge, Massachusetts: Harvard University Press, 1984); Coleman, *Death Is a Social Disease*, pp. 124–148; Terence D. Murphy, "Medical Knowledge and Statistical Methods in Early Nineteenth-Century France," *Medical History*, 25 (1981): 301–319; and Uhlrich Tröhler, "Quantification in British Medicine and Surgery, 1750–1830, with Special Reference to Its Introduction into Therapeutics" (Ph.D. diss., University of London, 1978).

48. James Jackson, Sr., to James Jackson, Jr., Boston, 15 January 1832, in James Jackson Putnam, *A Memoir of Dr. James Jackson* (Boston and New York: Houghton Mifflin, 1905), p. 332.

49. L. M. Whiting, "Investigation of Disease," *BMSJ*, 14 (1836): 181 and 188.

50. Ibid., p. 189.

51. C. L. Seeger, "On the Improvement of Medical Science," *BMSJ*, 14 (1836): 330.

52. David W. Cheever, "The Value and Fallacy of Statistics in the Observation of Disease," *BMSJ*, 63 (1860–61): 501.

53. "M. Louis on Typhoid Fever," *WL*, 1 (1842–43): 375.

54. Bennet Dowler, "Speculative and Practical Remarks on Absorption, the Enepidermic, Iatraleptic, Endermic, and Hypodermic Methods of Medication," *NOMSJ*, 17 (1860): 63.

55. "Outline of Remarks by A. Flint, M.D., of Buffalo, N.Y.," *BMSJ*, 24 (1841): 232.

56. Cheever, "The Value and Fallacy of Statistics," p. 483.

57. For example, Woodbridge Strong, "On the Present State of Medical Science, and on the Nature and Treatment of Typhus," *BMSJ*, 37 (1847–48): 249–260; and "Typhoid and Typhus Fever, Thirty-Two Years Ago," *WL*, 1 (1842–43): 420–421. Dale C. Smith examines the American discussion on the distinction between typhoid and typhus in "Gerhard's Distinction between Typhoid and Typhus and Its Reception in America, 1833–1860," *BHM*, 54 (1980): 368–385.

58. E. S., "Pinel, Broussais and Louis," *BMSJ*, 65 (1861–62): 291–292.

59. Putnam, *A Memoir of Dr. James Jackson*, p. 162.

60. Bennet Dowler, "Researches into the Types of Disease and Types of Therapy," *NOMSJ* 15 (1858): 594.

61. James Jackson, "Preface," in P. Ch. A. Louis, *Researches on the Effects of Bloodletting in Some Inflammatory Diseases, and on the Influence of Tartarized Antimony and Vesication in Pneumonitis*, trans. C. G. Putnam, with preface and appendix by James Jackson (Boston, 1836), pp. v–vi.

62. See "Dr. Jackson's Appendix to Louis on Bloodletting," *BMSJ*, 14 (1836): 14–17; "Fallacious Medical Statistics," *WLHR*, 12 (1851): 817–819; and "The True Value of Medical Experience," *BMSJ*, 19 (1839): 351–354. And see J. Worth Estes's reexamination of Louis's data in "Making Therapeutic Decisions with Protopharmacologic Evidence," *Transactions and Studies in the College of Physicians of Philadelphia*, s. 5, 1 (1979): 134–137.

63. Joseph LeCont[e], "On the Science of Medicine and the Causes Which Have Retarded Its Progress," *SMSJ*, n.s. 6 (1850): 461.

64. "M. Louis on Typhoid Fever," p. 376; and see [Robley] Dunglison, *An Introductory Lecture to the Course of Institutions of Medicine, &c in Jefferson Medical College, Delivered Nov. 4, 1844* (Philadelphia, 1844), pp. 19 and 25.

65. Alfred Stillé to Geo[rge] C. Shattuck, Philadelphia, 7 May 1842, Shattuck Papers, vol. 17.

66. H. I. B[owditch], "Medical and Physiological Commentaries," *BMSJ*, 23 (1840–41): 73. Louis shared this assessment of Paine's treatise; see P. C. A. Louis's letters to H. I. Bowditch of 1 October 1840 and 3 June 1841, MA—Countway. And see Martyn Paine, *Medical and Physiological Commentaries*, 2 vols. (New York and London, 1840), and a third volume bearing the same title (New York, 1841–44).

67. John Hamilton to Geo[rge] C. Shattuck, Dublin, 1 March 1841, Shattuck Papers, vol. 17. Hamilton had been sent a copy of Paine's *Commentaries* to review, and wrote to Shattuck because, as he explained, "I looked on you when here as an out and out disciple of Louis." Paine, Hamilton wrote, "seems to think this attack on Louis very necessary as a great many young American physicians came to America imbued with Louis notions greatly to the disservice of medicine in their native country. (This is so personal to you that I think you ought to call him out.)." As it happened, Bowditch performed that task instead of Shattuck.

68. M[artyn] P[aine], "Dr. Paine's Reply to H. I. B[owditch]," *BMSJ*, 23 (1840–41): 236.

69. B[owditch], "Medical and Physiological Commentaries," pp. 81 and 89.

70. "Dr. Dunglison's Introductory Lecture," *BMSJ*, 21 (1839): 357. Writing on Louis, Jackson, Jr., echoed, "He is one of the most scrupulous men I have ever seen in the admission of observations or circumstances as true or as *facts*— one difficulty is, however, that he seems hardly willing to allow any body's observation full credit except his own" (James Jackson, Jr., to James Jackson, Sr., Paris, 5 August 1831, Jackson Papers).

7. The Arbitration of Change

1. Report of the Committee on Ethics, Minutes of the Meetings of the Miami Medical Association, Madisonville, 29 March 1853, in William C. Langdon, Record Book, 1853–1900, OH—Cincinnati Hist. Soc.; and see Sam[ue]l Cartwright, *The Pathology and Treatment of Cholera: With an Appendix, Containing His Latest Instructions to Planters and Heads of Families (Remote from Medical Advice) in Regards to Its Prevention and Cure* (New Orleans, 1849), p. 24.

2. For example, see Notes Taken on Lectures Given by John Eberle on the Theory and Practice of Medicine, 1827–28, vol. 1, MD—NLM.

3. John. S. Williams, "Blood-Letting" (M.D. thesis, Transylvania University, 1839), KY—Transylvania U. Libe.

4. Joseph Ray, "Some of the Abuses of Bloodletting" (M.D. thesis, Cincinnati, 1831), OH—Cincinnati Pub. Libe.

5. Warren Stone, "On Inflammation," *NOMSJ*, 16 (1859): 765.

6. "Letters from Saml. D. Holt, M.D., upon Some Points of General Pathology. Letter No. 7" (Montgomery, Alabama, 25 November 1855), *SMSJ*, n.s. 12 (1856): 10.

7. G. T. B., "[Review of] William Turner, 'The Practice of Taking Blood in Diseases,'" *NOMSJ*, 8 (1851–52): 376–377; and see Richard Nickolls, "Bloodletting" (M.D. thesis, University of Nashville, 1858–59), TN—Vanderbilt Med. Libe., and D. S. H. Smith, "A Plea for Bloodletting," *New York Medical Journal*, 13 (1871): 722.

8. W. F. M'Cleeland, "Bloodletting," *Transactions of the Colorado Territorial Medical Society* (1874–75): 44; and see remarks of Charles O'Donovan, Baltimore Pathological Society Minutes, vol. 1, 1853–58, meeting of 29 March 1858, NC—Duke U. Libe.

9. D. Rice, "Can Typhoid Fever Be Broken Up or Shortened in Its Duration by Medical Means?" *BMSJ*, 73 (1865–66): 495.

10. Thomas Kennard, "Proceedings of the St. Louis Medical Society," *St. Louis Medical and Surgical Journal*, 17 (1859): 311–312.

11. Robert Southgate, "An Essay on Bloodletting, Read before the Medical Association of the State of Georgia, at Their Annual Meeting, Held at Rome, April 11th, 1860," *SMSJ*, 16 (1860): 484 and 496; and see Edward Montgomery, "A Plea for the Antiphlogistic Treatment of Disease," appendix to *Transactions of the Medical Association of the State of Missouri*, 6 (1872): 3–20.

12. C. H. Spillman, "Bloodletting Then and Now," *Medical and Surgical Reporter*, 16 (1867): 232.

13. N. W. Harris, "On Bloodletting As a Therapeutic Agent," *Medical Archives*, 3 (1869): 531–538; Harvey L. Byrd, "Blood-Letting in Disease," *Medical and Surgical Reporter*, 26 (1872): 25–26.

14. G. S. Scranton, Resident Student, Notes Taken on Lectures Given by Professor Hawthorne on Therapeutics, Case Book, Charity Hospital, New Orleans, Louisiana, 1873–74, LA—Matas.

15. See, for example, Minutes of the Academy of Medicine of Cincinnati, 1 April 1869–13 April 1874, remarks of Dr. Thornton at meeting of 24 January 1870, OH—Cincinnati Acad. Med.; Roberts Bartholow, "Clinical Lecture on the Treatment of Measles in the Adult, and the Use of the Sulphites in Zymotic Diseases," CLO, 26 (1865): 96–101; and Homer C. Bloom, "Progression vs. Fallacies of the Profession" (M.D. thesis, University of Pennsylvania, 1878), PA—U. PA Libe.

16. Bennet Dowler, "Researches into the Types of Disease and Types of Therapy," NOMSJ, 15 (1858): 589.

17. Quoted in Reginald C. McGrane, The Cincinnati Doctor's Forum (Cincinnati: Academy of Medicine of Cincinnati, 1957), p. 88. Since McGraine's research, the academy has lost many of its early minute books, including the one that recorded this 1862 meeting.

18. Ja[me]s Norcom to Benjamin Rush Norcom, Edenton, North Carolina, 21 November 1832, Dr. James Norcom and Family Papers, NC—State Archives; and see G. Bowen to S. P. Hildreth, n.p., 30 January 1842, Samuel P. Hildreth Papers, OH—Marietta Coll. Libe.; and "Prevailing Tendency of Diseases," BMSJ, 8 (1833): 82.

19. John A. Murphy, "Epidemic Dysentery of 1849–50: A Paper Read before the Medico-Chirurgical Society of Cincinnati," WLHR, 12 (1851): 70.

20. Elisha Bartlett to John O. Green, Lexington, 18 February 1844, NY—NY Acad. Med. On the role of typhoid's rise in therapeutic change, see C. H. Jordan, Daybook, North Carolina, 1849–54, entry in 1849, NC—State Archives; V. Kersey, "Abstract of the Reports to the Cambridge City Medical Association," WL, 15 (1854): 727; and Manning Simons, Notes Taken on Lectures Given at the Medical College of the State of South Carolina, 1866–67, lecture of 11 December 1866, SC—Waring.

21. On the association of typhoid fever and a "do-nothing" management, see, for example, Tho[mas]s D. Mitchell, "Typhoid Fever, an Objectionable Term," NOMSJ, 2 (1845–46): 391; idem, "The Remedial Powers of the Sulphate of Quinine," NOMSJ, 3 (1846–47): 23.

22. John. W. King, "Typhoid Fever As It Prevailed in the Southern States during the Autumn and Winter of theYears 1838 & 1839" (M.D. thesis, Transylvania University, 1841), KY—Transylvania U. Libe. On typhoid as a paradigmatic disease for therapeutic attitudes, see Lloyd G. Stevenson, "Exemplary Disease: The Typhoid Pattern," JHM, 37 (1982): 159–183.

23. Thus in the late 1860s a New York professor, speaking of venesection in pneumonia, could tell his students bluntly, "Louis proved it was beneficial" (F. E. Beckwith, Notes Taken on Lectures and Clinics Given at Bellevue Medical College, New York, 1 December 1868–4 February 1869, vol. 2, lecture by Clark, Frank Edwin Beckwith Notebooks, CT—Yale U. Libe.).

24. On the Edinburgh debate, see Lester S. King, "The Blood-Letting Controversy: A Study in the Scientific Method," BHM, 35 (1961): 1–13; and John Harley Warner, "Therapeutic Explanation and the Edinburgh Bloodletting Controversy: Two Perspectives on the Medical Meaning of Science in the Mid-Nineteenth Century," Medical History, 24 (1980): 241–258. The attitudes of American physicians toward the arguments of Bennett and Alison are briefly discussed in idem, " 'The Nature-Trusting Heresy': American Physicians and

the Concept of the Healing Power of Nature in the 1850's and 1860's," *Perspectives in American History*, 11 (1977–78): 310–313.

25. James F. Hibberd, "General Blood-Letting in the Treatment of Inflammation: Including a Reply to a Late Paper upon the Subject, by Prof. Lawson," *CLO*, 21 (1860): 225.

26. Ibid., p. 204.

27. Ibid., pp. 202–203.

28. Ibid., p. 203.

29. Ibid., p. 230.

30. Samuel D. Smith, "An Essay on Has the Type of Disease Changed" (M.D. thesis, University of Pennsylvania, 1863), PA—U. PA Libe. Henry Ingersoll Bowditch reviewed the Edinburgh debate in detail in his clinical lectures to students at the Massachusetts General Hospital in 1865 (lecture on the treatment of pneumonia, Lectures at the Hospital, 1865, MA—Countway).

31. "[Review of] *Watson's Practice of Physic . . . ,*" *Charleston Medical Journal and Review*, 14 (1859): 203. And see Stone, "On Inflammation," pp. 764–765.

32. L. M. Lawson, "Remarks on the Treatment of Inflammation, with Special Reference to Pneumonia," *AJMS*, 77 (1860): 28, 29, and 38.

33. "Northern Medical Association of Philadelphia. *Subject for Discussion.*—Bloodletting," *Medical and Surgical Reporter*, n.s. 4 (1860): 34.

34. "Routine Treatment," *BMSJ*, 55 (1856–57): 128; italics added. The debate had been reviewed in "Blood-Letting in Acute Internal Inflammations," *BMSJ*, 54 (1856): 285.

35. Bennet Dowler, "Speculative and Practical Researches on the Supposed Duality, Unity and Antagonism of Nature and Art in the Cure of Diseases," *NOMSJ*, 15 (1858): 789; Lawson, "Treatment of Inflammation," p. 18.

36. Ibid., pp. 299 and 303. And see L. M. Lawson, "[Letter] to the Editors of the Lancet and Observer" (Cincinnati, 14 April 1860), *CLO*, 21 (1860): 299.

37. Dowler, "Speculative and Practical Researches," p. 788. On Bennett's perceived influence on bloodletting in America, see, for example, J. L. Cabell, "Remarks on the Treatment of Acute Pneumonia," *Richmond Medical Journal*, 3 (1867): 303–313; and Edward Montgomery, "The Antiphlogistic or the Restorative Treatment, or Both," *Medical Archives*, 9 (1873): 257–268.

38. Dowler, "Researches into the Types of Diseases," p. 602.

39. Lawson, "Treatment of Inflammation," p. 36.

40. Ibid., p. 42; and see "The Blood Letting Discussion," *CLO*, 20 (1859): 247–249.

41. Hibberd, "General Blood-Letting," p. 225.

42. See J. N. Borland, "Report on the Cases of Pneumonia Treated in the Boston City Hospital from Its Opening, June 1, 1864, until February 8, 1868," *BMSJ*, 78 (1868): 250–251; "[Review of] Bennett's *Clinical Lectures*," *CLO*, 21 (1860): 315–316; "[Review of] Clinical Lectures on the Principles and Practice of Medicine. By John Hughes Bennett . . . ," *Charleston Medical Journal and Review*, 13 (1858): 513–522; and "[Review of] The Restorative Treatment of Pneumonia. By John Hughes Bennett . . . ," *BMSJ*, 75 (1866–67): 104.

43. S. D. Gross, "A Discourse on Bloodletting Considered As a Therapeutic Agent," *Transactions of the American Medical Association*, 26 (1875): 421; and see idem, "A Lost Art of Medicine," *Philadelphia Medical Times*, 5 (1874–75): 529–534; and "Editorial," *NOMSJ*, n.s. 3 (1875–76): 155–157.

44. See, for example, H. I. Bowditch's comments in discussion of W. A. Dunn, "The Therapeutics of Venesection," in Albert N. Blodgett, "Suffolk District Medical Society. Section for Clinical Medicine and Pathology," *BMSJ*, 106 (1882): 444–448. From the 1860s onward Bowditch persistently argued that the abandonment of venesection had gone too far; see, for example, his Introductory to the Course on Clinical Medicine, November 1861, Course of 1861–62, MA—Countway. That many practitioners agreed is evident in the supportive letters elicited by Bowditch's publication of an essay defending this view in the early 1870s: see letters to H. I. Bowditch from Williard Parker, New York, 20 March 1872; James A. Stetson, Quincy, Massachusetts, 22 April 1872; and W[illia]m G. White, Chelsea, Massachusetts, 7 March 1872, all in H. I. Bowditch, Autograph Letters and Portraits, MA—Countway.

45. "Discussion, in the College of Physicians and Surgeons of Lexington, on the Action of Calomel, in Health and Disease; At Their Sessions, June 6th and July 11th, 1837," *Transylvania Journal of Medicine*, 10 (1837): 457–475; Tho[ma]s D. Mitchell, "Calomel Considered As a Poison," *New Orleans Medical Journal*, 1 (1844–45): 29 and 32; John W. Kennedy, "The Maladministration of Cathartics" (M.D. thesis, Transylvania University, 1846), KY—Transylvania U. Libe.; Samuel Brown to Orlando Brown, Lexington, Kentucky, 20 January 1821, Orlando Brown Papers, KY—Filson. And see John S. Haller, Jr., "Sampson of the Materia Medica: Medical Theory and the Use and Abuse of Calomel in Nineteenth Century America," *Pharmacy in History*, 13 (1971): 27–34, 67–76.

46. "Abuse of Mercury in the Army," *BMSJ*, 68 (1863): 349. Calomel could still be specially ordered, and some other mercurials remained ordinarily available. "The 'calomel order,' " Hammond's biographer has noted, "proved to be one of the Surgeon General's worst mistakes" (Bonnie Ellen Blustein, "A New York Medical Man: William Alexander Hammond, M.D. [1828–1900]" [Ph.D. diss., University of Pennsylvania, 1979]). On the calomel controversy, see Gert Brieger, "Therapeutic Conflicts and the American Medical Profession in the 1860s," *BHM*, 41 (1967): 215–222.

47. E. B. Stevens, "Seventeenth Annual Session of the Ohio State Medical Society," *CLO*, 24 (1863): 420.

48. A Surgeon, "Calomel in the Army," *Chicago Medical Journal*, 20 (1863): 258; "The Surgeon-General," *Medical and Surgical Reporter*, 10 (1863): 124.

49. McGrane, *Cincinnati Doctors' Forum*, pp. 74–75; Stevens, "Seventeenth Annual Session," p. 420; "Meeting of the Medical Profession upon Surgeon General Hammond's Order No. 6," *Cincinnati Medical and Surgical News*, 4 (1863): 217–219.

50. For example, A Surgeon, "Calomel in the Army," p. 259.

51. Stevens, "Seventeenth Annual Session," p. 419.

52. "The Surgeon-General in a New Order," *CLO*, 24 (1863): 554 and 556.

53. "Our Surgeon-General Abroad," *Medical and Surgical Reporter*, 10 (1863): 223.

54. "The Case of Surg. Gen. Hammond," *CLO*, 25 (1864): 690.

55. "Meeting of the Medical Profession upon Surgeon General Hammond's Order No. 6," p. 218.

56. "The Surgeon-General in a New Order," p. 559.

57. "The Surgeon-General," p. 124.

58. "The Surgeon-General in a New Order," p. 557.

59. "Calomel and Tartar Emetic," *Medical and Surgical Reporter*, 10 (1863): 275–276.

60. "Calomel in the Army. The Surgeon-General's Order," *Chicago Medical Journal*, 20 (1863): 310–320.

61. J. F. Hibberd, "Circular No. 6, and the Profession" (Richmond, Indiana, June 1863), *CLO*, 24 (1863): 431 and 433.

62. Aretaeus, "Shall We Reject the Fathers?" *CLO*, 29 (1868): 432–436.

63. John Hughes Bennett, "Report of the Edinburgh Committee on the Action of Mercury, Podophylline, and Taraxacum on the Biliary Secretion," pt. 2, *British Medical Journal*, 1 (1869): 418 and 420.

64. Ibid., pp. 411–420; J. Hughes Bennett, "Report of the Edinburgh Committee on the Action of Mercury on the Liver," pt. 1, *British Medical Journal*, 2 (1868): 78–82; idem, "Report of Further Experiments Demonstrating that Mercury Has No Special Action on the Liver," *British Medical Journal*, 1871 (1): 1–2. Other members of the committee dissented from Bennett's conclusions and bitterly complained that he had misrepresented their position; for example, see Thomas R. Fraser, "Sketch of the Present State of Our Knowledge Respecting the Action of Mercury," *Edinburgh Medical Journal*, 16 (1871): 925.

65. J. C. M., "Letter from Edinburgh," *CLO*, 29 (1868): 559.

66. E. D. Fenner, "London Correspondence," *NOMNHG*, 6 (1859–60): 532.

67. "Action of Mercury on the Secretion of Bile," *BMSJ*, 61 (1859–60): 84–85.

68. T. M. Johnson, "Abstract of Proceedings of the Buffalo Medical Association," *Buffalo Medical and Surgical Journal*, 7 (1868): 413.

69. Ibid., p. 416.

70. Felix Coblens, Notes Taken on Lectures Given by L. P. Yandell, Jr., University of Louisville, Department of Medicine, 1874–75, KY—U. Louisville Med. Libe.

71. Cuyahoga County Medical Society, Minutes, remarks of Dr. Chalfont at meeting of 1 August 1876, OH—Dittrick.

72. "On the Cholagogue Action of Mercury," *BMSJ*, 81 (1869): 400. On the importance of physiological research for therapeutic theory contrasted with its irrelevance for therapeutic practice in the 1860s and 1870s, see John Harley Warner, "Physiological Theory and Therapeutic Explanation in the 1860s: The British Debate on the Medical Use of Alcohol," *BHM*, 54 (1980): 235–257.

73. E. P. Hurd, "On the Utility of Calomel in Infantile Intestinal Affections," *BMSJ*, 85 (1871): 363.

74. For example, Thomas Fairfax Keller, Notes Taken on Lectures Given by Daniel Drake, 1847, AL—State Archives.

75. Isaac Kay, "Clarke County Medical Society [Discussion on Mercury]," *CLO*, 32 (1871): 530.

76. On veratrum's earlier use, see, for example, Jonathan Greely Stevenson, Notes Taken on Lectures Given by James Jackson on the Theory and Practice of Physic, Boston, 1817–1819, MA—Countway; and Leroy Milton Yale, Notes Taken on Lectures Given by Jacob Bigelow on Materia Medica and by John Collins Warren on Anatomy and Surgery, Massachusetts Medical College, Boston, 1826–29, lecture by Bigelow of 12 January 1827, MA—Countway.

77. Wesley C. Norwood, "Veratrum Viride," *SMSJ*, n.s. 6 (1850): 333–340;

idem, "Observations on the Use of Veratrum Viride in Fevers, Convulsions, &c.," *SMSJ*, n.s. 7 (1851): 13–19; [idem] to A. Hester [editor], "Veratrum Viride, &c." (Abbeyville Court House, South Carolina, 18 November 1852), *NOMSJ*, 9 (1852–53): 600–604; idem, "Therapeutic Value of Veratrum Viride," *BMSJ*, 48 (1853): 430–431. A medical student from Abbeyville attending lectures in Charleston wrote an enthusiastic brief in support of Norwood's claims in 1853; see P. H. Bradley, "Veratrum Viride" (M.D. thesis, Medical College of the State of South Carolina, 1853), SC—Med. U. SC, Main Libe.

78. H. K. Pusey, "Use of Veratrum Viride," *CLO*, 20 (1859): 153.

79. "A Letter from an Old Fogy" (Pericksville, Ohio), *CLO*, 22 (1861): 291.

80. One southern editor commented on the lack of recognition veratrum had received in journals outside his region in 1853, and asserted, "How different would the case have been if the newly ascertained property of Veratrum Viride had been first announced in England, in France, or even in the depths of Germany!" ("Our Journal," *SMSJ*, n.s. 9 [1853]: 63).

81. Tho[ma]s Kennard, "Proceedings of the St. Louis Medical Society," *CLO*, 25 (1864): 523.

82. T. L. Wright, "On the Value of Blood-Letting in Symptomatic Fevers," *CLO*, 19 (1858): 465.

83. C. M'Dermont, "Proceedings of the Montgomery Co. Medical Society, April, 1858," *CLO*, 19 (1858): 344. The debate is recorded in Montgomery County Medical Society, Minutes, vol. 1, 15 September 1849–5 November 1880, meeting of 4 March 1858, Dayton Collection, OH—Dayton Pub. Libe.

84. Ibid., p. 345. On some of the members who took part in this debate, see W. J. Conklin, *President's Address. The Montgomery County Medical Society: Its Founders and Early Members* (Dayton: Montgomery County Medical Society, 1901).

85. Ephraim Cutter, "Veratrum Viride As an Arterial Sedative," *BMSJ*, 56 (1857): 509.

86. John S. Wilson, "A Brief Summary of My Experience with the Veratrum Viride," *SMSJ*, n.s. 9 (1853): 390.

87. Montgomery County Medical Society, Minutes, meeting of 4 March 1858.

88. M'Dermont, "Proceedings of the Montgomery Co. Medical Society," pp. 341, 345, and 346.

89. Ibid., p. 343.

90. Simon Baruch, Notes Taken on Lectures Given by Eli Geddings on the Institutes and Practice of Medicine, Medical College of South Carolina, 1860–61, entry for 18 February 1861, GA—Emory U. Libe.

91. For example, C. G. Comegys, remarks at meeting of 7 February 1870, Minutes of the Academy of Medicine of Cincinnati, 1 April 1869–13 April 1874; H. I. Bowditch, Lecture Notes for Clinical Course, 1862–63, No. 3, MA—Countway; John George Spenzer, Notes Taken on Lectures Given by John H. Lowman and John E. Darby on Materia Medica and Therapeutics, Medical Department, Western Reserve University, 1881–82, lecture of 21 January 1882, OH—Dittrick; W. B. Williams, "Veratrum Viride As a Therapeutic Agent" (M.D. thesis, University of Nashville, 1858–59), TN—Vanderbilt Med. Libe. For the opposing view that veratrum, whatever its virtues, was not a substitute for bloodletting, see Thomas J. Griffith, Notes Taken on Lectures Given by E. B. Stevens on Materia Medica, Miami Medical College, Cincinnati, Ohio, 1866–67, lecture of 15 January 1867, IN—IN U. Libe.

92. Wright, "On the Value of Blood-letting," quotations from pp. 465, 469, and 471.

93. Henry W. DeSaussure, Notes Taken on Lectures Given by Dr. Kinloch on Materia Medica, 1866–67, 21 February 1867, SC—Waring.

94. U. G. Mitchell Walker, "A Few Words in Defence of Veratrum Viride," NOMNHG, 4 (1857–58): 566.

95. "It should be used with caution, for it may produce death unless so used," Alonzo Clark told his students in New York in 1859. "It is a remedy of terrible power, and should not be used if anything else will readily produce the desired effect" (Titus Munson Coan, Notes Taken on Lectures Given by Alonzo Clark, College of Physicians and Surgeons, New York, 1859–60, NY—NY Hist. Soc.).

96. "Vermont Medical Society [Discussion on Veratrum Viride]," BMSJ, 72 (1865): 493–494; Smyrna Medical Society, By-Laws and Minutes, 1876–79, remarks of Dr. G. W. Crosthwait at meeting of 6 February 1877, discussion on pneumonia, TN—TN State Libe. Enthusiasm for veratrum had certainly diminished by the late 1860s, and a New York City medical professor was correct when he told his class in 1869, "The fashion for veratrum viride in Pneumonia has gone" (F. E. Beckwith, Notes Taken on Lectures and Clinics, Bellevue Medical College, 1868–69, vol. 2, lecture of McLane, Frank Edwin Beckwith Notebooks, CT—Yale U. Libe.).

8. Physiological Therapeutics and the Dissipation of Therapeutic Gloom

1. D. G. Kolb, "The Disadvantages of Therapeutics" (M.D. thesis, Medical College of the State of South Carolina, 1859), SC—Med. U. SC, Main Libe.

2. John H. Fairfield, "On Conservative Medicine" (M.D. thesis, University of Pennsylvania, 1880), PA—U. PA Libe.; and see undated discussion in Minutes of the Savannah Medical Club, December 1889–90, NC—Duke U. Libe.

3. John P. Spooner, "The Different Modes of Treating Disease, or the Different Action of Medicine on the System in an Abnormal State," BMSJ, 66 (1862): 245.

4. Henry I. Bowditch, Public Hygiene in America: Being the Centennial Discourse Delivered before the International Medical Congress, Philadelphia, September, 1876 (Boston, 1877), pp. 17 and 28.

5. Henry Ingersoll Bowditch, Introductory to the Course on Clinical Medicine for November 1861, 1861–62, lecture of 28 November 1861, MA—Countway.

6. James Jackson, Sr., to James Jackson, Jr., Waltham, Massachusetts, 12 June 1833 (and see letter dated Boston, 20 November 1832), James Jackson Papers, MA—Countway.

7. T. L. Wright, "Transcendental Medicine.—An Enquiry Concerning the Manner of Morbific and Remedial Agents Independently of Empiricism," CLO, 38 (1877): 1016–17.

8. David W. Cheever, "The Value and Fallacy of Statistics in the Observation of Disease," BMSJ, 63 (1860–61): 455–456.

9. Ibid., p. 516.

10. Robert T. Edes, "Practical Medicine As a Science. The Annual Address Delivered before the Norfolk Dist. Med. Society, May 11, 1870," BMSJ, 84 (1871): 294.

11. Ibid., p. 291.

12. George L. Goodale, "The Tendency of Modern Therapeutics," *Transactions of the Maine Medical Association* (1869–70): 199, 200, 208, and 211. And see William W. Wellington, *"Modern Medicine: Its Need and Its Tendency.* The Annual Discourse before the Massachusetts Medical Society, May 25th, 1870," *BMSJ*, 83 (1870): 168 and 170; italics removed.

13. Samuel S. Wallian, "The Therapeutics of the Future," *New York Medical Journal*, 39 (1884): 267.

14. Paul F. Eve, "Gentlemen of the Course," [address given ca. 1876], Paul Fitzsimmons Eve Papers, TN—TN State Libe.; and see J. R. Black, "The Bearing of Hygiene on Therapeutics," *Transactions of the American Medical Association*, 29 (1878): 608.

15. Willard Parker to Paul Eve, New York, 10 January 1876, Eve Papers.

16. Bowditch, *Public Hygiene*, pp. 5, 5–6, and 29. While the Louisiana State Board of Health was founded earlier, it remained in effect a municipal board for the city of New Orleans when the Massachusetts State Board was established. Bowditch's work and motivation are analyzed in Barbara Gutmann Rosenkrantz, *Public Health and the State: Changing Views in Massachusetts, 1842–1936* (Cambridge, Massachusetts: Harvard University Press, 1972), especially pp. 156–163.

17. Henry I. Bowditch, *Preventive Medicine and the Physician of the Future* (Boston, 1874), pp. 34 and 35.

18. Ibid., p. 35. This attitude was clearly expressed in the stance of some public health officials regarding the therapeutic relevance of bacteriology. The one therapy that killed bacteria without also killing human tissue was education. See, for example, Charles V. Chapin, *What Changes Has the Acceptance of the Germ Theory Made for Measures for the Prevention and Treatment of Consumption?* (Providence, 1888).

19. Quoted in E. W. Gray, "The Relation of Physiology to the Practice of Medicine," *Transactions of the American Medical Association*, 25 (1874): 165; and see "Preface to the Second Edition," in John William Draper, *Human Physiology, Statical and Dynamical; or, The Conditions and Course of the Life of Man* (New York, 1865), pp. v-viii, especially p. vi. On Draper and the kinship to Comtian positivism of his medical optimism, see Donald Fleming, *John William Draper and the Religion of Science* (New York: Octagon Books, 1972).

20. This shift is analyzed in John Harley Warner, "From Specificity to Universalism in Medical Therapeutics: Transformation in the Nineteenth-Century United States," in *The History of Therapy*, ed. Yosio Kawakita (Tokyo: Taniguchi Foundation, forthcoming).

21. Claude Bernard, *An Introduction to the Study of Experimental Medicine*, trans. Henry Copley Greene (New York: Macmillan, 1927; first pub. Paris, 1865), p. 19.

22. Ibid., p. 139.

23. Ibid., pp. 136, 139, and 210. See Joseph Schiller, "Claude Bernard et la statistique," in *Claude Bernard et les problèmes scientifiques de son temps* (Paris: Editions du Cédre, 1967), pp. 155–171.

24. This point is developed in John Harley Warner, "Physiological Theory and Therapeutic Explanation in the 1860s: The British Debate on the Medical Use of Alcohol," *BHM*, 54 (1980): 235–257; and idem, "Therapeutic Explanation and the Edinburgh Bloodletting Controversy: Two Perspectives on the Medical

Meaning of Science in the Mid-Nineteenth Century," *Medical History*, 24 (1980): 241–258.

25. For example, see Bennet Dowler, "Speculative and Practical Researches on the Supposed Duality, Unity, and Antagonism of Nature and Art in the Cure of Diseases," *NOMSJ*, 15 (1858): 787–805; and idem, "Speculative and Practical Remarks on Absorption, the Enepidermic, Iatraleptic, Endermic, and Hypodermic Methods of Medication," *NOMSJ*, 17 (1860): 56–73. A brief description of Dowler's work is Karlem Riess, "The Rebel Physiologist–Bennet Dowler," *JHM*, 16 (1961): 39–48. Edward C. Atwater discusses experimental physiology in America through the 1860s in " 'Squeezing Mother Nature': Experimental Physiology in the United States before 1870," *BHM*, 52 (1978): 313–335.

26. See Paul Bert, "Claude Bernard," in Bernard, *Introduction*, p. xviii. On Americans' relation to Bernard, see E. Harris Olmsted, "Historical Phases in the Influence of Bernard's Scientific Generalizations in England and America," in *Claude Bernard and Experimental Medicine*, ed. Francisco Grande and Maurice B. Visscher (Cambridge, Massachusetts: Schenkman, 1967), pp. 24–34.

27. "How to Study Medicine.–No. III. Pathology and Physiology–A Plea for Autopsies and for Vivisections," *BMSJ*, 79 (1868–69): 75 and 76. A useful study showing how central vivisection became to the American medical profession is William Gary Roberts, "Man before Beast: The Response of Organized Medicine to the American Antivivisection Movement" (A.B. thesis, Harvard University, 1979).

28. [H. C. Wood], "The Principles of Modern Therapeutics," *BMSJ*, 110 (1884): 597 and 598.

29. Edward H. Clarke, "Recent Progress in Materia Medica. An Introductory Lecture Delivered at the Mass. Med. College, at the Opening of the Winter Course of Instruction in Harvard University," *BMSJ*, 71 (1864–65): 321.

30. Z. Collins McElroy, "The Matter of the First Phases of Life, and the Action of So-Called Remedies in Living Beings," *CLO*, 33 (1873): 450.

31. Roberts Bartholow, "Experimental Investigations into the Actions and Uses of the Bromide of Potassium," *CLO*, 26 (1865): 658.

32. [Wood], "Principles of Modern Therapeutics," p. 598.

33. Ibid., p. 597. On the variable meanings of *science* in American medicine and the need to scrutinize them, see John Harley Warner, "Science in Medicine," in *Historical Writing on American Science*, ed. Sally Gregory Kohlstedt and Margaret Rossiter, *Osiris*, n.s. 1 (1985): 37–58.

34. Gray, "The Relation of Physiology to the Practice of Medicine," p. 153.

35. Roberts Bartholow, "The Present State of Therapeutics. An Address Delivered at the Opening of the Fifty-Sixth Course of Lectures in Jefferson Medical School," *Medical Record*, 16 (1879): 337.

36. Ibid.

37. Gray, "The Relation of Physiology to the Practice of Medicine," p. 160.

38. A. Patton, "Specific Methods in the Treatment and Investigation of Diseases, *CLO*, 38 (1877): 116.

39. E. B. Thompson to Mary Eleanor Thompson, New Orleans, 30 December 1866, Benson-Thompson Family Papers, NC—Duke U. Libc.

40. G. S. Scranton, Resident Student, Notes Taken on Lectures Given by

Professor Hawthorne on Therapeutics, Case Book, Charity Hospital, New Orleans, 1873–74, LA—Matas; W. W. Seely, Commencement Address Given at the Medical College of Ohio, [ca. 1882], clipping pasted in Medical College of Ohio, Faculty Minutes, 1852–1902, OH—U. Cincinnati Libe.; John George Spenzer, Notes Taken on Lectures Given by John H. Lowman and John E. Darby on Materia Medica and Therapeutics, Medical Department, Western Reserve University, 1881, lecture of 7 September 1881, OH—Dittrick; Notes Taken on Lectures Given by John A. McCorkle, Long Island College Hospital, 1882, MD—NLM.

41. Patton, "Specific Methods," pp. 119–120.

42. Wright, "Transcendental Medicine," p. 1017.

43. Typically, one reviewer appraised H. C. Wood's goal to be "the founding of a new system of therapeutics upon a scientific basis" (A., "[Review of] A Treatise on Therapeutics, Comprising Materia Medica and Toxicology. By H. C. Wood, Jr. . . . ," BMSJ, 90 [1874]: 577).

44. Patton, "Specific Methods," p. 116.

45. "The modern physiological school of therapeutics," Wood confessed as late as 1884, "[has] no known law of therapeutics,—unless it is that of antagonisms" ([Wood], "Principles of Modern Therapeutics," p. 597). The work sponsored by the British Medical Association was presented in John Hughes Bennett, "Report of the Committee of the British Medical Association to Investigate the Antagonism of Medicines," British Medical Journal, 2 (1874): 436–439, 464–466, 485–486, 518–520, 547–548, 581–583, 615–617, 674–678, 771, 805–806, and British Medical Journal, 1 (1875): 97–98.

46. "[Review of] A Treatise on the Practice of Medicine for the Use of Students and Practitioners. By Roberts Bartholow . . . 1882," NOMSJ, n.s. 10 (1882–83): 682.

47. Roberts Bartholow, On the Antagonism between Medicines and between Remedies and Diseases. Being the Cartwright Lectures for the Year 1880 (New York, 1881), p. 114.

48. Ibid.; and see Bartholow's remarks in Minutes of the Cincinnati Academy of Medicine, 1 April 1869–13 April 1874, meeting of 3 May 1869, and in Minutes of the Cincinnati Academy of Medicine, 20 April 1874–15 May 1876, meeting of 26 October 1874, OH—Cincinnati Acad. Med.; and Roberts Bartholow, "The Principle of Physiological Antagonism As Applied to the Treatment of the Febrile State," in A Series of American Clinical Lectures, ed. E. C. Seguin, vol. 2, no. 1 (New York, 1876), 1–21. Bartholow stated clearly the necessity of coupling animal experimentation with clinical inquiry in order to bring about therapeutic progress in "The Physiological Effects and Therapeutical Uses of Atropia and Its Salts," Transactions of the American Medical Association, 20 (1869): 640.

49. James T. Whittaker, "Doctrines of Therapy. Address Introductory to the Course of Theory and Practice in the Medical College of Ohio, October 5, 1885," Cincinnati Lancet and Clinic, 15 (1885): 559.

50. Roberts Bartholow, "Introductory Lecture on Experimental Therapeutics," quoted in "Opening of the Schools," CLO, 33 (1872): 636.

51. Joel Seaverns, "Recent Advances in Medicine and Their Influence on Therapeutics. The Annual Address Delivered before the Norfolk District Med. Society, May 10, 1871," BMSJ, 85 (1871): 118.

52. Alfred Stillé, Therapeutics and Materia Medica, vol. 1 (Philadelphia, 1874), p. 31; and see George A. Pierson, Notes Taken on Lectures Given by Alfred Stillé on the Theory and Practice of Medicine, University of Pennsyl-

vania, 1874, 2 vols., PA—U. PA Archives. On the link between advocacy of the healing power of nature and an animus against experimental laboratory science, see John Harley Warner, " 'The Nature-Trusting Heresy': American Physicians and the Concept of the Healing Power of Nature in the 1850's and 1860's," *Perspectives in American History*, 11 (1977–78): 291–324.

53. T[homas] C. M[inor], "[Review of] *Materia Medica and Therapeutics. By Roberts Bartholow . . . 1876*," *CLO*, 37 (1876): 841.

54. Ibid., p. 842.

55. Elisha Bartlett, *An Essay on the Philosophy of Medical Science* (Philadelphia, 1844), pp. 113–114.

56. A. Stillé to G. C. Shattuck, Philadelphia, 24 October 1844, Shattuck Papers, vol. 18, MA—MA Hist. Soc.

57. Roberts Bartholow, "The Degree of Certainty in Therapeutics," *Transactions of the Medical and Chirurgical Faculty of the State of Maryland* (1876): 33–50; Elisha Bartlett, *An Enquiry into the Degree of Certainty in Medicine* (Philadelphia, 1848); P.-J.-G. Cabanis, *An Essay on the Certainty of Medicine*, trans. R. La Roche (Philadelphia, 1823; first pub. Paris, 1797). Typical of his attitude toward French clinicians was Roberts Bartholow's "Therapeutical Notes," *Cincinnati Medical Repertory*, 1 (1868): 15.

58. Bartholow, "Degree of Certainty," p. 34.

59. Ibid., p. 45.

60. Quoted in ibid.

61. Bartholow, "Degree of Certainty," p. 45.

62. Ibid., p. 49.

9. Cui Bono?

1. The complexities of the reconstruction witnessed in the American medical profession from the 1870s through the early twentieth century have attracted on the whole more sophisticated analysis than has the antebellum period. Among the most enlightening studies are Donald Fleming, *William H. Welch and the Rise of Modern Medicine* (Boston: Little, Brown, 1954); George Rosen, *The Structure of American Medical Practice, 1875–1941* (Philadelphia: University of Pennsylvania Press, 1983); Charles E. Rosenberg, "Between Two Worlds: American Medicine in 1879," in *Centenary of Index Medicus, 1879–1979*, ed. John B. Blake (Bethesda: National Library of Medicine, 1980), pp. 3–30; S. E. D. Shortt, "Physicians, Science, and Status: Issues in the Professionalization of Anglo-American Medicine in the Nineteenth Century," *Medical History*, 27 (1983): 51–68; and Paul Starr, *The Social Transformation of American Medicine* (New York: Basic Books, 1982).

2. E. W. Gray, "The Relation of Physiology to the Practice of Medicine," *Transactions of the American Medical Association*, 25 (1874): 159; and see "[Review of] Wood's Therapeutics," *BMSJ*, 93 (1875): 646.

3. F. Forchheimer, "Valedictory Address to the Medical College of Ohio Class of 1881," quoted in "College Commencements," *Cincinnati Lancet and Clinic*, n.s. 6 (1881): 221.

4. Samuel Kneeland, "Preparatory Medical Education," *BMSJ*, 80 (1869): 181.

5. See the emphasis on "vigilance" over drugging in Minutes of the Union District Medical Association, 1880–96, meeting at Rushville, Indiana, 28 October 1880, OH—Miami U. Libe.

6. On the relationship between these debates on the code of ethics and

the newly emerging conception of professional identity, see Barbara Gutmann Rosenkrantz, "The Search for Professional Order in 19th-Century American Medicine," in *Sickness and Health in America: Readings in the History of Medicine and Public Health*, ed. Ronald L. Numbers and Judith Walzer Leavitt, 2nd ed. (Madison: University of Wisconsin Press, forthcoming). Arguments against the code stemming from a New York debate were elaborated in Alfred C. Post et al., *An Ethical Symposium: Being a Series of Papers Concerning Medical Ethics and Etiquette from the Liberal Standpoint* (New York, 1883).

7. Roberts Bartholow, *Cui Bono? and What Nature, What Art Does in the Cure of Disease. Two Introductory Lectures Delivered in the Medical College of Ohio, Sessions of 1872–3 and 1873–4* (Cincinnati, 1873), p. 17.

8. See Roberts Bartholow, *A Practical Treatise on Materia Medica and Therapeutics* (New York, 1876); and Horatio C. Wood, *A Treatise on Therapeutics. Comprising Materia Medica and Toxicology, with Especial Reference to the Application of the Physiological Action of Drugs to Clinical Medicine* (Philadelphia, 1874). By 1884 both textbooks were in their fifth editions. Thomas N. Bonner traces the growing number of American physicians who studied in Germany during this period in *American Doctors and German Universities: A Chapter in International Intellectual Relations, 1870–1914* (Lincoln: University of Nebraska Press, 1963).

9. Quotations are respectively from Geo[rge] B. Wood and Franklin Bache, *The Dispensatory of the United States of America*, 15th ed. (Philadelphia, 1883), p. viii; and "Review of *The Dispensatory of the United States. By Geo. B. Wood and Franlin Bache* (1883)," *NOMSJ*, n.s. 11 (1883–84): 154. The New Orleans reviewer praised H. C. Wood's revisions, though he thought them "a little too *hypothetical*" (p. 154). On H. C. Wood, see George B. Roth, "An Early American Pharmacologist: Horatio C. Wood (1841–1920)," *Isis*, 30 (1939): 37–44.

10. B., "Letter from Boston" (10 March 1870), *CLO*, 31 (1870): 234; and see Edward H. Clarke, "Recent Progress in Materia Medica. An Introductory Lecture Delivered at the Mass. Med. College, at the Opening of the Winter Couse of Instruction in Harvard University," *BMSJ*, 71 (1864–65): 309–321; and Edward B. Stevens, "A Report on New Remedies," *CLO*, 25 (1864): 449.

11. Samuel Nickels, "Modern Therapeutics. Introductory Lecture at Medical College of Ohio, Tuesday, Oct. 4, 1881," *Cincinnati Lancet and Clinic*, n.s. 7 (1881): 324, 325, and 330; italics added. And see Thomas J. Griffith, Notes Taken on Lectures Given by Professor Palmer at the Department of Medicine and Surgery, University of Michigan, 10 October 1865–15 March 1866, lecture of 17 November 1865, IN—IN U. Libe.

12. J. R. Chadwick, Notes Taken on Lectures Given by Edward Hammond Clarke on Materia Medica, Boston, 1869, MA—Countway; and see Nickels, "Modern Therapeutics," pp. 324–325.

13. Gray, "The Relation of Physiology to the Practice of Medicine," p. 160.

14. Roberts Bartholow, "Clinical Lecture on the Treatment of Measles in the Adult, and the Use of the Sulphites in Zymotic Diseases," *CLO*, 26 (1865): 96.

15. Robert[s] Bartholow, " 'The Chlorides' in Pneumonia," *CLO*, 25 (1864): 516; also see Frank Edwin Beckwith, Notes Taken on Lectures and Clinics Delivered at the Bellevue Medical College, vol. 2, 1 December 1868–4 February 1869, lecture of Professor Flint, Jr., 16 December 1868, CT—Yale U. Libe.; C. P. Kirley, Notes Taken on Lectures Given by John A. Octerlony on Materia

Medica and Therapeutics and Clinical Medicine at the Lousville City Hospital, Louisville Medical College, 1874, KY—U. Louisville Med. Libe.; and Notes Taken on Lectures Given by William Pepper on the Practice of Medicine at the University of Pennsylvania, 1886–88, PA—U. PA Archives.

16. Michel Mandel to J. E. Hawkins, Opeloma, Louisiana, 11 June 1880, J. E. Hawkins Papers, LA—LSU; and see Charles A. V. Lutz, "Medical Thermometry" (M.D. thesis, University of Pennsylvania, 1877), PA—U. PA Libe.

17. Roberts Bartholow, "The Degree of Certainty in Therapeutics," *Transactions of the Medical and Chirurgical Faculty of the State of Maryland* (1876): 47; see also Thomas C. Butler, "The Introduction of Chloral Hydrate into Medical Practice," *BHM*, 44 (1970): 168–172; and M. P. Earles, "Introduction of Chloral Hydrate into Medicine," *Pharmacological Journal*, 202 (1969): 457–459.

18. Joel Seaverns, "Recent Advances in Medicine and Their Influence on Therapeutics. The Annual Address Delivered before the Norfolk District Med. Society, May 10, 1871," *BMSJ*, 85 (1871): 118; and see Charles H. Merkheim, "Chloral—The New Hypnotic" (M.D. thesis, University of Pennsylvania, 1870), PA—U. PA Libe.

19. Edward H. Clarke, "Hydrate of Chloral, with Cases Illustrating Its Action," *BMSJ*, 82 (1870): 449. On early studies of the relationship between the chemical structure of drugs and the physiological actions they brought about, see William F. Bynum, "Chemical Structure and Pharmacological Action: A Chapter in the History of 19th Century Molecular Pharmacology," *BHM*, 44 (1970): 518–538; and John Parascandola, "Structure-Activity Relationships—The Early Mirage," *Pharmacy in History*, 13 (1971): 3–10.

20. S., "Medical Improvement," *BMSJ*, 9 (1833–34): 238.

21. "Report of Committee on Practice of Medicine to Medical Society of Wabashaw County, Minnesota," *CLO*, 33 (1872): 451. This was an especially common criticism of pathological knowledge. Thus the editors of one medical journal recognized that many readers would respond to their review about current knowledge regarding cholera by asking how all this better prepared them to treat the disease. "We fear they will still have good cause to exclaim, *Cui bono?*" ("Editorial," *NOMSJ*, 19 [1866–67]: 544).

22. Alfred George Tebault, Notes on Medical Lectures Taken at the University of Virginia, Lecture Notebook, No. 4, n.d. [but internally dated as ca. 1885–95], Alfred George Tebault Papers, VA—U. VA Libe.

23. On attitudes toward vivisection, see James Turner, *Reckoning with the Beast: Animals, Pain, and Humanity in the Victorian Mind* (Baltimore and London: Johns Hopkins University Press, 1980), especially pp. 96–121. The best study of the antivivisection movement, restricted to the British context, is Richard D. French, *Antivivisection and Medical Science in Victorian Society* (Princeton: Princeton University Press, 1975).

24. T[homas] C. M[inor], "[Review of] *The Action of Medicines*. By Isaac Ott . . . 1878," *CLO*, 40 (1878): 206.

25. T[homas] C. M[inor], "[Review of] *Materia Medica and Therapeutics*. By Roberts Bartholow . . . 1876," *CLO*, 37 (1876): 842. The shrinking distinctions between humans and animals that the period after Darwin witnessed certainly made the proposition that some principles discovered by experimentation on animals in the laboratory could be valid as well at the human patient's bedside increasingly plausible, at least to some medical thinkers.

26. The best analyses of the debate and ensuing reforms are Henry K. Beecher and Mark D. Altschule, *Medicine at Harvard: The First 300 Years*

(Hanover, New Hampshire: University Press of New England, 1977), pp. 87–125; and Kenneth M. Ludmerer, "Reform at the Harvard Medical School, 1869–1909," *BHM*, 55 (1981): 343–370.

27. Michael F. Nigro, Jr., "Reform at the Harvard Medical School in 1871" (A.B. thesis, Harvard University, 1966), p. 6.

28. James C. White, "An Introductory Lecture Delivered before the Medical Class of Harvard University, Nov. 2, 1870," *BMSJ*, 83 (1870): 279. White earlier advocated reform in his unsigned essays "Censorial Duties—Medical Education," *BMSJ*, 75 (1866–67): 105–107; "Election at Harvard University," *BMSJ*, 74 (1866): 508–509; and "Medical Education—New Professorships in the Medical Department of Harvard University," *BMSJ*, 74 (1866): 63–65.

29. White, "An Introductory Lecture," pp. 286–287.

30. Ibid., p. 287.

31. Henry Jacob Bigelow, *Medical Education in America: Being the Annual Address Read before the Massachusetts Medical Society, June 7, 1871* (Cambridge, Massachusetts, 1871), p. 12. On Bigelow, see [William Sturgis Bigelow], *A Memoir of Henry Jacob Bigelow, A.M., M.D., LL.D.* (Boston, 1894).

32. Eliot remained more aloof from the question of the immediate relevance of reforms to medical practice. A scientist rather than a physician, he was more committed to the ideal of science than to the promise of utility. Much the same was true of Henry P. Bowditch, who returned from study in Germany in basic science to teach experimental physiology and pursue his own research at Harvard. He was the first medical school faculty member explicitly freed from the need to practice by being given a full-time position of this sort by the school. On Bowditch's motivation, see W. Bruce Fye, "Why a Physiologist?—The Case of Henry P. Bowditch," *BHM*, 56 (1982): 19–29. To be sure, the argument of relevance was sometimes used by reformers driven by a primary allegiance to science to justify greater scientific content in medical school programs. It is nonetheless clear that therapeutic relevance was the single most potent argument for augmenting the curriculum's scientific content and that the principal line of battle was drawn between those who did and those who did not believe that experimental science was the proper basis for therapeutic action.

33. Bigelow, *Medical Education*, pp. 12 and 41.

34. Ibid., pp. 30–31.

35. Ibid., pp. 27 and 38.

36. Ibid., pp. 43 and 45. The link between concern for practical knowledge and opposition to vivisection was also clear in Oliver Wendell Holmes's thought; see John T. Morse, Jr., *Life and Letters of Oliver Wendell Holmes*, vol. 1 (Cambridge, Massachusetts: 1897), p. 181; and Eleanor M. Tilton, *Amiable Autocrat: A Biography of Dr. Oliver Wendell Holmes* (New York: Henry Schuman, 1947), p. 294.

37. Bigelow, *Medical Education*, pp. 9–10.

38. Roberts Bartholow, "The Present State of Therapeutics. An Address Delivered at the Opening of the Fifty-Sixth Course of Lectures in Jefferson Medical School," *Medical Record*, 16 (1879): 340.

39. On physiologists' perceptions of late-nineteenth-century American medicine and its institutions as a promising context in which to objectify their scientific protocols, see Gerald L. Geison, "Divided We Stand: Physiologists and Clinicians in the American Context," in *The Therapeutic Revolution: Essays in the Social History of American Medicine*, ed. Morris J. Vogel and Charles E. Rosenberg (Philadelphia: University of Pennsylvania Press, 1979),

pp. 67–90; and John Harley Warner, "Physiology," in *The Education of American Physicians: Historical Essays*, ed. Ronald L. Numbers (Berkeley, Los Angeles, and London: University of California Press, 1980), pp. 48–71. A more probing development of similar themes in the context of biological chemistry is Robert E. Kohler, *From Medical Chemistry to Biochemistry: The Making of a Biochemical Discipline* (Cambridge: Cambridge University Press, 1982).

40. On the early reception of the germ theory in America, see Phyllis Allen, "Americans and the Germ Theory of Disease" (Ph.D. diss., University of Pennsylvania, 1949). And see Margaret Warner, "Hunting the Yellow Fever Germ: The Principle and Practice of Etiological Proof in Late Nineteenth-Century America," *BHM*, 59 (1985): 361–382. On the persistent tensions that attended the image and application of bacteriology in medical practice, see John Martin Dent, "Two Views of Bacteriology at Harvard" (A.B. thesis, Harvard University, 1982); and Russell C. Maulitz, " 'Physician versus Bacteriologist': The Ideology of Science in Clinical Medicine," *The Therapeutic Revolution*, ed. Vogel and Rosenberg, pp. 91–107; and see Russell C. Maulitz, "Pathology," in *Education of American Physicians*, ed. Numbers, pp. 122–142.

41. A useful analysis of the concept of "internal antisepsis" is John K. Crellin, "Internal Antisepsis or the Dawn of the Germ Theory," *JHM*, 36 (1981): 9–18.

42. Seaverns. "Recent Advances in Medicine," p. 115; and see "Antiseptic Therapeutics," *BMSJ*, 111 (1884): 257–258; Roberts Bartholow, "Investigations into the Use of the Sulphites in Zymotic Diseases," *CLO*, 26 (1865): 521–529; and the debate on the internal therapeutic use of carbolic acid in Minutes of the Cincinnati Academy of Medicine, 5 April 1869–13 April 1874, meeting of 7 June 1869, OH—Cincinnati Acad. Med.

43. Seaverns, "Recent Advances in Medicine," p. 120.

44. Bartholow, "Degree of Certainty in Therapeutics," p. 41. And see John M. Keating, "The Presence of the Micrococcus in the Blood of Malignant Measles; Its Importance in Treatment," *BMSJ*, 107 (1882): 105; and George Spenzer, Notes Taken on Lectures Given by John H. Lowman and John E. Darby on Materia Medica and Therapeutics, Medical Department, Western Reserve University, 1881, lecture on alcohol of 29 November 1881, OH—Dittrick. Koch's discovery of the tubercle bacillus was also used to legitimize "germicides" already in use; for example, M. James, "Treatment of Consumption Indicated by the Discoveries of Koch and Others of Its Parasitic Origin," *NOMSJ*, n.s. 10 (1882–83): 141–144.

45. "The Germ Theory of Disease and Its Relation to Therapeutics," *BMSJ*, 112 (1885): 234.

46. John Ashburton Cutter, "Clinical Morphology versus Bacteriology, with Some Therapeutic Deductions," *Medical Bulletin*, 11 (1889): 316.

47. Ibid., pp. 314–315.

48. Henry Koplik, Notes Taken on Lectures Given by Alois Epstein, Karl Shroeder, Carl Gerhardt, Emanuel Mendel, Robert Koch, and Edward A. Martin, Berlin and Prague, 1885–86, vol. 2, bacteriological notes beginning Munich, May 1886, NY—NY Acad. Med.

49. Particularly poignant in expressing the frustration generated by early bacteriology's failure to deliver on its therapeutic promise is the course of lectures that Harold Clarence Ernst gave on bacteriology starting in 1886 at Harvard Medical School; see his Lectures on Bacteriology, 1886–96, Harold C. Ernst Papers, MA—Countway. These lectures represented the first instruction

in bacteriology as part of the regular course in an American medical school. And see Charles V. Chapin, *The Present State of the Germ-Theory of Disease* (Providence, 1885), p. 43.

50. For example, Seaverns, "Recent Advances in Medicine," especially p. 113.

51. Eric E. Sattler, "The Present Status of the Tubercle-Bacillus Question," *Cincinnati Lancet and Clinic*, n.s. 12 (1884): 415.

52. Samuel S. Wallian, "The Therapeutics of the Future," *New York Medical Journal*, 39 (1884): 266.

53. See Lloyd G. Stevenson, "Science Down the Drain. On the Resistance of Certain Sanitarians to Animal Experimentation, Bacteriology, and Immunology," *BHM*, 29 (1955): 1–26. And see Regina Markell Morantz, "Feminism, Professionalism, and Germs: The Thought of Mary Putnam Jacobi and Elizabeth Blackwell," *American Quarterly*, 34 (1982): 459–478.

54. A. Jacobi, "Inaugural Address, Delivered before the New York Academy of Medicine," *Medical Record*, 27 (1885): 169, 172, and 174.

55. Erwin H. Ackerknecht, *Rudolf Virchow: Doctor, Statesman, Anthropologist* (Madison: University of Wisconsin Press, 1953), pp. 105–118. Virchow was skeptical of the therapeutic relevance of his own ideas on cellular pathology as well; see idem, "Cellular Theory and Therapeutics," *Clio Medica*, 5 (1970): 1–5.

56. Jonathan R. Quinan to Dr. [W. S.] Forward, [illegible: Lyon Cay, North Carolina?], 19 June 1884, William Strump Forward Papers, NC—SHC.

57. Alfred Stillé to Henry I. Bowditch, Philadelphia, 25 February 1882, Bowditch Scrapbook, vol. 4, MA—Countway.

A Note on Sources for the
History of Therapeutics

The particular primary sources I have cited in this study by and large
have no singular virtue to recommend them to the attention of the
historian interested in exploring deeper into medical therapeutics in
nineteenth-century America. In some instances I have selected the
most forceful example I know of to make my point, as in using Elisha
Bartlett's *Philosophy of Medical Science* (1844) to illustrate the American commitment to Parisian empiricism. With some exceptions this
study could have argued the same points drawing upon a substantially
different evidential foundation; more often than not, the examples I
cite could readily be replicated on the basis of research in other archives
or publications. I have generally kept supporting references in the notes
to a minimum, and the reader who cares will find fuller documentation
in my "The Therapeutic Perspective: Medical Knowledge, Practice,
and Professional Identity in America, 1820–1885" (Ph.D. diss., Harvard
University, 1984). In any event, it is difficult indeed to identify primary
records of nineteenth-century medicine that do not in some way inform
the history of therapeutics as I have approached it. Therefore although
the historian interested in therapeutics will find something useful in
the sources I happen to cite in the notes, he or she will gain more by
considering the types of sources I have exploited and their peculiar
values and limitations.

Published nineteenth-century medical literature is at its most useful and most reliable when used as a source of knowledge about therapeutic theory and principle, about assumptions on the nature of
therapeutic knowledge, and about professional programs for proper behavior and change. Formal addresses, including the oratory that opened
and closed each session at medical schools, introduced each professor's
course of lectures, and annually gave the presidents of medical societies
the opportunity of displaying their classical learning, are especially

telling. They reveal what physicians held to be important and what they saw as threatening. In perhaps no other context is the symbolic function of medical therapeutics for the regular profession so clear. This means, however, that even more than most medical literature, such discourses must not be taken at face value, especially when they purport to describe something like therapeutic activity. They are best regarded as liturgical literature that accompanied professional rituals and should be read with the caveats appropriate to that genre in mind.

Textbooks on therapeutics, materia medica, and the practice of medicine are perhaps the most treacherous source for the history of therapeutics. As representations of a single person's views, often appearing in an exaggerated form that served internal consistency, they have considerable value. Danger lies in assuming that they represent the views of their readers rather than just their authors. Knowing that a particular textbook was widely used suggests that the ideas it espoused were prevalent among American physicians, but it says very little about the extent to which those ideas were accepted or applied. Manuscript records left by physicians so often controvert the proposition that they adhered to textbook instructions that texts have little evidential authority. The time lags between principle and practice grew especially long in the case of textbooks. Sometimes these volumes were in the vanguard, but frequently they represented older teachings that few regarded as extensively applicable to contemporary practice. Like other monographic literature, textbooks can be read as valid sources for what one person believed therapeutics ought to be like; when they are taken to be more than this, their validity becomes doubtful.

Medical journal literature is the richest source of knowledge about therapeutic theory and principle. It presents a diversity of views from a broader cross section of the upper levels of the profession than the sources already mentioned. The chief pitfall in using journal literature as a gauge of therapeutic principle (aside from confusing principle with practice) is the risk of missing critical discussion by presuming incorrectly where in journals pertinent information will be contained. For many purposes, a journal's index—even the most complete one—is virtually worthless. While it leads to articles on some types of topics, it is misleading as a guide to movements in therapeutic thought. For example, if the historian wants to understand the extent, locus, and animus of regular physicians' discussion on bloodletting between the 1840s and 1870s, he or she will get a disastrously skewed notion of what was in fact going on if the only articles examined are those identified either by key words in the index or by obviously pertinent titles. Much valuable information is in places that cannot be systematically predicted, such as articles on individual cases or diseases, or even obituaries.

Accordingly I would make the unpleasant proposal that anyone who is serious about understanding therapeutic debate or such a topic as physicians' assumptions about therapeutic epistemology or the limitations of therapeutic knowledge must literally read page by page through selected runs of journals from the period under study. This is the approach I have taken for the 1820s through the 1880s with the journals published in the three cities selected to highlight regional variability—Boston, Cincinnati, and New Orleans. Particularly through the 1860s these journals reflected strong regional variations in medical thought and practice, and care must be taken not to represent a caricature drawn principally from one region's sources as "American" therapeutics. Beyond the fine-grained sketch of therapeutic preoccupations and diversity that arises from a comprehensive reading of selected journals, articles from other journals accessible through indexes, especially papers written by articulate and well-known physicians, are principally valuable as a source of powerful programmatic statements that supplement and help crystallize knowledge gleaned elsewhere about the major currents in therapeutics.

Manuscript materials from over sixty repositories have been consulted in the course of this study, impressing me strongly with the staggering abundance of such sources to be found in archives in virtually all parts of the United States that are useful for illuminating therapeutic thought. As with other categories of sources, before generalization is warranted the researcher must closely study enough manuscript materials of any particular type from a variety of contexts so that he or she can confidently evaluate the novelty or typicalness of any newly examined source. Most types of narrative manuscript sources are so widely available that this is not an insurmountable problem.

Several categories of manuscript sources are especially prevalent. The notes that students took on medical school lectures survive in perhaps greater profusion than any other major type. (Professors' notes on their lectures are not rare, but neither are they common.) I have come to regard student notes as generally a more useful source than textbooks for knowledge about what the practitioner was taught. At least in the case of the larger medical schools, notes taken by a number of students on the same series of lectures often can be assembled. Because such sources, read comparatively, display variability among students, they can provide greater awareness of the (sometimes bizarre) variations on the professor's message the individual students received and to some extent carried with them into practice. In addition lecture notes present the diversity among various professors' teachings both at any given time and across time. Often, too, statements made in the classroom had a directness that was tempered by the more polished, internally consistent rhetoric of the textbook.

Manuscript medical theses also provide intriguing insights into the ways the instruction given in medical schools had been transformed by the time it had filtered down to the students who were to take these notions with them to the bedside. Recurrent patterns in theses written at a single school offer one particularly useful indicator of what the students believed the professors wanted to hear, be it advocacy of a particular therapeutic theory, condemnation of a practice, or a tirade against a competing professor and his therapeutic views. Unlike lecture notebooks, theses are concentrated in a few large collections rather than being dispersed in many archives, although a few can be found in most collections that have any strength in medical materials. Exceptionally rich collections I have drawn on are deposited at the Library of Congress (Joseph M. Toner Papers), the Van Pelt Library of the University of Pennsylvania, the Health Sciences Library at Vanderbilt University, the Waring Historical Library of the Medical University of South Carolina, and the Archives of Transylvania University. An analytical study of the changing nature of the M.D. thesis as a genre of professional literature over time could be extremely fruitful; to my knowledge this enterprise has yet to be undertaken.

Manuscript medical society minutes reveal intraprofessional therapeutic debate with a candor difficult to duplicate through other records. While many societies regularly published their minutes in journals, the secretary ordinarily cleaned them up before they went into print. Thus, for example, the often flexible divisions that existed between orthodox and sectarian medicine appear more rigid in published records than in the manuscript versions. The image that a medical society wished to present to outsiders often clouded precisely those characteristics that the historian finds most telling. The uncensored verbal assaults by one physician on another that occurred in society debates and the care taken to keep such discord from the public ear can be especially valuable in elucidating the professional meaning of change in therapeutic principle and practice. Medical school faculty minutes are similarly useful in correcting the advertised images presented in schools' catalogs and in revealing professional values in operation, but the insights they provide into therapeutic theory, practice, and change are much more meager.

Correspondence that discusses therapeutic principle and practice ordinarily was generated in one of several discrete contexts. The most common sort of useful correspondence is that between medical students (usually attending classes, but sometimes in apprenticeship) and their parents (or whoever was paying their bills). Such letters disclose much about how future practitioners regarded their didactic and clinical training and how they assessed its place in their preparation for life and career. The correspondence of American students abroad provides the most incisive evidence for understanding how European medicine appeared to American eyes and is indispensable in evaluating the place of European teachings in the transformation of American therapeutics. To an extent students told their parents what they wanted to hear, especially regarding the intensity of their own exertion, yet their opinions about their instructors and instruction and their voicing of their anxieties about facing practice do provide insights not readily accessible elsewhere. When as was often the case the student's father was also a physician, the correspondence frequently includes a running commentary by the elder practitioner on the student's reports of therapeutic teachings.

A young physician setting up practice could also generate revealing correspondence. If the family members with whom he exchanged letters were not physicians, the medical content of letters tended to dwindle quickly; but if his father, brother, or uncle was a physician, the younger practitioner often described the patients he was seeing, how he was managing them, his anxieties about the care he was giving (and about his socioeconomic situation), and most valuably of all, the rationale behind his therapeutic choices. At times this information elicited advice, correction, or counterexamples from medical kin. Severe epidemic disease or its approach especially encouraged the physician to be reflective in his letters about the therapeutic power and frailty of the profession.

Physicians' diaries were eclectic documents that often recorded the management of interesting cases. Aside from true case books, it is in diaries that records of patient resistance to treatment, for example, are to be found. Diaries are uniquely valuable as a source of knowledge about social interactions between orthodox physicians and irregular practitioners. The content of diaries also provides one indicator of what occupied physicians' attention, as is illustrated by the fact that a diary not infrequently doubled as a meteorological journal.

All these types of narrative sources contain some information about therapeutic practice. The overarching difficulty, however, is distinguishing between accounts of actual practice and those of principle. Some published writings, most notoriously textbooks on practice, are virtually worthless as mirrors of therapeutic activity. Whether the principle they taught had a strong or a faint correlation to bedside prescribing habits cannot be assessed by a knowledge of the textbook alone or even by a sense of how widely it was consulted. The unflinching preservation of venesection in principle contrasted with its decline in practice should be sufficient to make the most sanguine historical user of textbooks on practice read skeptically.

Most published sources were by their very nature normative, even when their stated task was to be objectively descriptive. The historian simply has no way of knowing whether published statements on practice reflected actual behavior or merely principle without further confirming evidence such as case records. However, instances in which the ways physicians characterized practice diverge from the knowledge the historian can derive from records of *actual* practice are sufficiently numerous to make narrative records suspect as indicators of therapeutic activity.

Two exceptions are important. Clinical lecture notes, though scarcely nonnormative reportage on everyday hospital practice, nonetheless present explicit correlations between behavior and principle that are scarce elsewhere. Published clinical lectures are similarly useful, but I have been more inclined to give attention to less formal, extemporaneous manuscript notes. Correspondence among physicians is also a helpful source of knowledge about practice, though it is hardly free from rationalization. I have paid particular attention to letters in which a physician presented the case at hand, described his treatment, and asked for advice on how to proceed.

The kinds of records from which the historian can draw information about actual therapeutic practice and the strengths and limitations of each are discussed in Chapter 4. These include pharmacy prescription registers, physicians' daybooks and financial records, private practice case records, and hospital case history books. Financial records of practice (ubiquitous in archival collections) are by far the most common but yield the least detailed information about treatment. Pharmacy records are common enough, especially from the 1850s onward, to reward a major study that would examine, among other factors, regional differences in prescribing habits. Private practice case books are rare and often represent only a small segment of a physician's practice.

The singular virtues and shortcomings of hospital case history records are also evaluated in Chapter 4. In this study I have relied principally on the records of the Massachusetts General Hospital (from 1823 to 1885) and the Commercial Hospital of Cincinnati (from 1837 to 1881). I am aware of and have examined only two other extensive collections of hospital medical case records books that span any substantial portion of the period under study, namely those of the New York Hospital (1809–1890) at New York Hospital–Cornell Medical

Center and those of the Pennsylvania Hospital in Philadelphia, both on microfilm. Isolated volumes from other hospitals survive, such as those from the Roper Hospital (1859–1862) in Charleston (deposited at the Waring Historical Library) and those from the Charity Hospital (1882–1884) in New Orleans (deposited at Louisiana State University). I would be overjoyed to learn of other substantial sets of antebellum hospital case records, especially from the South. From the 1870s onward, preserved collections of hospital case books are far more common. The historian interested in the place of hospital patient care in the community or in the functioning of the hospitals themselves should note that although I have drawn only lightly on hospital records other than case histories, institutional records for the period I examine here are available in much richer abundance than actual case history records. Thus, for example, although to my knowledge case records including therapeutic information from the Charity Hospital in New Orleans do not exist for most of this period, a basement closet in that hospital's records department contains several hundred volumes of nineteenth-century patient records, including detailed demographic and diagnostic information, which certainly could reward close study.

Some of the most enlightening secondary sources are identified in notes to the text. A more complete bibliography on medical therapeutics, listing historical writings of variable sophistication, is included in my dissertation. To itemize all the sources that have been of use to me in preparing this study would do little to assist the reader and would require an additional volume. Ordinarily I have made bibliographic entries for the historical writings that have been most important in shaping my approach to the history of therapeutics only if they bear directly on nineteenth-century American medical practice. Accordingly, while part of my heavy reliance on Charles Rosenberg's work is evident in the notes, my indebtedness to the writings of Donald Fleming, Perry Miller, and Owsei Temkin is not apparent. To keep the notes lean I have excluded most of the works I have used that lay open the intellectual and social contexts of nineteenth-century America in which the changes described here occurred. I have also excluded most of a sizable literature on nineteenth-century European medicine, on American medicine outside the chronological confines of this work, and on the history of the nonmedical sciences, even though these have had obvious heuristic and explanatory value for me.

Index